Nutrition and Metabolism: An Integrated Approach

Nutrition and Metabolism: An Integrated Approach

Evelyn Howard

⬚SYRAWOOD
PUBLISHING HOUSE

New York

Published by Syrawood Publishing House,
750 Third Avenue, 9th Floor,
New York, NY 10017, USA
www.syrawoodpublishinghouse.com

Nutrition and Metabolism: An Integrated Approach
Evelyn Howard

International Standard Book Number: 978-1-64740-027-9 (Hardback)

This book contains information obtained from authentic and highly regarded sources. All chapters are published with permission under the Creative Commons Attribution Share Alike License or equivalent. A wide variety of references are listed. Permissions and sources are indicated; for detailed attributions, please refer to the permissions page. Reasonable efforts have been made to publish reliable data and information, but the authors, editors and publisher cannot assume any responsibility for the validity of all materials or the consequences of their use.

Trademark Notice: Registered trademark of products or corporate names are used only for explanation and identification without intent to infringe.

Cataloging-in-Publication Data

Nutrition and metabolism : an integrated approach / Evelyn Howard.
   p. cm.
Includes bibliographical references and index.
ISBN 978-1-64740-027-9
1. Nutrition. 2. Metabolism. 3. Nutrient interactions. 4. Diet. I. Howard, Evelyn.
TX353 .N88 2020
641.3--dc23

TABLE OF CONTENTS

PREFACE

The science of interpreting the interaction of nutrients and other substances in food with respect to various processes needed to sustain life in organisms is known as nutrition. Some of the processes which are studied within this discipline in relation to food are health, maintenance, reproduction, growth and disease of an organism. The set of chemical reactions which are essential for the sustenance of life is known as metabolism. There are three major purposes of metabolism. The first purpose is the elimination of nitrogenous wastes. The second one is the conversion of food to energy for running cellular processes. The third purpose of metabolism is the conversion of food to building blocks for proteins, lipids, nucleic acids etc. This book provides comprehensive insights into the fields of nutrition and metabolism. It consists of contributions made by international experts. Coherent flow of topics, student-friendly language and extensive use of examples make this book an invaluable source of knowledge.

A foreword of all Chapters of the book is provided below:

Chapter 1 - The field of science which deals with the study of the interaction of nutrients along with other substances in food with respect to growth, reproduction, maintenance, health and disease of an organism is called nutrition. This is an introductory chapter which will introduce briefly all the significant aspects of nutrition.; **Chapter 2** - The group of chemical reactions in organisms responsible for conversion of food to energy, conversion of food to building blocks for lipids, nucleic acids and proteins, and elimination of nitrogenous wastes is known as metabolism. This chapter discusses in detail the concepts related to metabolism such as metabolic rate and metabolic fuel.; **Chapter 3** - The different types of nutrients include minerals, carbohydrates, proteins, lipids and vitamins. Some of the major minerals are sodium, potassium, chloride, calcium, phosphorus, magnesium and sulfur. The topics elaborated in this chapter will help in gaining a better perspective about these different nutrients.; **Chapter 4** - The biological process through which food is converted into small water-soluble food molecules which can be absorbed into the blood is known as digestion. The chapter closely examines the processes related to the digestion and absorption of carbohydrates, proteins, lipids and vitamins to provide an extensive understanding of the subject.; **Chapter 5** - Nutritional deficiency occurs when the body does not receive the required amount of nutrients from food. It can cause a number of different diseases such as osteoporosis, rickets, goiter, anemia and beriberi. The topics elaborated in this chapter will help in gaining a better perspective about the deficiency of different nutrients and the diseases caused by their deficiency.

I would like to thank the entire editorial team who made sincere efforts for this book and my family who supported me in my efforts of working on this book. I take this opportunity to thank all those who have been a guiding force throughout my life.

Evelyn Howard

Chapter 1

Nutrition: An Introduction

The field of science which deals with the study of the interaction of nutrients along with other substances in food with respect to growth, reproduction, maintenance, health and disease of an organism is called nutrition. This is an introductory chapter which will introduce briefly all the significant aspects of nutrition.

Nutrition, nourishment, or aliment, is the supply of materials - food - required by organisms and cells to stay alive. In science and human medicine, nutrition is the science or practice of consuming and utilizing foods.

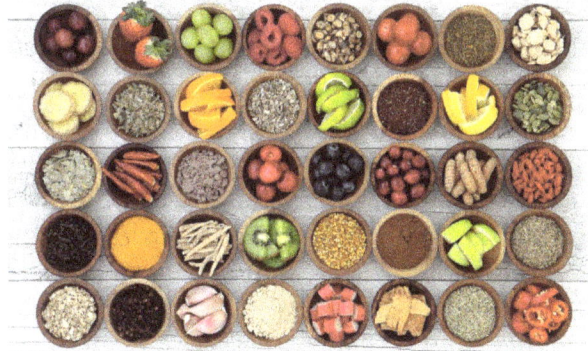

Nutrition has become more focused on metabolism and metabolic pathways - biochemical steps through which substances inside us are transformed from one form to another.

Nutrition also focuses on how diseases, conditions, and problems can be prevented or reduced with a healthy diet.

Similarly, nutrition involves identifying how certain diseases and conditions may be caused by dietary factors, such as poor diet (malnutrition), food allergies, and food intolerances.

Types of Nutrition

A nutrient is a source of nourishment, a component of food, for instance, protein, carbohydrate, fat, vitamin, mineral, fiber and water.

- Macronutrients are nutrients we need in relatively large quantities.
- Micronutrients are nutrients we need in relatively small quantities.

Macronutrients can be further split into energy macronutrients (that provide energy), and macronutrients that do not provide energy.

Macronutrients

There are three macronutrients – carbohydrates, fats, and proteins. They provide 'structural materials' (e.g., amino acids, lipids) and energy (joules or kilocalories). When necessary, or as a result of disease, proteins can be broken down to generate energy, but carbohydrates and fats are used preferentially for energy.

Carbohydrates

Carbohydrates and fats consist of carbon, hydrogen, and oxygen. Carbohydrates range from simple monosaccharides (e.g., glucose, fructose, galactose) through a range of saccharides, depending on the number of sugars present (e.g., disaccharides such as sucrose or table sugar) to highly complex polysaccharides (starch). Carbohydrates are found mainly in starchy foods (e.g., grain and potatoes), fruits, milk, and yogurt. Other foods such as vegetables, beans, nuts, and seeds also contain carbohydrates, but in smaller amounts.

About half (45–65%) of our daily energy intakes should be sourced from carbohydrates. Cells and tissues use glucose for energy, but glucose is essential for proper functioning of the brain and central nervous system, kidneys, and muscles including the heart. Glucose is stored in muscles and the liver as glycogen for later use, being restored to the blood through glycogenolysis.

Traditionally,simple carbohydrates were thought to raise blood glucose levels more rapidly than complex carbohydrates. Infact, some simple carbohydrates (e.g., fructose) follow different metabolic pathways (e.g., fructolysis), which result in only partial conversion to glucose, while many complex carbohydrates (e.g., potato starches) – so-called high glycemic index (GI) or high glucose loading (GL) foods – are digested at the same rate as simple carbohydrates. Glucose stimulates the production of insulin by beta cells in the pancreas, driving up take by the muscles. Dysfunction in the production of insulin and the response of receptors to insulin leads to impaired glucose tolerance and, ultimately, diabetes. Fiber consists largely of cellulose, which is not digested, but helps maintain gut function by bulking out waste and providing a food source (prebiotics) for gut bacteria (microbiome). Low fiber intakes are associated with constipation and increased risk of colon cancer. Diets high in fiber, however, not only reduce symptoms associated with poor gut function, but also help lower cholesterol, and decrease the risk of obesity and cardiovascular disease (CVD). High-fiber foods include fruits, vegetables, and whole grain products.

There are, however, two types of fiber: soluble and insoluble. As suggested by its name, soluble fiber forms a gel with water during digestion, increasing the size of and softening stools, slowing digestion. Formation of this gel reduces the rate of glucose uptake, smoothing out peaks and troughs in glucose and insulin, and helping to reduce the risk of diabetes. In contrast, soluble fiber is found in oat bran, barley, nuts, seeds, beans, lentils, peas, and some fruits and vegetables, and adds bulk to stools, shortening gut transit by stimulating peristalsis, the rhythmic muscular contractions of the intestines.

Fats

Fats (triglycerides) consist of fatty acid monomers, some of which are essential, bound to a glycerol backbone. They are classified as saturated or unsaturated, depending on the detailed structure present, specifically the number of double bonds. Although saturated fats from animal sources and, for example, coconut have been a staple food for millennia, unsaturated fats (e.g., vegetable oil) are still considered to be healthier, despite recent evidence suggesting saturated fats might not be as detrimental as previously thought. Most saturated fats are solid at room temperature while unsaturated fats are typically liquids (e.g., olive or rapeseed oils).

Trans fats are unsaturated with one or more trans-isomer bond; these are rare in nature and typically created during industrial processing, specifically hydrogenation. Unsaturated fats can be classified as monounsaturated (one double-bond) or polyunsaturated (many double-bonds). Depending on the location of the double bonds, unsaturated fatty acids may be classified as omega-3 or omega-6 fatty acids.

Most fatty acids are nonessential, but omega-3 and omega-6 fatty acids can only be obtained from the diet and should be obtained at a ratio of 1:1–1:5. In general, Western diets are deficient in omega-3 and have excess omega-6, which are thought to promote many diseases, including CVD, cancer, and inflammatory and autoimmune diseases (e.g., asthma). Omega-3 and -6 are substrates for prostaglandins, which have a variety of roles in the human body. Fatty acids, such as conjugated linoleic acid, catalpic acid, eleostearic acid, and punicic acid, in addition to providing energy, are potent immune modulators.

Protein

In addition to carbon, hydrogen, and oxygen, proteins contain nitrogen and, in the case of methionine and cysteine, also sulfur. Proteins are structural molecules as well as enzymes. The body cannot store amino acids and requires a continuous source to produce new, and replace damaged, proteins. Of the 20 amino acids utilized by humans, 9 are essential (histidine, isoleucine, leucine, lysine, methionine, phenylalanine, threonine, tryptophan, and valine) and must be sourced from the diet, as the body cannot synthesize them de novo. Complete protein sources contain all the essential amino acids while an incomplete protein source lacks one or more of the essential amino acids. In combination, incomplete sources of protein may provide all the essential amino acids.

Micronutrients

Micronutrients are, generally, minerals and vitamins. Dietary minerals are inorganic elements, besides carbon, hydrogen, nitrogen, and oxygen, which are present in most organic molecules. Some minerals are absorbed much more readily as salts (ionic form), and some foods are fortified with minerals to increase uptakes (e.g., iodine in salt, iron in breakfast cereals).

Macrominerals are required in relatively large amounts (RDA greater than 150 mg/day) and have roles in structure (e.g., bone) and function (e.g., electrolyte) and include calcium (e.g., muscle function, digestive health, bone, signaling); chlorine (common electrolyte); magnesium (e.g., ATP processing, bone, peristalsis); phosphorus (e.g., bone, ATP); potassium (common electrolyte, heart and nerve health); sulfur (three essential amino acids); and sodium (common electrolyte). Excessive sodium consumption can deplete calcium and magnesium and is associated with increased risk of hypertension and osteoporosis.

Some elements are only required in trace amounts (RDA < 200 mg day1), usually because they have a role in enzymes, such as cobalt (biosynthesis of vitamin B_{12} co-enzymes); copper (redox enzymes including cytochrome c oxidase); chromium (sugar metabolism); iodine (e.g., biosynthesis of thyroxine); iron (range of enzymes, hemoglobin and other proteins); manganese (processing of oxygen); molybdenum (xanthine oxidase and related oxidases); nickel (urease); selenium (peroxidases); and zinc (enzymes such as dehydrogenase). Deficient or excess intakes of minerals can have serious health consequences.

As with minerals, most vitamins (vital amines) are essential nutrients (e.g., vitamin C). The only exception is vitamin D, which can be synthesized in the skin. Vitamin deficiencies may result in diseases including goiter, scurvy, osteoporosis, certain forms of cancer, and poor psychological health. However, excess of some vitamins are also dangerous to health (e.g., vitamin A).

Antinutrients

- Antinutrients are natural or synthetic compounds that interfere with the absorption of nutrients. Examples include the following:

- Protease inhibitors, which inhibit trypsin, pepsin, and other proteases in the gut, preventing digestion and absorption of proteins and amino acids.

- Lipase inhibitors (e.g., tetrahydrolipstatin), which interfere with enzymes, such as lipases, which catalyze hydrolysis of some lipids and fats.

- Amylase inhibitors in beans, which prevent the action of enzymes that break the glycosidic bonds of starches and other complex carbohydrates, preventing the release of simple sugars and absorption by the body.

- Phytic acid in the hulls of nuts, seeds, and grains, which has a strong binding affinity for calcium, magnesium, iron, copper, and zinc, preventing their absorption.

- Oxalic acid and oxalates, which are present in many plants, particularly members of the spinach family, bind calcium to prevent its absorption.

Many traditional preparation methods (e.g., fermentation) reduce antinutrients, such as phytic acid, increase the nutritional quality of plant foods, and are widely used in societies where cereals and legumes are a significant part of the diet. For example, cassava is fermented to reduce levels of both toxins and antinutrients. Glucosinolates (e.g., broccoli, Brussels sprouts, cabbage, and cauliflower), although widely recognized for their putative health benefits, also interfere with the uptake of iodine and flavonoids, and chelate metals (e.g., iron and zinc) thus reducing their absorption.

Bioactive Compounds

Bioactive compounds are those food components that have an effect on the body as a whole or specific tissues or cells. They are distinct from nutrients because bio active compounds are not essential and, currently, there are no recommended daily intake values. However, it is well established that a range of compounds from plant and animal sources has a positive influence on human health. These compounds include non-pro-vitamin A carotenoids and polyphenols, phytosterols, fatty acids and peptides.

The mechanisms of action for the various compounds, especially as related to reduced risk of disease in individuals, are not fully understood. Some act as antioxidants while others stimulate defense mechanisms that enhance the response to oxidative stress, preventing widespread damage or enhancing repair. There is insufficient evidence to recommend intakes, efficacy, and safety of these substances, especially as isolate supplements, but it is generally agreed that, consumed as part of a balanced diet, the benefits are significant.

Diet and Disease

Many compounds have different biological effects within our bodies, and diet and disease are intimately associated. Apart from the diseases associated with malnutrition or an inadequate supply of a specific compound, leading to deficiency (e.g., scurvy and beriberi), the long-term effects of under nutrition in the developed world are also becoming apparent.

Low birth weight infants experience increased rates of CVD in adulthood, and there is increasing evidence to support an association with obesity and metabolic disorders, such as diabetes. Animal and increasingly human studies suggest that malnourished mothers whether deprived of energy or individual nutrients have offspring that are more susceptible to chronic disease. Cancer incidence is significantly higher in subpopulations that consume a greater proportion of animal-derived fats and few if any vegetables, fruits, grains, and cereal. Nutritional disorders in Europe are typical of affluent societies, but age-related chronic diseases occur less frequently and later in life in the populations of Mediterranean countries (Spain, Southern France, Greece, and Italy) than those in Northern Europe (UK and Germany). Thus, given sufficient food, it is important to maintain a balance in which the right amounts of each food component are absorbed and available for use.

Understanding how our bodies respond to what we eat and make the most of what is available is central to unraveling the relationship between food and disease and health. Common to all nutritionally related diseases may be inappropriate changes in gene expression. Studies of diet–gene interactions have been under way for a number of years and have produced many interesting results. Until relatively recently, however, researchers have been limited in their investigations; one or at most a handful of genes, maybe one or two biochemical pathways, and single or simple groups of nutrients rather than whole foods. Nutrigenetics and a nutrigenomics have provided background information and new tools that enable researchers to take a much more global and realistic perspective.

Malnutrition

Malnutrition arises from eating a diet that is insufficient in or has excess calories, protein, carbohydrates, vitamins, or minerals. Not enough nutrients leads to under nutrition but the termmal nutrition is often, wrongly, used in place of under nutrition. Under nutrition during pregnancy or infancy can result in permanent problems with physical and mental development. Starvation, extreme under nourishment, is associated with reduced stature, thin arms and legs (lack of muscle bulk), low energy levels, and swollen legs and abdomen, but symptoms of malnutrition can be as apparently minor as increased frequency of infections and tiredness. Symptoms related to micronutrient deficiencies depend on the substance that is lacking. One of the commonest micronutrient deficiencies globally is iron.

In developing countries, over nutrition is beginning to be as much of a problem as it is in many developed countries. Over nutrition is a form of malnutrition, often in combination with a sedentary lifestyle, that increase an individual's risk of (mechanical) disability and disease (e.g., cancer and CVD),reducing quality of life, productivity, and life expectancy. Factors contributing to malnutrition of all types include poverty, socio economic status, agricultural productivity(e.g., availability of land, adverse weather, farming skills, lack of technology or resources), and food security (e.g., global warming, conflict, etc. that lead to disruption in global food and resource supply, disease (e.g., colony collapse disorder, wheat stem rust)).

Chronic Diseases

Life-stage, lifestyle, and genetics affect our risk of developing chronic diseases. As we age, our bodies are less effective at avoiding disease. The resulting breakdown in structure and function leads to an increased risk of chronic disease including cancer, CVD, type II diabetes, cataract and macula degeneration, arthritis, etc. Poor diet can accelerate this process while 80% of case- controlled studies support the hypothesis that a diet rich in fruits and vegetables, or more specifically bioactive compounds, can reduce the risks.

Diet has a role in the maintenance of health and development of disease. Understanding this relationship has proven very difficult, and what is obvious is that the benefits of some dietary choices are not the same for everyone. Maintaining an appropriate weight for height, moderating consumption of alcohol, not smoking, and taking regular exercise determine whether the majority of the population is at high or low risk of developing chronic disease. However, individual genetic differences in response to diet have been evident for years, e.g., cholesterol and saturated fat intake, salt intake, and hypertension. Some genetic diseases have no association with diet (e.g., sickle cell disease) while others may create specific dietary needs (e.g., cystic fibrosis, phenylketonuria) or may be exacerbated by some foods (e.g., lactose intolerance, celiac and food allergy). Others carry a high risk of developing disease (e.g., BRCA1/2 and breast cancer), which may or may not be affected by diet or other lifestyle choices.

Nutrigenetics examines single gene/single food compound interaction. One of the best-described examples is the relationship between folate and the gene for MTHFR – 5,10-methylenetetrahydrofolate reductase. Nutrigenomics, on the other hand, aims to examine the response of individuals and populations to food/food components using postgenomics technologies ('omics'). The huge advantage in this approach is that the studies can examine people (i.e., populations, subpopulations – based on genes or disease – and individuals), food, life-stage, and lifestyle. For example, to understand the role of vitamin E in the prevention of CVD, nutrigenomics enables researchers to examine lipid and lipoprotein genotypes; glucose metabolism (i.e., the insulin– glucagon regulatory mechanism); triglyceride regulation (which retinoids and, therefore, some carotenoids, may act on); and fatty acid metabolism simultaneously. The various techniques, however, also reveal genes, proteins, and metabolites, which might not have predicted as relevant.

There are, however, fewer than 100 genes – compared with c.25 000 in the human genome – with polymorphisms that appear to confer a significant disadvantage that may be overcome through dietary modification, and our understanding of whole genome– food relationships is still limited. In addition, there are a number of wider issues to consider, not least the ethical, legal, and societal aspects of the research. Genotypes that confer a substantial disadvantage are not usually preserved in a population and those that do, although unrelated to diet, have been shown to offer some other benefit. The fact that the most common polymorphism for MTHFR is present in 15–20% of the European population should at least raise the question why it and the others have persisted so successfully if they only bestow a disadvantage or whether the disadvantage arises only because of modern dietary behaviors. Secondly, we do not know how or which of these genes interact with one another or the consequences of modifying the response of a few on the majority, and the impact on our immediate or long-term health.

Allergy and Intolerance

The public perception is that food allergy is a common condition, affecting up to one in three of the population (i.e., up to 20 million in the UK). Allergy in general is increasing and with it also food allergy. The numbers of foods causing an allergic reaction and the frequency of severe reactions (anaphylaxis) are also increasing, but only around 1–2% of adults are food allergic although rates are higher among children (c.5–8% of under 16).

Food allergy is an immune response to a protein or portion of a protein found in food. The allergic reaction can occur at a point of contact (e.g., the lips or tongue) as well as throughout the body (systemic). Symptoms differ greatly between individuals and might present differently in the same person, depending on the route and duration of exposure.

Food allergy develops in two stages: sensitization occurs when the immune system encounters an unrecognized molecule (almost always a protein). At this stage, individuals have indication they are potentially allergic. An allergic reaction is triggered only when the individual eats the same food or is exposed to the allergen (protein) in a different food.

Clinical experience suggests that food allergies are limited to a relative small group of foods including cow's milk, egg, soy, peanut, tree nuts, cereals, crustaceans and fish, and seeds. One theory suggests that the modern obsession with cleanliness explains why allergies are becoming more important. The reduced incidence of previously common infections and increased use of antibiotics may have shifted the immune system toward sensitization. In truth, however, although we know how people become allergic, the why remains elusive.

At present there is no cure for food allergy. The only treatment is avoidance of the problem food(s), but even this can be problematic meaning food allergy can have a detrimental impact beyond simply what can and cannot be eaten.

Food Intolerance

Not all reactions to food are an allergy; it can be food intolerance (e.g.,lactose intolerance)or symptoms of a disease (e.g., celiac).Food intolerance, unlike food allergy, can have a number of different causes. It is also much more common than food allergy. The onset of symptoms is usually slower and persists for several hours or longer. Intolerance to several foods or groups of foods is not uncommon, making identification of the cause much more challenging. Those with food intolerance(s) can sometimes tolerate small amounts of the food that induces symptoms, but too much or too frequent consumption leads to symptoms, which can also vary significantly between individuals or depending on the route of exposure. Symptoms include fatigue, gastrointestinal disturbance (e.g., diarrhea, vomiting, bloating, irritable bowel, etc.), and skin-related symptoms (e.g., urticaria, eczema, etc.). Causes of intolerance can be genetic (e.g.,enzyme defects/deficiency, lactose intolerance and gluten in tolerance(celiac disease)),which means substance in the food cannot be digested correctly, pharmacological (e.g.,caffeine intolerance), or toxicity (e.g., histamine). However, apart from celiac disease and lactose intolerance, there are no reliable or validated tests to identify food intolerance.

Chapter 2

Understanding Metabolism

The group of chemical reactions in organisms responsible for conversion of food to energy, conversion of food to building blocks for lipids, nucleic acids and proteins, and elimination of nitrogenous wastes is known as metabolism. This chapter discusses in detail the concepts related to metabolism such as metabolic rate and metabolic fuel.

Metabolism is the sum of the chemical reactions that take place within each cell of a living organism and that provide energy for vital processes and for synthesizing new organic material.

Living organisms are unique in that they can extract energy from their environments and use it to carry out activities such as movement, growth and development, and reproduction. But how do living organisms—or, their cells—extract energy from their environments, and how do cells use this energy to synthesize and assemble the components from which the cells are made?

The answers to these questions lie in the enzyme-mediated chemical reactions that take place in living matter (metabolism). Hundreds of coordinated, multistep reactions, fueled by energy obtained from nutrients and solar energy, ultimately convert readily available materials into the molecules required for growth and maintenance.

Unity of Life

At the cellular level of organization, the main chemical processes of all living matter are similar, if not identical. This is true for animals, plants, fungi, or bacteria; where variations occur (such as, for example, in the secretion of antibodies by some molds), the variant processes are but variations on common themes. Thus, all living matter is made up of large molecules called proteins, which provide support and coordinated movement, as well as storage and transport of small molecules, and, as catalysts, enable chemical reactions to take place rapidly and specifically under mild temperature, relatively low concentration, and neutral conditions (i.e., neither acidic nor basic). Proteins are assembled from some 20 amino acids, and, just as the 26 letters of the alphabet can be assembled in specific ways to form words of various lengths and meanings, so may tens or even hundreds of the 20 amino-acid "letters" be joined to form specific proteins. Moreover, those portions of protein molecules involved in performing similar functions in different organisms often comprise the same sequences of amino acids.

There is the same unity among cells of all types in the manner in which living organisms preserve their individuality and transmit it to their offspring. For example, hereditary information is encoded in a specific sequence of bases that make up the DNA (deoxyribonucleic acid) molecule in the nucleus of each cell. Only four bases are used in synthesizing DNA: adenine, guanine, cytosine, and thymine. Just as the Morse code consists of three simple signals—a dash, a dot, and a space—the precise arrangement of which suffices to convey coded messages, so the precise arrangement of the bases in DNA contains and conveys the information for the synthesis and assembly of cell components. Some primitive life-forms, however, use RNA (ribonucleic acid; a nucleic acid differing from DNA in containing the sugar ribose instead of the sugar deoxyribose and the base uracil instead of the base thymine) in place of DNA as a primary carrier of genetic information. The replication of the genetic material in these organisms must, however, pass through a DNA phase. With minor exceptions, the genetic code used by all living organisms is the same.

The chemical reactions that take place in living cells are similar as well. Green plants use the energy of sunlight to convert water (H_2O) and carbon dioxide (CO_2) to carbohydrates (sugars and starches), other organic (carbon-containing) compounds, and molecular oxygen (O_2). The process of photosynthesis requires energy, in the form of sunlight, to split one water molecule into one-half of an oxygen molecule (O_2; the oxidizing agent) and two hydrogen atoms (H; the reducing agent), each of which dissociates to one hydrogen ion (H^+) and one electron. Through a series of oxidation-reduction reactions, electrons (denoted e^-) are transferred from a donating molecule (oxidation), in this case water, to an accepting molecule (reduction) by a series of chemical reactions; this "reducing power" may be coupled ultimately to the reduction of carbon dioxide to the level of carbohydrate. In effect, carbon dioxide accepts and bonds with hydrogen, forming carbohydrates ($Cn[H_2O]n$).

Living organisms that require oxygen reverse this process: they consume carbohydrates and other organic materials, using oxygen synthesized by plants to form water, carbon dioxide, and energy. The process that removes hydrogen atoms (containing electrons) from the carbohydrates and passes them to the oxygen is an energy-yielding series of reactions.

In plants, all but two of the steps in the process that converts carbon dioxide to carbohydrates are the same as those steps that synthesize sugars from simpler starting materials in animals, fungi, and bacteria. Similarly, the series of reactions that take a given starting material and synthesize certain molecules that will be used in other synthetic pathways are similar, or identical, among all cell types. From a metabolic point of view, the cellular processes that take place in a lion are only marginally different from those that take place in a dandelion.

Biological Energy Exchanges

The energy changes associated with physicochemical processes are the province of thermodynamics, a subdiscipline of physics. The first two laws of thermodynamics state, in essence, that energy can be neither created nor destroyed and that the effect of physical and chemical changes is to increase the disorder, or randomness (i.e., entropy), of the universe. Although it might be supposed that biological processes—through which organisms grow in a highly ordered and complex manner, maintain order and complexity throughout their life, and pass on the instructions for order to succeeding generations—are in contravention of these laws, this is not so. Living organisms neither consume nor create energy: they can only transform it from one form to another. From the environment they absorb energy in a form useful to them; to the environment they return an equivalent amount of energy in a biologically less useful form. The useful energy, or free energy, may be defined as energy capable of doing work under isothermal conditions (conditions in which no temperature differential exists); free energy is associated with any chemical change. Energy less useful than free energy is returned to the environment, usually as heat. Heat cannot perform work in biological systems because all parts of cells have essentially the same temperature and pressure.

Carrier of Chemical Energy

At any given time, a neutral molecule of water dissociates into a hydrogen ion (H^+) and a hydroxide ion (OH^-), and the ions are continually re-forming into the neutral molecule. Under normal conditions (neutrality), the concentration of hydrogen ions (acidic ions) is equal to that of the hydroxide ions (basic ions); each are at a concentration of 10^{-7} mole per litre, which is described as a pH of 7.

All cells either are bounded by membranes or contain organelles that have membranes. These membranes do not permit water or the ions derived from water to pass into or out of the cells or organelles. In green plants, sunlight is absorbed by chlorophyll and other pigments in the chloroplasts of the cells, called photosystem II. When a water molecule is split by light energy, one-half of an oxygen molecule and two hydrogen atoms (which dissociate to two electrons and two hydrogen ions, H^+) are formed. When excited by sunlight, chlorophyll loses one electron to an electron carrier molecule but quickly recovers it from a hydrogen atom of the split water molecule, which sends H^+ into solution in the process. Two oxygen atoms come together to form a molecule of oxygen gas (O_2). The free electrons are passed to photosystem I, but, in doing so, an excess concentration of positively charged hydrogen ions (H^+) appears on one side of the membrane in the chloroplast, whereas an excess of negatively charged hydroxide ions (OH^-) builds up on the other side. The free energy released as H^+ ions move through a specific "pore" in the membrane, to equalize the concentrations of ions, is sufficient to make some biological processes work, such as the uptake of certain nutrients by bacteria and the rotation of the whiplike protein-based propellers that enable such bacteria to move. Equally important, however, is that this gradient across the membrane powers the formation of adenosine triphosphate (ATP) from inorganic phosphate (HPO_4^{2-}, abbreviated Pi) and adenosine diphosphate (ADP). ATP is the major carrier of biologically utilizable energy in all forms of living matter. The interrelationships of energy-yielding and energy-requiring metabolic reactions may be considered largely as processes that couple the formation of ATP with its breakdown.

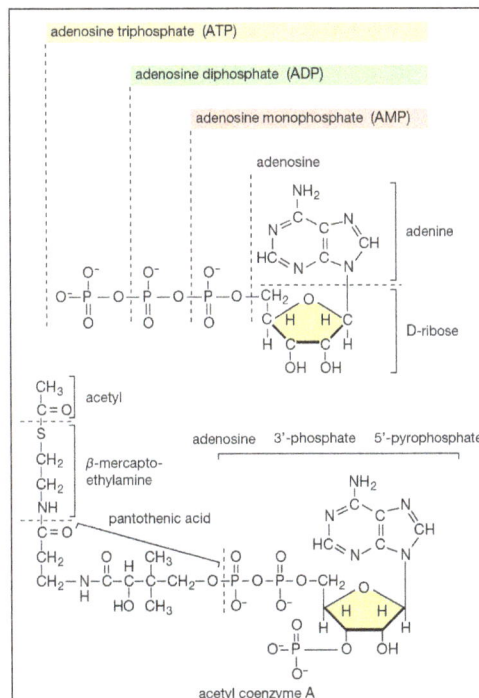

Biological energy carriers

Synthesis of ATP by green plants is similar to the synthesis of ATP that takes place in the mitochondria of animal, plant, and fungus cells, and in the plasma membranes of bacteria that use oxygen (or other inorganic electron acceptors, such as nitrate) to accept electrons from the removal of hydrogen atoms from a molecule of food. Through these processes most of the energy stored in food materials is released and converted into the molecules that fuel life processes. It must also be remembered, however, that many living organisms (usually bacteria and protozoa) cannot tolerate oxygen; they form ATP from inorganic phosphate and ADP by substrate-level phosphorylations (the addition of a phosphate group) that do not involve the establishment and collapse of proton gradients across membranes. It must also be borne in mind that the fuels of life and the cellular "furnace" in which they are "burned" are made of the same types of material: if the fires burn too brightly, not only the fuel but also the furnace is consumed. It is therefore essential to release energy at small, discrete, readily utilizable intervals. The relative complexity of the catabolic pathways (by which food materials are broken down) and the complexity of the anabolic pathways (by which cell components are synthesized) reflect this need and offer the possibility for simple feedback systems to control the rate at which materials travel along these sequences of enzymic reactions.

Catabolism

The release of chemical energy from food materials essentially occurs in three phases. In the first phase (phase I), the large molecules that make up the bulk of food materials are broken down into small constituent units: proteins are converted to the 20 or so different amino acids of which they are composed; carbohydrates (polysaccharides such as starch in plants and glycogen in animals) are degraded to sugars such as glucose; and fats (lipids) are broken down into fatty acids and glycerol. The amounts of energy liberated in phase I are relatively small: only about 0.6 percent of the free, or useful, energy of proteins and carbohydrates, and about 0.1 percent of that of fats, is released during this phase. Because this energy is liberated largely as heat, it cannot be used by the cell. The purpose of the reactions of phase I, which can be grouped under the term digestion and which, in animals, occur mainly in the intestinal tract and in tissues in which reserve materials are prepared, or mobilized, for energy production, is to prepare the foodstuffs for the energy-releasing processes.

Incomplete Oxidation

In the second phase of the release of energy from food (phase II), the small molecules produced in the first phase—sugars, glycerol, a number of fatty acids, and about 20 varieties of amino acids—are incompletely oxidized (in this sense, oxidation means the removal of electrons or hydrogen atoms), the end product being (apart from carbon dioxide and water) one of only three possible substances: the two-carbon compound acetate, in the form of a compound called acetyl coenzyme A; the four-carbon compound oxaloacetate; and the five-carbon compound α-oxoglutarate. The first, acetate in the form of acetyl coenzyme A, constitutes by far the most common product—it is the product of two-thirds of the carbon incorporated into carbohydrates and glycerol; all of the carbon in most fatty acids; and approximately half of the carbon in amino acids. The end product of several amino acids is α-oxoglutarate; that of a few others is oxaloacetate, which is formed either directly or indirectly (from fumarate). These processes occur in animals, plants, bacteria, fungi, and other organisms capable of oxidizing their food materials wholly to carbon dioxide and water.

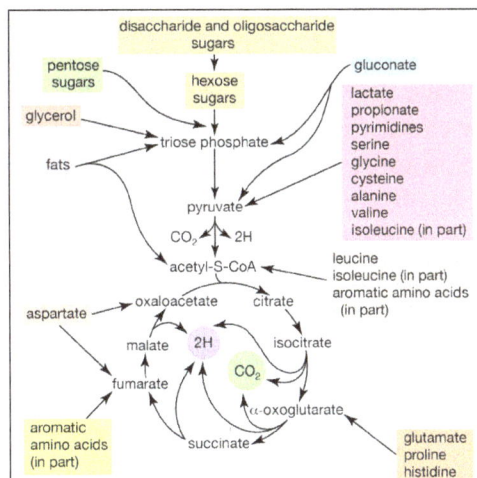

Pathways for the catabolism of nutrients by Escherichia coli.

Complete Oxidation

Total oxidation of the relatively few products of phase II occurs in a cyclic sequence of chemical reactions known as the tricarboxylic acid (TCA) cycle, or the Krebs cycle, after its discoverer, Sir Hans Krebs; it represents phase III of energy release from foods. Each turn of this cycle is initiated by the formation of citrate, with six carbon atoms, from oxaloacetate (with four carbons) and acetyl coenzyme A; subsequent reactions result in the reformation of oxaloacetate and the formation of two molecules of carbon dioxide. The carbon atoms that go into the formation of carbon dioxide are no longer available to the cell. The concomitant stepwise oxidations—in which hydrogen atoms or electrons are removed from intermediate compounds formed during the cycle and, via a system of carriers, are transferred ultimately to oxygen to form water—are quantitatively the most important means of generating ATP from ADP and inorganic phosphate. These events are known as terminal respiration and oxidative phosphorylation.

Some microorganisms, incapable of completely converting their carbon compounds to carbon dioxide, release energy by fermentation reactions, in which the intermediate compounds of catabolic routes either directly or indirectly accept or donate hydrogen atoms. Such secondary changes in intermediate compounds result in considerably less energy being made available to the cell than occurs with the pathways that are linked to oxidative phosphorylation; however, fermentation reactions yield a large variety of commercially important products. Thus, for example, if the oxidation (removal of electrons or hydrogen atoms) of some catabolic intermediate is coupled to the reduction of pyruvate or of acetaldehyde derived from pyruvate, the products formed are lactic acid and ethyl alcohol, respectively.

Anabolism

Catabolic pathways effect the transformation of food materials into interconvertible intermediates. Anabolic pathways, on the other hand, are sequences of enzyme-catalyzed reactions in which the component building blocks of large molecules, or macromolecules (e.g., proteins, carbohydrates, and fats), are constructed from the same intermediates. Thus, catabolic routes have clearly defined beginnings but no unambiguously identifiable end products; anabolic routes, on the other hand, lead to clearly distinguishable end products from diffuse beginnings. The two types of pathway are linked through reactions of phosphate transfer, involving ADP, AMP, and ATP, and also through electron transfers, which enable reducing equivalents (i.e., hydrogen atoms or electrons), which have been released during catabolic reactions, to be utilized for biosynthesis. But, although catabolic and anabolic pathways are closely linked, and although the overall effect of one type of route is obviously the opposite of the other, they have few steps in common. The anabolic pathway for the synthesis of a particular molecule generally starts from intermediate compounds quite different from those produced as a result of catabolism of that molecule; for example, microorganisms catabolize aromatic (i.e., containing a ring, or cyclic, structure) amino acids to acetyl coenzyme A and an intermediate compound of the TCA cycle. The biosynthesis of these amino acids, however, starts with a compound derived from pyruvate and an intermediate compound of the metabolism of pentose (a general name for sugars with five carbon atoms). Similarly, histidine is synthesized from a pentose sugar but is catabolized to α-oxoglutarate.

Even in cases in which a product of catabolism is used in an anabolic pathway, differences emerge; thus, fatty acids, which are catabolized to acetyl coenzyme A, are synthesized not from acetyl coenzyme A directly but from a derivative of it, malonyl coenzyme A. Furthermore, even enzymes that catalyze apparently identical steps in catabolic and anabolic routes may exhibit different properties. In general, therefore, the way down (catabolism) is different from the way up (anabolism). These differences are important because they allow for the regulation of catabolic and anabolic processes in the cell.

In eukaryotic cells (i.e., those with a well-defined nucleus, characteristic of organisms higher than bacteria) the enzymes of catabolic and anabolic pathways are often located in different cellular compartments. This also contributes to the manner of their cellular control; for example, the formation of acetyl coenzyme A from fatty acids, referred to above, occurs in animal cells in small sausage-shaped components, or organelles, called mitochondria, which also contain the enzymes for terminal respiration and for oxidative phosphorylation. The biosynthesis of fatty acids from acetyl coenzyme A, on the other hand, occurs in the cytoplasm.

Integration of Catabolism and Anabolism

Fine Control

Possibly the most important means for controlling the flux of metabolites through catabolic and anabolic pathways, and for integrating the numerous different pathways in the cell, is through the regulation of either the activity or the synthesis of key (pacemaker) enzymes. It was recognized in the 1950s, largely from work with microorganisms, that pacemaker enzymes can interact with small molecules at more than one site on the surface of the enzyme molecule. The reaction between an enzyme and its substrate—defined as the compound with which the enzyme acts to form a product—occurs at a specific site on the enzyme known as the catalytic, or active, site; the proper fit between the substrate and the active site is an essential prerequisite for the occurrence of a reaction catalyzed by an enzyme. Interactions at other, so-called regulatory sites on the enzyme, however, do not result in a chemical reaction but cause changes in the shape of the protein; the changes profoundly affect the catalytic properties of the enzyme, either inhibiting or stimulating the rate of the reaction. Modulation of the activity of pacemaker enzymes may be effected by metabolites of the pathway in which the enzyme acts or by those of another pathway; the process may be described as a "fine control" of metabolism. Very small changes in the chemical environment thus produce important and immediate effects on the rates at which individual metabolic processes occur.

Most catabolic pathways are regulated by the relative proportions of ATP, ADP, and AMP in the cell. It is reasonable to suppose that a pathway that serves to make ATP available for energy-requiring reactions would be less active if sufficient ATP were already present, than if ADP or AMP were to accumulate. The relative amounts of the adenine nucleotides (i.e., ATP, ADP, and AMP) thus modulate the overall rate of catabolic pathways. They do so by reacting with specific regulatory sites on pacemaker enzymes necessary for the catabolic pathways, which do not participate in the anabolic routes that effect the opposite reactions. Similarly, it is reasonable to suppose that many anabolic processes, which require energy, are inhibited by ADP or AMP; elevated levels of these nucleotides may be regarded therefore as cellular distress signals indicating a lack of energy.

Since one way in which anabolic pathways differ from catabolic routes is that the former result in identifiable end products, it is not unexpected that the pacemaker enzymes of many anabolic pathways—particularly those effecting the biosynthesis of amino acids and nucleotides —are regulated by the end products of these pathways or, in cases in which branching of pathways occurs, by end products of each branch. Such pacemaker enzymes usually act at the first step unique to a particular anabolic route. If branching occurs, the first step of each branch is controlled. By this so-called negative feedback system, the cellular concentrations of products determine the rates of their formation, thus ensuring that the cell synthesizes only as much of the products as it needs.

Coarse Control

A second and less immediately responsive, or "coarse," control is exerted over the synthesis of pacemaker enzymes. The rate of protein synthesis reflects the activity of appropriate genes, which contain the information that directs all cellular processes. Coarse control is therefore exerted on genetic material rather than on enzymes. Preferential synthesis of a pacemaker enzyme is particularly required to accommodate a cell to major changes in its chemical milieu. Such changes occur in multicellular organisms only to a minor extent, so that this type of control mechanism is less important in animals than in microorganisms. In the latter, however, it may determine the ease with which a cell previously growing in one nutrient medium can grow after transfer to another. In cases in which several types of organism compete in the same medium for available carbon sources, the operation of coarse controls may well be decisive in ensuring survival.

Alterations in the differential rates of synthesis of pacemaker enzymes in microorganisms responding to changes in the composition of their growth medium also manifest the properties of negative feedback systems. Depending on the nature of the metabolic pathway of which a pacemaker enzyme is a constituent, the manner in which the alterations are elicited may be distinguished. Thus, an increase in the rates at which enzymes of catabolic routes are synthesized results from the addition of inducers—usually compounds that exhibit some structural similarity to the substrates on which the enzymes act. A classic example of an inducible enzyme of this type is β-galactosidase. Escherichia coli growing in nutrient medium containing glucose do not utilize the milk sugar, lactose (glucose-4-β-D-galactoside); however, if the bacteria are placed in a growth medium containing lactose as the sole source of carbon, they synthesize β-galactosidase and can therefore utilize lactose. The reaction catalyzed by the enzyme is the hydrolysis (i.e., breakdown involving water) of lactose to its two constituent sugars, glucose and galactose; the preferential synthesis of the enzyme thus allows the bacteria to use the lactose for growth and energy. Another characteristic of the process of enzyme induction is that it continues only as long as the inducer (in this case, lactose) is present; if cells synthesizing β-galactosidase are transferred to a medium containing no lactose, synthesis of β-galactosidase ceases, and the amount of the enzyme in the cells is diluted as they divide, until the original low level of the enzyme is reestablished.

In contrast, the differential rates of synthesis of pacemaker enzymes of anabolic routes are usually not increased by the presence of inducers. Instead, the absence of small molecules that act to repress enzyme synthesis accelerates enzyme formation. Similar to the fine control processes described above is the regulation by coarse control of many pacemaker enzymes of amino-acid biosynthesis. Like the end product inhibitors, the repressors in these cases also appear to be the amino-acid end products themselves. It is useful to regard the acceleration of the enzyme-forming machinery as the consequence, metaphorically, of either placing a foot on the accelerator or removing it from the brake.

Fragmentation of Complex Molecules

Food materials must undergo oxidation in order to yield biologically useful energy. Oxidation does not necessarily involve oxygen, although it must involve the transfer of electrons from a donor molecule to a suitable acceptor molecule; the donor is thus oxidized and the recipient reduced. Many microorganisms either must live in the absence of oxygen (i.e., are obligate anaerobes) or can live in its presence or its absence (i.e., are facultative anaerobes).

If no oxygen is available, the catabolism of food materials is effected via fermentations, in which the final acceptor of the electrons removed from the nutrient is some organic molecule, usually generated during the fermentation process. There is no net oxidation of the food molecule in this type of catabolism; that is, the overall oxidation state of the fermentation products is the same as that of the starting material.

Organisms that can use oxygen as a final electron acceptor also use many of the steps in the fermentation pathways in which food molecules are broken down to smaller fragments; these fragments, instead of serving as electron acceptors, are fed into the TCA cycle, the pathway of terminal respiration.

In this cycle all of the hydrogen atoms (H) or electrons (e^-) are removed from the fragments and are channeled through a series of electron carriers, ultimately to react with oxygen. All carbon atoms are eliminated as carbon dioxide (CO_2) in this process. The sequence of reactions involved in the catabolism of food materials may thus be conveniently considered in terms of an initial fragmentation (fermentation), followed by a combustion (respiration) process.

Catabolism of Glucose

Glycolysis

Quantitatively, the most important source of energy for cellular processes is the six-carbon sugar glucose ($C_6H_{12}O_6$). Glucose is made available to animals through the hydrolysis of polysaccharides, such as glycogen and starch, the process being catalyzed by digestive enzymes. In animals, the sugar thus set free passes from the gut into the bloodstream and from there into the cells of the liver and other tissues. In microorganisms, no such specialized tissues are involved.

The fermentative phase of glucose catabolism (glycolysis) involves several enzymes; the action of each is summarized below. In living cells, many of the compounds that take part in metabolism exist as negatively charged moieties, or anions.

In order to obtain a net yield of ATP from the catabolism of glucose, it is first necessary to invest ATP. During the first step given below, the alcohol group at position 6 of the glucose molecule readily reacts with the terminal phosphate group of ATP, forming glucose 6-phosphate and ADP. For convenience, the phosphoryl group (PO_3^{2-}) is represented by Ⓟ. Because the decrease in free energy is so large, this reaction is virtually irreversible under physiological conditions.

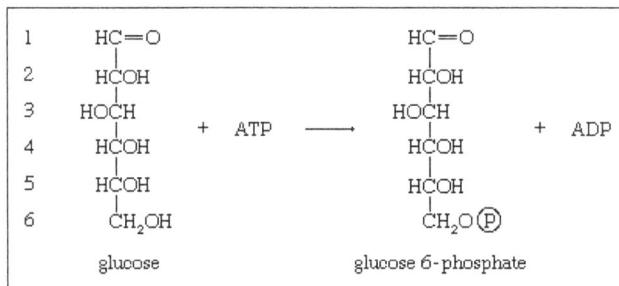

In animals, this phosphorylation of glucose, which yields glucose 6-phosphate, is catalyzed by two different enzymes. In most cells a hexokinase with a high affinity for glucose—i.e., only small amounts of glucose are necessary for enzymatic activity—effects the reaction. In addition, the liver contains a glucokinase, which requires a much greater concentration of glucose before it reacts. Glucokinase functions only in emergencies, when the concentration of glucose in the blood rises to abnormally high levels.

Certain facultative anaerobic bacteria also contain hexokinases but apparently do not use them to phosphorylate glucose. In such cells, external glucose can be utilized only if it is first phosphorylated to glucose 6-phosphate via a system linked to the cell membrane that involves a compound called phosphoenolpyruvate, which serves as an obligatory donor of the phosphate group; i.e., ATP cannot serve as the phosphate donor in the reaction.

The reaction in which glucose 6-phosphate is changed to fructose 6-phosphate is catalyzed by phosphoglucoisomerase reaction given below. In the reaction, a secondary alcohol group ($-C|HOH$) at the second carbon atom is oxidized to a keto-group (i.e., $-C|=O$), and the aldehyde group ($-CHO$) at the first carbon atom is reduced to a primary alcohol group ($-CH_2OH$). Reaction Below is readily reversible, as is indicated by the double arrows.

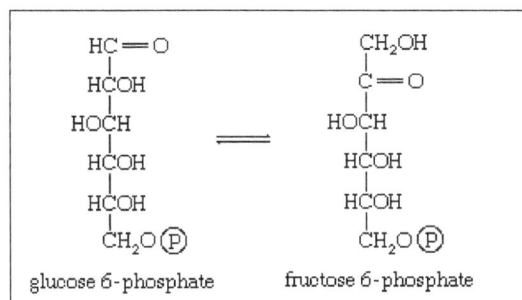

The formation of the alcohol group at the first carbon atom permits the repetition of the reaction effected in the first step of the reaction; that is, a second molecule of ATP is invested. The product is fructose 1,6-diphosphate. Again, as in the hexokinase reaction, the decrease in free energy of the reaction, which is catalyzed by phosphofructokinase, is sufficiently large to make this reaction virtually irreversible under physiological conditions; ADP is also a product.

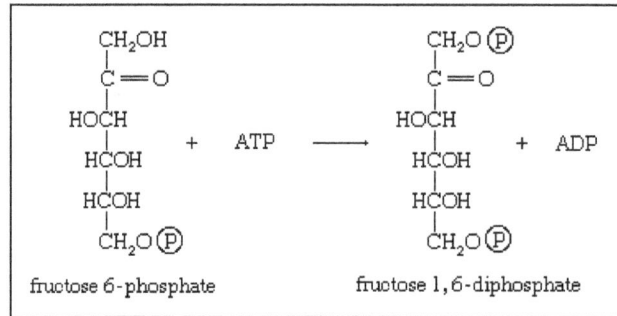

The first three steps of glycolysis have thus transformed an asymmetrical sugar molecule, glucose, into a symmetrical form, fructose 1,6-diphosphate, containing a phosphoryl group at each end; the molecule next is split into two smaller fragments that are interconvertible. This elegant simplification is achieved via the following two steps discussed below.

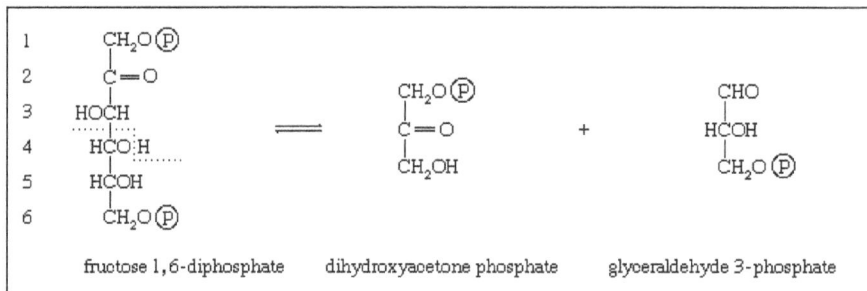

Aldolase Reaction

In the above step of reaction, an enzyme catalyzes the breaking apart of the six-carbon sugar fructose 1,6-diphosphate into two three-carbon fragments. The molecule is split between carbons 3 and 4. Reversal of this cleavage—i.e., the formation of a six-carbon compound from two three-carbon compounds—is possible. Because the reverse reaction is an aldol condensation—i.e., an aldehyde (glyceraldehyde 3-phosphate) combines with a ketone (dihydroxyacetone phosphate)—the enzyme is commonly called aldolase. The two three-carbon fragments produced in above step, dihydroxyacetone phosphate and glyceraldehyde 3-phosphate, are also called triose phosphates. They are readily converted to each other by a process below. The enzyme that catalyzes the interconversion below is triose phosphate isomerase.

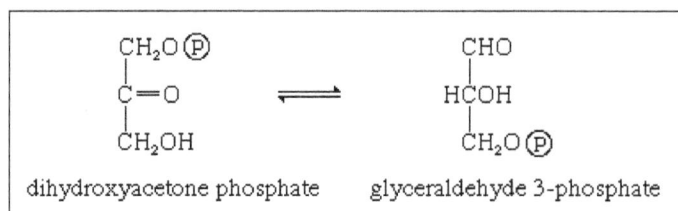

Formation of ATP

The second stage of glucose catabolism comprises the following four reactions, in which a net gain of ATP is achieved through the oxidation of one of the triose phosphate compounds formed in the above reaction. One molecule of glucose forms two molecules of the triose phosphate; both three-carbon fragments follow the same pathway, and following four reactions must occur twice to complete the glucose breakdown.

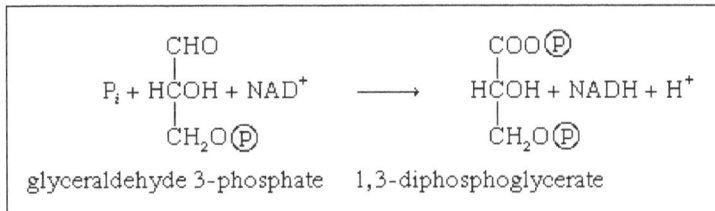

$$
\begin{array}{ccc}
\text{CHO} & & \text{COO}\,\textcircled{P} \\
| & & | \\
P_i + \text{HCOH} + \text{NAD}^+ \longrightarrow & \text{HCOH} + \text{NADH} + \text{H}^+ \\
| & & | \\
\text{CH}_2\text{O}\,\textcircled{P} & & \text{CH}_2\text{O}\,\textcircled{P} \\
\text{glyceraldehyde 3-phosphate} & & \text{1,3-diphosphoglycerate}
\end{array}
$$

The above reaction, in which glyceraldehyde 3-phosphate is oxidized, is one of the most important reactions in glycolysis. It is during this step that the energy liberated during oxidation of the aldehyde group ($-$CHO) is conserved in the form of a high-energy phosphate compound—namely, as 1,3-diphosphoglycerate, an anhydride of a carboxylic acid and phosphoric acid. The hydrogen atoms or electrons removed from the aldehyde group during its oxidation are accepted by a coenzyme (so called because it functions in conjunction with an enzyme) involved in hydrogen or electron transfer. The coenzyme, nicotinamide adenine dinucleotide (NAD$^+$), is reduced to form NADH + H$^+$ in the process. The NAD$^+$ thus reduced is bound to the enzyme glyceraldehyde 3-phosphate dehydrogenase, catalyzing the overall reaction.

The 1,3-diphosphoglycerate produced in the above reaction reacts with ADP in a reaction catalyzed by phosphoglycerate kinase, with the result that one of the two phosphoryl groups is transferred to ADP to form ATP and 3-phosphoglycerate. This reaction given below is highly exergonic (i.e., it proceeds with a loss of free energy); as a result, the oxidation of glyceraldehyde 3-phosphate (in the above reaction), is irreversible. In summary, the energy liberated during oxidation of an aldehyde group ($-$CHO in glyceraldehyde 3-phosphate) to a carboxylic acid group ($-$COO$^-$ in 3-phosphoglycerate) is conserved as the phosphate bond energy in ATP during the reactions above and below. This reaction occurs twice for each molecule of glucose. Thus, the initial investment of ATP is recovered.

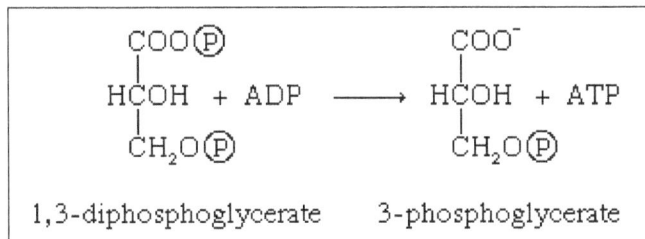

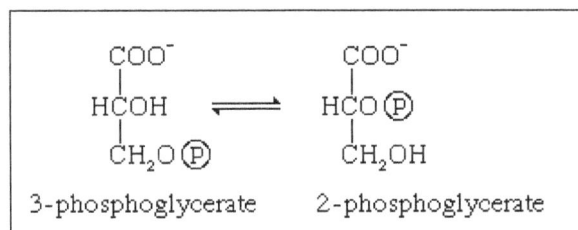

$$
\begin{array}{ccc}
\text{COO}\,\textcircled{P} & & \text{COO}^- \\
| & & | \\
\text{HCOH} + \text{ADP} \longrightarrow & \text{HCOH} + \text{ATP} \\
| & & | \\
\text{CH}_2\text{O}\,\textcircled{P} & & \text{CH}_2\text{O}\,\textcircled{P} \\
\text{1,3-diphosphoglycerate} & & \text{3-phosphoglycerate}
\end{array}
$$

$$
\begin{array}{ccc}
\text{COO}^- & & \text{COO}^- \\
| & & | \\
\text{HCOH} \rightleftharpoons & \text{HCO}\,\textcircled{P} \\
| & & | \\
\text{CH}_2\text{O}\,\textcircled{P} & & \text{CH}_2\text{OH} \\
\text{3-phosphoglycerate} & & \text{2-phosphoglycerate}
\end{array}
$$

The 3-phosphoglycerate in the above step now forms 2-phosphoglycerate in a reaction catalyzed by phosphoglyceromutase. During the reaction given below the enzyme enolase reacts with 2-phosphoglycerate to form phosphoenolpyruvate (PEP), water being lost from 2-phosphoglycerate in the process. Phosphoenolpyruvate acts as the second source of ATP in glycolysis. The transfer of the phosphate group from PEP to ADP, catalyzed by pyruvate kinase, is also highly exergonic and is thus virtually irreversible under physiological conditions.

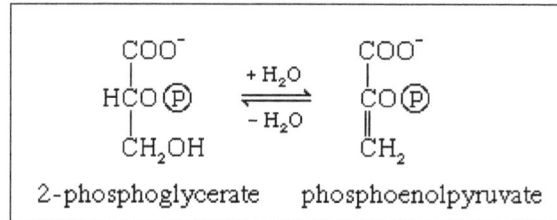

$$
\begin{array}{ccc}
\text{COO}^- & & \text{COO}^- \\
| & \xrightarrow{+\,H_2O} & | \\
\text{HCO}\,\textcircled{P} & \xleftarrow{-\,H_2O} & \text{CO}\,\textcircled{P} \\
| & & \| \\
\text{CH}_2\text{OH} & & \text{CH}_2 \\
\text{2-phosphoglycerate} & & \text{phosphoenolpyruvate}
\end{array}
$$

Reaction given below occurs twice for each molecule of glucose entering the glycolytic sequence. Thus, the net yield is two molecules of ATP for each six-carbon sugar. No further molecules of glucose can enter the glycolytic pathway, however, until the NADH + H$^+$ produced above, in which glyceraldehyde 3-phosphate is oxidized, is reoxidized to NAD$^+$. In anaerobic systems this means that electrons must be transferred from (NADH + H$^+$) to some organic acceptor molecule, which thus is reduced in the process. Such an acceptor molecule could be the pyruvate formed in reaction.

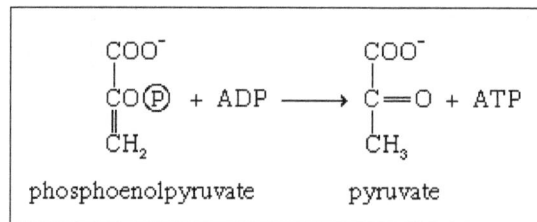

$$
\begin{array}{ccc}
\text{COO}^- & & \text{COO}^- \\
| & & | \\
\text{CO}\,\textcircled{P} \;+\; \text{ADP} & \longrightarrow & \text{C}=\text{O} \;+\; \text{ATP} \\
\| & & | \\
\text{CH}_2 & & \text{CH}_3 \\
\text{phosphoenolpyruvate} & & \text{pyruvate}
\end{array}
$$

In certain bacteria (e.g., so-called lactic acid bacteria) or in muscle cells functioning vigorously in the absence of adequate supplies of oxygen, pyruvate is reduced to lactate via a reaction catalyzed by lactate dehydrogenase; i.e., NADH gives up its hydrogen atoms or electrons to pyruvate, and lactate and NAD$^+$ are formed.

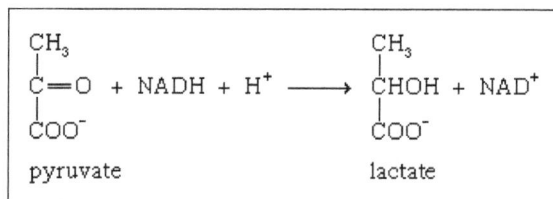

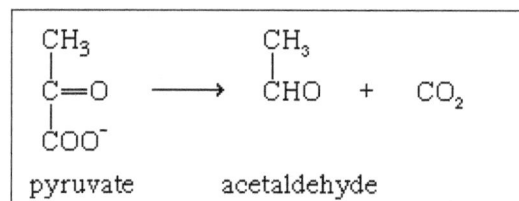

$$
\begin{array}{ccc}
\text{CH}_3 & & \text{CH}_3 \\
| & & | \\
\text{C}=\text{O} \;+\; \text{NADH} + \text{H}^+ & \longrightarrow & \text{CHOH} \;+\; \text{NAD}^+ \\
| & & | \\
\text{COO}^- & & \text{COO}^- \\
\text{pyruvate} & & \text{lactate}
\end{array}
$$

$$
\begin{array}{ccc}
\text{CH}_3 & & \text{CH}_3 \\
| & & | \\
\text{C}=\text{O} & \longrightarrow & \text{CHO} \;+\; \text{CO}_2 \\
| & & \\
\text{COO}^- & & \\
\text{pyruvate} & & \text{acetaldehyde}
\end{array}
$$

Alternatively, in organisms such as brewers' yeast, pyruvate is first decarboxylated to form acetaldehyde and carbon dioxide in a reaction catalyzed by pyruvate decarboxylase.

$$
\begin{array}{ccc}
\underset{\mid}{CH_3} & & \underset{\mid}{CH_3} \\
\overset{\mid}{C}\!\!=\!\!O & \longrightarrow & \overset{\mid}{C}HO \quad + \quad CO_2 \\
\overset{\mid}{C}OO^- & & \\
\text{pyruvate} & & \text{acetaldehyde}
\end{array}
$$

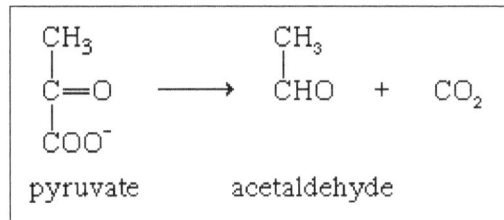

Acetaldehyde then is reduced (by NADH + H$^+$) in a reaction catalyzed by alcohol dehydrogenase, yielding ethanol and oxidized coenzyme (NAD$^+$).

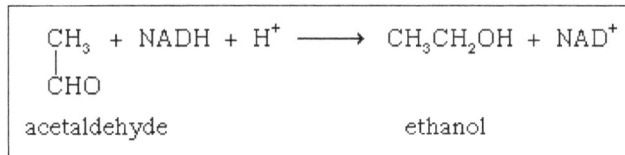

$$
\begin{array}{l}
\underset{\mid}{CH_3} + NADH + H^+ \longrightarrow CH_3CH_2OH + NAD^+ \\
\overset{\mid}{C}HO \\
\text{acetaldehyde} \qquad\qquad\qquad\qquad \text{ethanol}
\end{array}
$$

Many variations of above three reactions occur in nature. In the heterolactic (mixed lactic acid) fermentations carried out by some microorganisms, a mixture of reactions regenerates NAD$^+$ and results in the production, for each molecule of glucose fermented, of a molecule each of lactate, ethanol, and carbon dioxide. In other types of fermentation, the end products may be derivatives of acids such as propionic, butyric, acetic, and succinic; decarboxylated materials derived from them (e.g., acetone); or compounds such as glycerol.

Phosphogluconate Pathway

Many cells possess, in addition to all or part of the glycolytic pathway that comprises all of the above reactions, other pathways of glucose catabolism that involve, as the first unique step, the oxidation of glucose 6-phosphate instead of the formation of fructose 6-phosphate Above. This is the phosphogluconate pathway, or pentose phosphate cycle. During the following reaction, hydrogen atoms or electrons are removed from the carbon atom at position 1 of glucose 6-phosphate in a reaction catalyzed by glucose 6-phosphate dehydrogenase. The product of the reaction is 6-phosphogluconate.

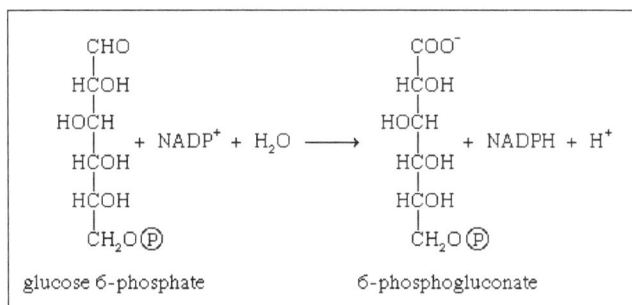

$$
\begin{array}{ccc}
\underset{\mid}{CHO} & & \underset{\mid}{COO^-} \\
\underset{\mid}{H\overset{\mid}{C}OH} & & \underset{\mid}{H\overset{\mid}{C}OH} \\
\underset{\mid}{HO\overset{\mid}{C}H} & + NADP^+ + H_2O \longrightarrow & \underset{\mid}{HO\overset{\mid}{C}H} + NADPH + H^+ \\
\underset{\mid}{H\overset{\mid}{C}OH} & & \underset{\mid}{H\overset{\mid}{C}OH} \\
\underset{\mid}{H\overset{\mid}{C}OH} & & \underset{\mid}{H\overset{\mid}{C}OH} \\
CH_2O\,\text{\textcircled{P}} & & CH_2O\,\text{\textcircled{P}} \\
\text{glucose 6-phosphate} & & \text{6-phosphogluconate}
\end{array}
$$

The reducing equivalents (hydrogen atoms or electrons) are accepted by nicotine adenine dinucleotide phosphate (NADP$^+$), a coenzyme similar to but not identical with NAD$^+$. A second molecule of NADP$^+$ is reduced as 6-phosphogluconate is further oxidized; the reaction is catalyzed by 6-phosphogluconate dehydrogenase. The products of the reaction also include ribulose 5-phosphate and carbon dioxide. (The numbers at the carbon atoms in the following reaction indicate that carbon 1 of 6-phosphogluconate forms carbon dioxide).

$$
\begin{array}{ll}
\begin{array}{ll}
1 & COO^- \\
2 & HCOH \\
3 & HOCH \\
4 & HCOH \\
5 & HCOH \\
6 & CH_2O\,\textcircled{P}
\end{array} + NADP^+
\longrightarrow
\begin{array}{ll}
2 & CH_2OH \\
3 & C=O \\
4 & HCOH \\
5 & HCOH \\
6 & CH_2O\,\textcircled{P}
\end{array} + CO_2 + NADPH + H^+ \\
\\
\text{6-phosphogluconate} \qquad\qquad \text{ribulose 5-phosphate}
\end{array}
$$

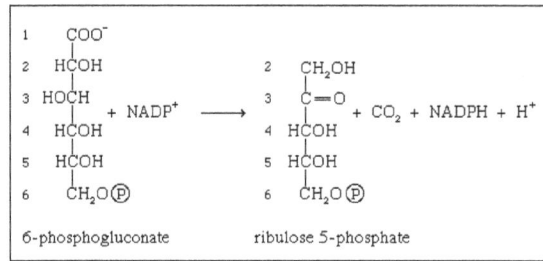

Ribulose 5-phosphate can undergo a series of reactions in which two-carbon and three-carbon fragments are interchanged between a numbers of sugar phosphates. This sequence of events can lead to the formation of two molecules of fructose 6-phosphate and one of glyceraldehyde 3-phosphate from three molecules of ribulose 5-phosphate (i.e., the conversion of three molecules with five carbons to two with six and one with three). Although the cycle is the main pathway in microorganisms for fragmentation of pentose sugars, it is not of major importance as a route for the oxidation of glucose. Its primary purpose in most cells is to generate reducing power in the cytoplasm, in the form of reduced $NADP^+$. This function is especially prominent in tissues—such as the liver, the mammary gland, adipose tissue, and the cortex (outer region) of the adrenal gland—that actively carry out the biosynthesis of fatty acids and other fatty substances (e.g., steroids). A second function of the above two reactions is to generate from glucose 6-phosphate the pentoses that are used in the synthesis of nucleic acids.

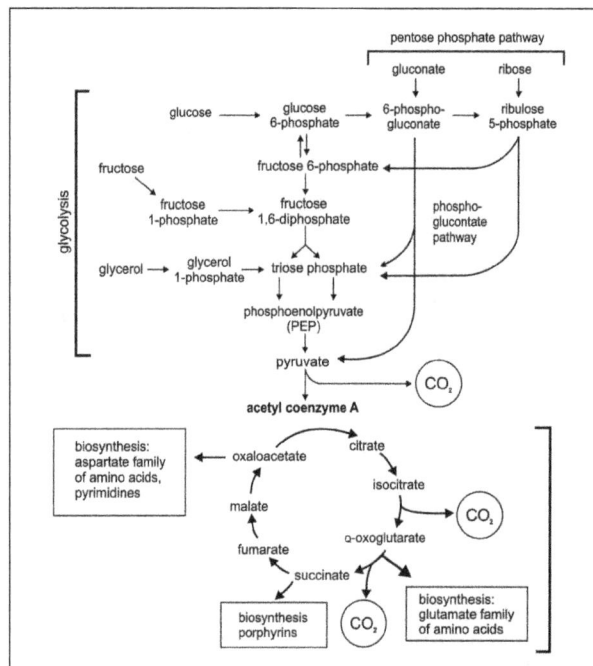

Pathways for the utilization of carbohydrates.

In photosynthetic organisms, some of the reactions of the phosphogluconate pathway are part of the major route for the formation of sugars from carbon dioxide. In this case, the reactions occur in a direction opposite to that in which they occur in nonphotosynthetic tissues.

A different route for the catabolism of glucose also involves 6-phosphogluconate; it is of considerable importance in microorganisms lacking some of the enzymes necessary for glycolysis. In this route, 6-phosphogluconate is not oxidized to ribulose 5-phosphate via the above reaction but, in an enzyme-catalyzed reaction, loses water, forming the compound 2-keto-3-deoxy-6-phosphoglu-conate (KDPG).

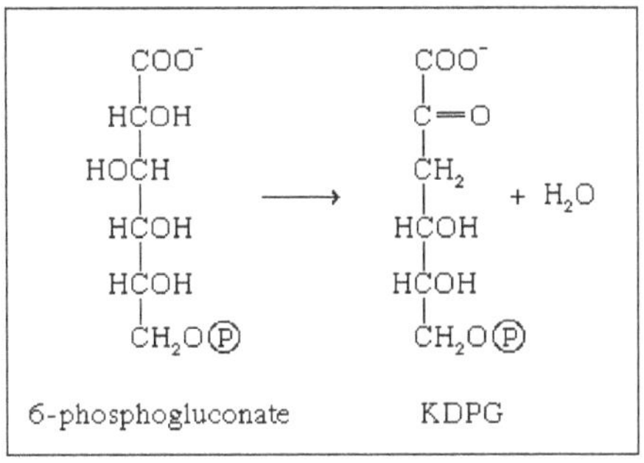

This is then split into pyruvate and glyceraldehyde-3-phosphate, both of which are intermediates of the glycolytic pathway.

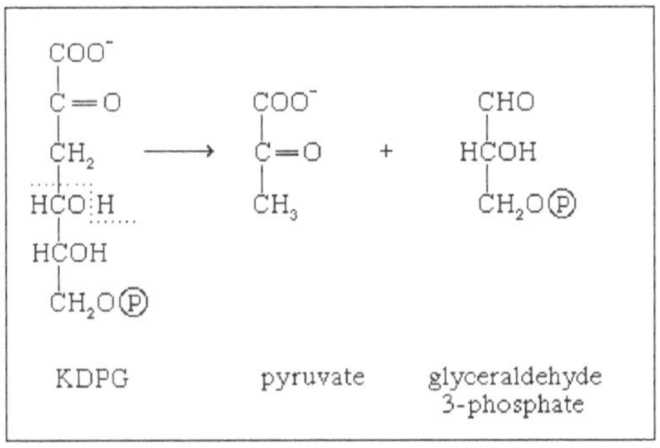

Catabolism of Sugars other than Glucose

Release of Glucose from Glycogen

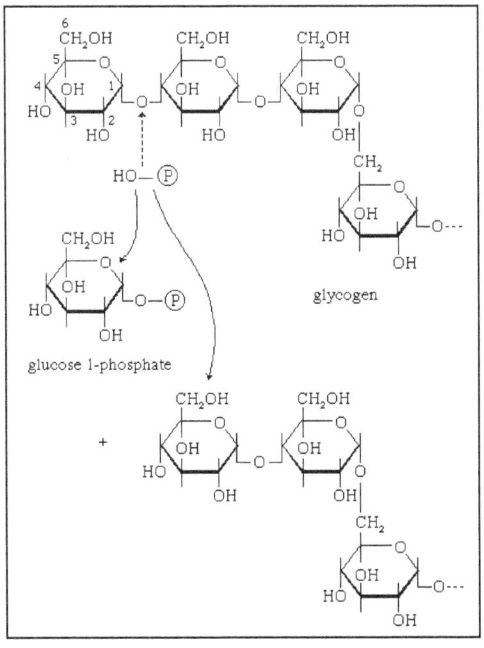

The main storage carbohydrate of animal cells is glycogen, in which chains of glucose molecules—linked end-to-end, the C1 position of one glucose being linked to the C4 position of the adjacent one—are joined to each other by occasional linkages between a carbon at position 1 on one glucose and a carbon at position 6 on another. Two enzymes cooperate in releasing glucose molecules from glycogen. Glycogen phosphorylase catalyzes the splitting of the 1,4-bonds by adding the elements of phosphoric acid at the point shown by the broken arrow in the following reaction rather than water, as in the digestive hydrolysis of polysaccharides such as glycogen and starch. The products of the following reaction are glucose 1-phosphate and chains of sugar molecules shortened by one unit; the chains are degraded further by repetition of the following reaction. When a bridge linking two chains, at C1 and C6 carbon atoms of adjacent glucose units, is reached, it is hydrolyzed in a reaction involving the enzyme α (1 → 6) glucosidase. After the two chains are separated, reaction given below can occur again. The glucose 1-phosphate thus formed from glycogen or, in plants, from starch is converted to glucose 6-phosphate by phosphoglucomutase. Glucose 6-phosphate can then undergo further catabolism via glycolysis or via either of the routes involving formation of 6-phosphogluconate.

Fragmentation of other Sugars

Other sugars encountered in the diet are likewise transformed into products that are intermediates of central metabolic pathways. Lactose, or milk sugar, is composed of one molecule of galactose linked to one molecule of glucose. Sucrose, the common sugar of cane or beet, is made up of glucose linked to fructose. Both sucrose and lactose are hydrolyzed to glucose and fructose or galactose, respectively. Glucose is utilized as already described, but special reactions must occur before the other sugars can enter the catabolic routes. Galactose, for example, is phosphorylated in a manner analogous to step above of glycolysis. The reaction, catalyzed by a galactokinase, results in the formation of galactose 1-phosphate. This product is transformed to glucose 1-phosphate by a sequence of reactions requiring as a coenzyme uridine triphosphate (UTP). Fructose may also be phosphorylated in animal cells through the action of hexokinase above, in which case fructose 6-phosphate is the product, or in liver tissue via a fructokinase that gives rise to fructose 1-phosphate. ATP supplies the phosphate group in both cases.

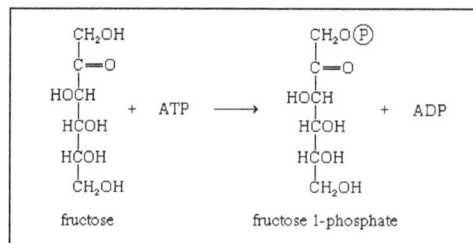

$$
\begin{array}{llll}
CH_2OH & & CH_2O\,\textcircled{P} & \\
| & & | & \\
C=\!\!\!=\!O & & C=\!\!\!=\!O & \\
| & & | & \\
HOCH & & HOCH & \\
| & +\ ATP \longrightarrow & | & +\ ADP \\
HCOH & & HCOH & \\
| & & | & \\
HCOH & & HCOH & \\
| & & | & \\
CH_2OH & & CH_2OH & \\
\text{fructose} & & \text{fructose 1-phosphate} &
\end{array}
$$

Fructose 1-phosphate is also formed when facultative anaerobic microorganisms use fructose as a carbon source for growth; in this case, however, the source of the phosphate is phosphoenolpyruvate rather than ATP. Fructose 1-phosphate can be catabolized by one of two routes. In the liver, it is split by an aldolase enzyme abundant in that tissue (but lacking in muscle); the products are dihydroxyacetone phosphate and glyceraldehyde. It will be recalled that dihydroxyacetone phosphate is an intermediate compound of glycolysis. Although glyceraldehyde is not an intermediate of glycolysis, it can be converted to one (glyceraldehyde 3-phosphate) in a reaction involving the conversion of ATP to ADP.

$$\begin{array}{c}
CH_2O\,\textcircled{P} \\
| \\
C=O \\
| \\
HOCH \\
| \\
HCOH \\
| \\
HCOH \\
| \\
CH_2OH
\end{array}
\quad\rightleftharpoons\quad
\begin{array}{c}
CH_2O\,\textcircled{P} \\
| \\
C=O \\
| \\
CH_2OH
\end{array}
\quad+\quad
\begin{array}{c}
CHO \\
| \\
HCOH \\
| \\
CH_2OH
\end{array}$$

fructose 1-phosphate   dihydroxyacetone   glyceraldehyde
                                    phosphate

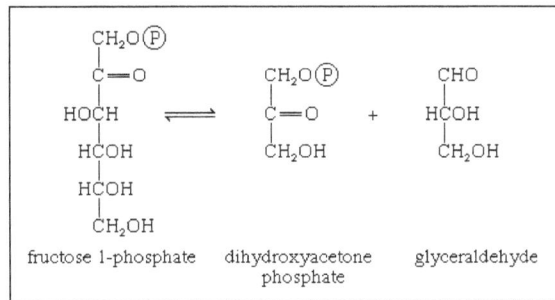

In many organisms other than mammals, fructose 1-phosphate does not have to undergo the above reaction in order to enter central metabolic routes. Instead, a fructose 1-phosphate kinase, distinct from the phosphofructokinase that catalyzes step Above of glycolysis, effects the direct conversion of fructose 1-phosphate and ATP to fructose 1,6-diphosphate and ADP.

Catabolism of Lipids (Fats)

Although carbohydrates are the major fuel for most organisms, fatty acids are also a very important energy source. In vertebrates at least half of the oxidative energy used by the liver, kidneys, heart muscle, and resting skeletal muscle is derived from the oxidation of fatty acids. In fasting or hibernating animals or in migrating birds, fat is virtually the sole source of energy.

Neutral fats or triglycerides, the major components of storage fats in plant and animal cells, consist of the alcohol glycerol linked to three molecules of fatty acids. Before a molecule of neutral fat can be metabolized, it must be hydrolyzed to its component parts. Hydrolysis is effected by intracellular enzymes or gut enzymes, and it forms phase I of fat catabolism. Letters x, y, and z represent the number of $-CH_2-$ groups in the fatty acid molecules.

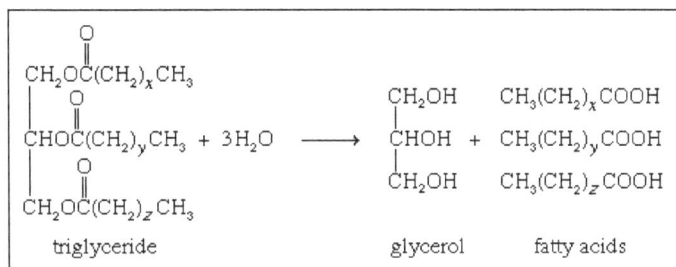

$$\begin{array}{c}
\quad\;\; O \\
\quad\;\; \| \\
CH_2OC(CH_2)_xCH_3 \\
\quad\;\; O \\
\quad\;\; \| \\
CHOC(CH_2)_yCH_3 \; + \; 3H_2O \\
\quad\;\; O \\
\quad\;\; \| \\
CH_2OC(CH_2)_zCH_3
\end{array}
\quad\longrightarrow\quad
\begin{array}{c}
CH_2OH \\
| \\
CHOH \\
| \\
CH_2OH
\end{array}
\quad+\quad
\begin{array}{c}
CH_3(CH_2)_xCOOH \\
CH_3(CH_2)_yCOOH \\
CH_3(CH_2)_zCOOH
\end{array}$$

triglyceride   glycerol   fatty acids

As is apparent from the above reaction, the three molecules of fatty acid released from the triglyceride need not be identical. A fatty acid usually contains 16 or 18 carbon atoms but may also be unsaturated—that is, containing one or more double bonds ($-CH=CH-$). Only the fate of saturated fatty acids—of the type $CH_3(CH_2)nCOOH$ (n most commonly is an even number)—is dealt with here.

Fate of Glycerol

It requires but two reactions to channel glycerol into a catabolic pathway. In a reaction catalyzed by glycerolkinase, ATP is used to phosphorylate glycerol; the products are glycerol 1-phosphate and ADP. Glycerol 1-phosphate is then oxidized to dihydroxyacetone phosphate, an intermediate of glycolysis. The reaction is catalyzed by either a soluble (cytoplasmic) enzyme, glycerolphosphate dehydrogenase, or a similar enzyme present in the mitochondria. In addition to their different locations, the two dehydrogenase enzymes differ in that a different coenzyme accepts the electrons removed from glycerol 1-phosphate. In the case of the cytoplasmic enzyme, NAD^+ accepts the electrons (and is reduced to $NADH + H^+$); in the case of the mitochondrial enzyme, flavin adenine dinucleotide (FAD) accepts the electrons (and is reduced to $FADH_2$).

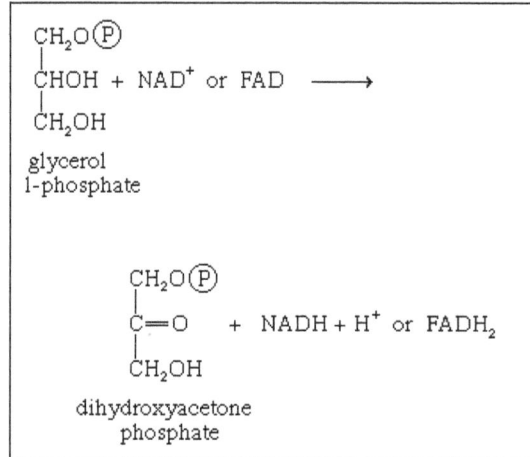

$$
\begin{array}{l}
CH_2O\textcircled{P} \\
| \\
CHOH + NAD^+ \text{ or } FAD \longrightarrow \\
| \\
CH_2OH \\
\text{glycerol} \\
\text{1-phosphate}
\end{array}
$$

$$
\begin{array}{l}
CH_2O\textcircled{P} \\
| \\
C{=}O \quad + \quad NADH + H^+ \text{ or } FADH_2 \\
| \\
CH_2OH \\
\text{dihydroxyacetone} \\
\text{phosphate}
\end{array}
$$

Fate of Fatty Acids

Formation of Fatty Acyl Coenzyme a Molecules

As with sugars, the release of energy from fatty acids necessitates an initial investment of ATP. A problem unique to fats is a consequence of the low solubility in water of most fatty acids. Their catabolism requires mechanisms that fragment them in a controlled and stepwise manner. The mechanism involves a coenzyme for the transfer of an acyl group (e.g., $CH_3Cl{=}O$)—namely, coenzyme A. The functional portion of this complex molecule is the sulfhydryl ($-SH$) group at one end. The coenzyme is often identified as $CoA-SH$ (the reaction given below). The organized and stepwise degradation of fatty acids linked to coenzyme A is ensured because the necessary enzymes are sequestered in particulate structures. In microorganisms these enzymes are associated with cell membranes, in higher organisms with mitochondria.

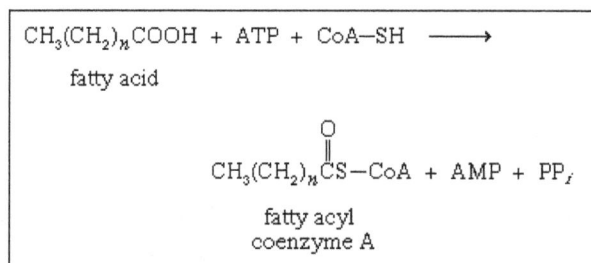

$$
\begin{array}{l}
CH_3(CH_2)_n COOH + ATP + CoA-SH \longrightarrow \\
\quad \text{fatty acid}
\end{array}
$$

$$
\begin{array}{l}
\qquad\qquad O \\
\qquad\qquad \| \\
CH_3(CH_2)_n CS-CoA + AMP + PP_i \\
\qquad \text{fatty acyl} \\
\qquad \text{coenzyme A}
\end{array}
$$

Fatty acids are linked to coenzyme A ($CoA-SH$) in one of two main ways. In higher organisms, enzymes in the cytoplasm called thiokinases catalyze the linkage of fatty acids with $CoA-SH$ to form a compound that can be called a fatty acyl coenzyme A in the above reaction. This step requires ATP, which is split into AMP and inorganic pyrophosphate (PPi) in the process.

In this series of reactions, n indicates the number of hydrocarbon units ($-CH_2-$) in the molecule. Because most tissues contain highly active pyrophosphatase enzymes, which catalyze the virtually irreversible hydrolysis of inorganic pyrophosphate (PPi) to two molecules of inorganic phosphate (Pi), the above reaction proceeds overwhelmingly to completion—i.e., from left to right.

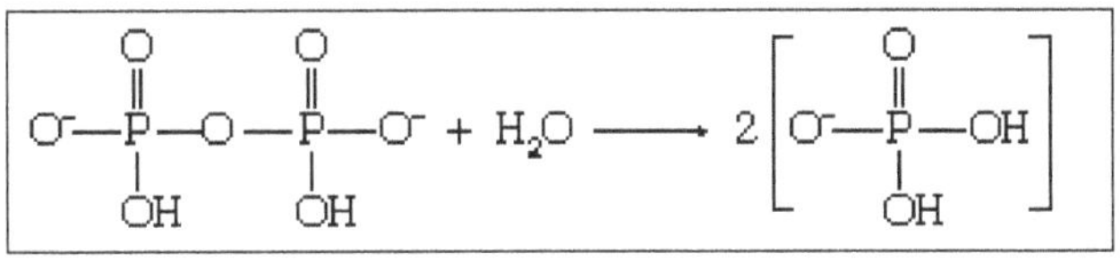

Although fatty acids are activated in this way, the acyl coenzyme A derivatives that are formed must be transported to the enzyme complex that effects their oxidation. Activation occurs in the cytoplasm, but, in animal cells, oxidation takes place in the mitochondria. The transfer of fatty acyl coenzyme A across the mitochondrial membrane is effected by the enzyme carnitine, a nitrogen-containing small hydroxy acid of the formula $(CH_3)_3NCH_2CH(OH)CH_2COO^-$. The –OH group within the carnitine molecule accepts the acyl group of fatty acyl coenzyme A, forming acyl carnitine, which can cross the inner membrane of the mitochondrion and there return the acyl group to coenzyme A.

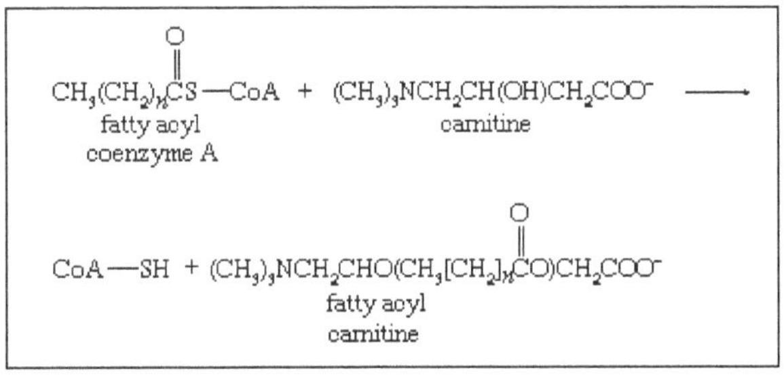

These reactions are catalyzed by the enzyme carnitine acyl transferase. Defects in this enzyme or in the carnitine carrier are inborn errors of metabolism. In obligate anaerobic bacteria the linkage of fatty acids to coenzyme A may require the formation of a fatty acyl phosphate—i.e., the phosphorylation of the fatty acid by using ATP; ADP is also a product.

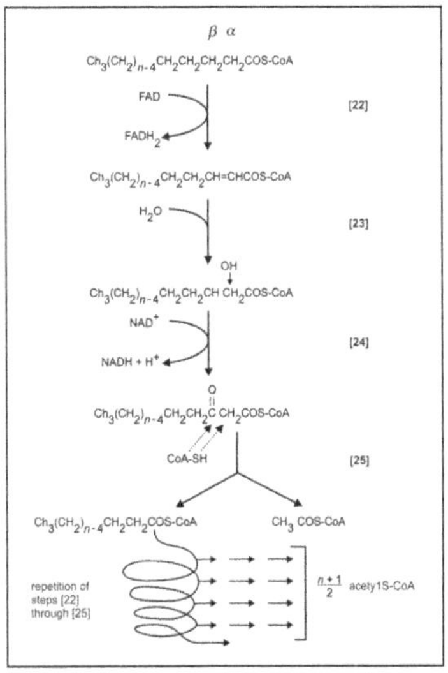

Fragmentation of acyl coenzyme

$$CH_3(CH_2)_nCOOH + ATP \longrightarrow CH_3(CH_2)_nCOO\textcircled{P} + ADP$$

fatty acid → fatty acyl phosphate

The fatty acyl moiety [$CH_3(CH_2)nCOO^-$] is then transferred to coenzyme A, forming a fatty acyl coenzyme A compound and Pi.

Fragmentation of Fatty Acyl Coenzyme a Molecules

Initially (in the reaction given below), two hydrogen atoms are lost from the fatty acyl coenzyme A, resulting in the formation of an unsaturated fatty acyl coenzyme A (i.e., with a double bond, $-CH=CH-$) between the α- and β-carbons of the acyl moiety.

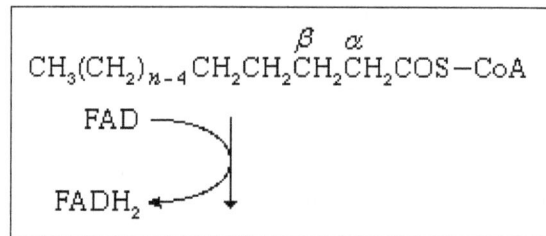

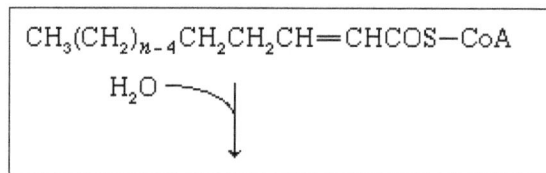

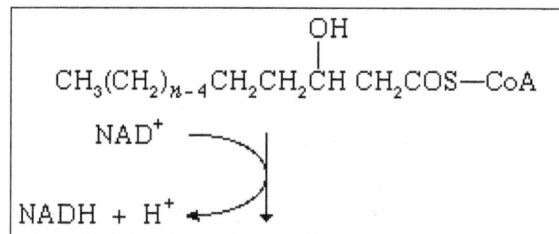

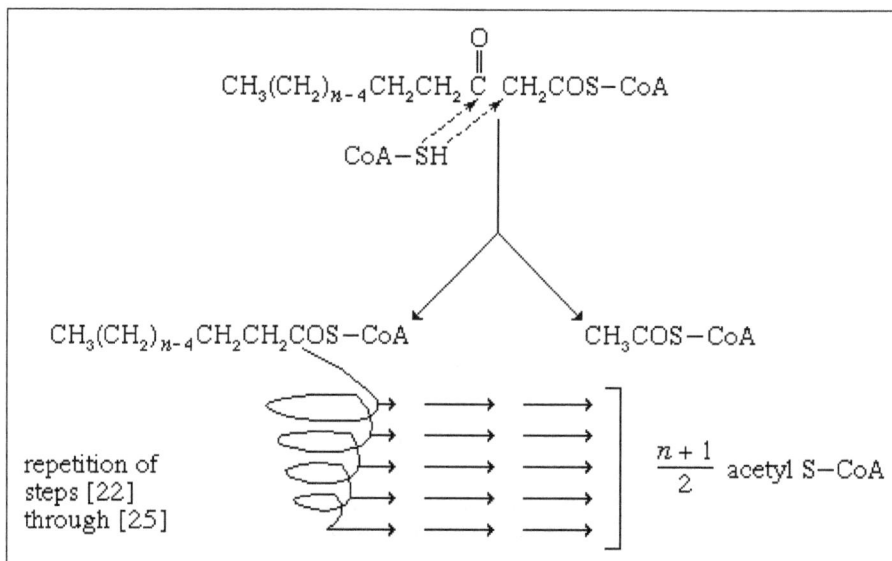

(The α-carbon is the one closest to the carboxyl [$-COOH$] group of a fatty acid, the next closest is the β-, and so on to the end of the hydrocarbon chain.) The hydrogen atoms are accepted by the coenzyme FAD (flavin adenine dinucleotide), which is reduced to $FADH_2$. The product α,β-unsaturated fatty acyl coenzyme A, is enzymatically hydrated; i.e., water is added across the double bond. The product, called a β-hydroxyacyl coenzyme A, can again be oxidized in an enzyme-catalyzed reaction; the electrons removed are accepted by NAD^+. The product is called a β-ketoacyl coenzyme A.

The next enzymatic step enables the energy invested in the above reaction in which coenzyme CoA−SH is formed, is to be conserved. The β-ketoacyl coenzyme A that is the product of reaction above, is split, not by water but by coenzyme A. The process, called thiolysis (as distinct from hydrolysis), yields the two-carbon fragment acetyl coenzyme A and a fatty acyl coenzyme A.

The shortened fatty acyl coenzyme A molecule now undergoes the sequence of reactions again, beginning with the dehydrogenation reaction, and another two-carbon fragment is removed as acetyl coenzyme A. With each passage through the process of fatty acid oxidation, the fatty acid loses a two-carbon fragment as acetyl coenzyme A and two pairs of hydrogen atoms to specific acceptors. The 16-carbon fatty acid, palmitic acid, for example, undergoes a total of seven such cycles, yielding eight molecules of acetyl coenzyme A and 14 pairs of hydrogen atoms, seven of which appear in the form of $FADH_2$ and seven in the form of $NADH + H^+$. The reduced coenzymes, $FADH_2$ and reduced NAD^+, are reoxidized when the electrons pass through the electron transport chain, with concomitant formation of ATP. In anaerobes, organic molecules, not oxygen, are electron acceptors, and, thus, the yield of ATP is reduced. In all organisms, however, the acetyl coenzyme A formed from the breakdown of fatty acids joins that arising from the catabolism of carbohydrates and many amino acids.

Fatty acids with an odd number of carbon atoms are relatively rare in nature but may arise during microbial fermentations or through the oxidation of amino acids such as valine and isoleucine. They may be fragmented through repeated cycles of the above four reactions until the final five-carbon acyl coenzyme A is split into acetyl coenzyme A and propionyl coenzyme A, which has three carbon atoms. In many bacteria, this propionyl coenzyme A can be transformed either to acetyl coenzyme A and carbon dioxide or to pyruvate. In other microorganisms and in animals, propionyl coenzyme A has a different fate: carbon dioxide is added to propionyl coenzyme A in a reaction requiring ATP. The product, methylmalonyl coenzyme A, has four carbon atoms; the molecule undergoes a rearrangement, forming succinyl coenzyme A, which is an intermediate of the TCA cycle.

Catabolism of Proteins

The amino acids derived from proteins function primarily as the precursors, or building blocks, for the cells own proteins and (unlike lipids and carbohydrates) are not primarily a source of energy. Many microorganisms, on the other hand, can grow by using amino acids as the sole carbon and nitrogen source. Under these conditions these microorganisms derive from the amino acids all of their required energy and all of the precursors of the macromolecules that comprise the components of their cells. Moreover, it has been calculated that a man of average weight (70 kilograms, or 154 pounds) turns over about 0.4 kilogram of protein per day. About 0.1 kilogram is degraded and replaced by dietary amino acids; the remaining 0.3 kilogram is recycled as part of the dynamic state of cell constituents. The cells of plants contain and metabolize many amino acids in addition to the 20 or so that are normally found in proteins.

Before proteins can enter cells, the bonds linking adjacent amino acids (peptide bonds) must be hydrolyzed; this process releases the amino acids constituting the protein. The utilization of dietary proteins thus requires the operation of extracellular digestive enzymes; i.e., enzymes outside the cell. Many microorganisms secrete such enzymes into the nutrient media in which they are growing; animals secrete them into the gut. The turnover of proteins within cells, on the other hand, requires the functioning of intracellular enzymes that catalyze the splitting of the peptide bonds linking adjacent amino acids; little is known about the mechanism involved.

Amino acids may be described by the general formula $RCH(NH_2)COOH$, or $RCH(NH_3^+)COO^-$, in which R represents a specific chemical moiety. The catabolic fate of amino acids involves (1) removal of nitrogen, (2) disposal of nitrogen, and (3) oxidation of the remaining carbon skeleton.

Removal of Nitrogen

The removal of the amino group $(-NH_2)$ generally constitutes the first stage in amino acid catabolism. The amino group usually is initially transferred to the anion of one of three different α-keto acids (i.e., of the general structure $RCOCOO^-$): pyruvate, which is an intermediate of carbohydrate fragmentation; or oxaloacetate or α-oxoglutarate, both intermediates of the TCA cycle. The products are alanine, aspartate, and glutamate (the following three reactions).

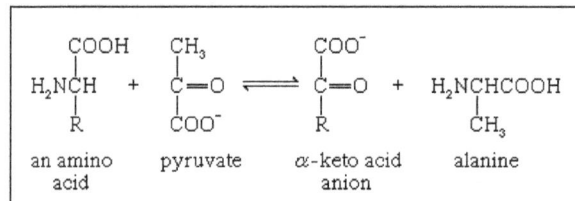

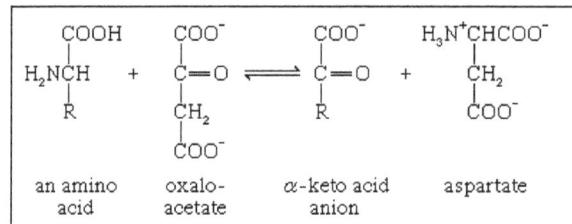

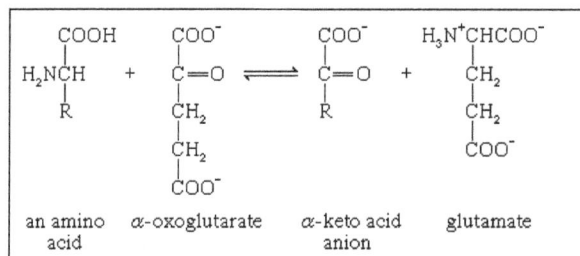

Since the effect of these reactions is to produce n amino acids and n keto acids from n different amino acids and n different keto acids, no net reduction in the nitrogen content of the system has yet been achieved. The elimination of nitrogen occurs in a variety of ways.

In many microorganisms, ammonia (NH_3) can be removed from aspartate via a reaction catalyzed by aspartase; the other product, fumarate, is an intermediate of the TCA cycle.

$$\underset{\text{aspartate}}{\overset{\displaystyle H_3N^+CHCOO^-}{\underset{\displaystyle CH_2COO^-}{|}}} \rightleftharpoons NH_3 + \underset{\text{fumarate}}{\overset{\displaystyle {}^-OOCCH}{\underset{\displaystyle CHCOO^-}{\|}}}$$

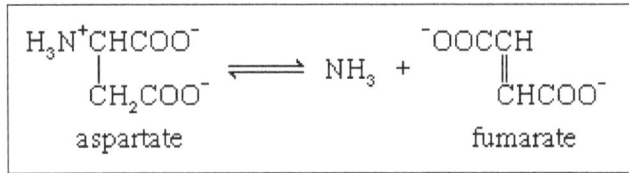

A quantitatively more important route is that catalyzed by glutamate dehydrogenase, in which the glutamate thus formed is oxidized to α-oxoglutarate, another TCA cycle intermediate. Either NADP$^+$ or both NADP$^+$ and NAD$^+$ may serve as the hydrogen or electron acceptor, depending on the organism, and some organisms synthesize two enzymes, one of which prefers NADP$^+$ and the other NAD$^+$. In the following reaction, NAD(P)$^+$ is used to indicate that either NAD$^+$, NADP$^+$, or both may serve as the electron acceptor.

The occurrence of the transfer reactions either the above two or, more importantly, the reaction given below, allows the channeling of many amino acids into a common pathway by which nitrogen can be eliminated as ammonia.

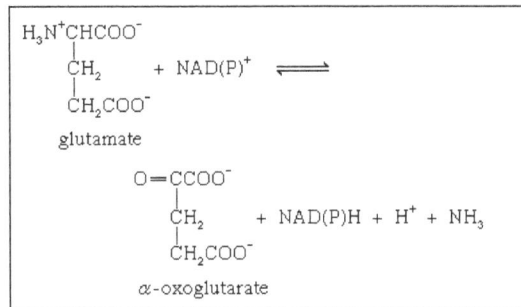

$$\underset{\text{glutamate}}{\overset{\displaystyle H_3N^+CHCOO^-}{\underset{\displaystyle CH_2COO^-}{\underset{\displaystyle |}{\overset{\displaystyle |}{CH_2}}}}} + NAD(P)^+ \rightleftharpoons$$

$$\underset{\alpha\text{-oxoglutarate}}{\overset{\displaystyle O=CCOO^-}{\underset{\displaystyle CH_2COO^-}{\underset{\displaystyle |}{\overset{\displaystyle |}{CH_2}}}}} + NAD(P)H + H^+ + NH_3$$

Disposal of Nitrogen

In animals that excrete ammonia as the main nitrogenous waste product (e.g., some marine invertebrates, crustaceans), it is derived from nitrogen transfer reactions and oxidation via glutamate dehydrogenase. Because ammonia is toxic to cells, however, it is detoxified as it forms. This process involves an enzyme-catalyzed reaction between ammonia and a molecule of glutamate; ATP provides the energy for the reaction, which results in the formation of glutamine, ADP, and inorganic phosphate. This reaction is catalyzed by glutamine synthetase, which is subject to a variety of metabolic controls. The glutamine thus formed gives up the amide nitrogen in the kidney tubules. As a result, glutamate is formed once again, and ammonia is released into the urine.

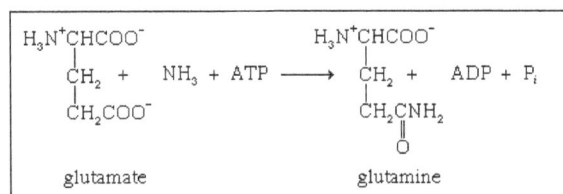

$$\underset{\text{glutamate}}{\overset{\displaystyle H_3N^+CHCOO^-}{\underset{\displaystyle CH_2COO^-}{\underset{\displaystyle |}{\overset{\displaystyle |}{CH_2}}}}} + NH_3 + ATP \longrightarrow \underset{\text{glutamine}}{\overset{\displaystyle H_3N^+CHCOO^-}{\underset{\displaystyle CH_2CNH_2}{\underset{\displaystyle \underset{O}{\|}}{\underset{\displaystyle |}{\overset{\displaystyle |}{CH_2}}}}}} + ADP + P_i$$

In terrestrial reptiles and birds, uric acid rather than glutamate is the compound with which nitrogen combines to form a nontoxic substance for transfer to the kidney tubules. Uric acid is formed by a complex pathway that begins with ribose 5-phosphate and during which a so-called purine skeleton is formed; in the course of this process, nitrogen atoms from glutamine and the amino acids aspartic acid and glycine are incorporated into the skeleton. These nitrogen donors are derived from other amino acids via amino group transfer and the reaction catalyzed by glutamine synthetase.

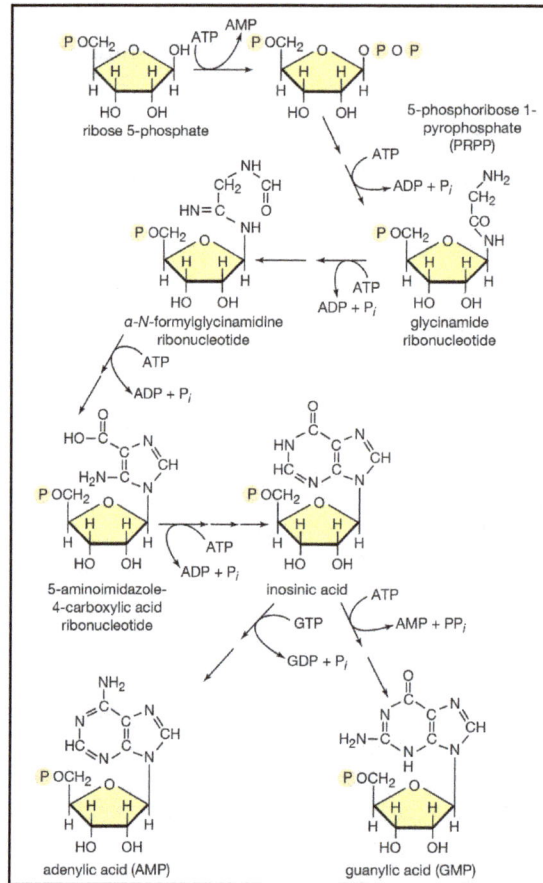

Biosynthesis of purine nucleotides: Biosynthesis of purine nucleotides.
Not all of the intermediate compounds formed are shown.

In most fishes, amphibians, and mammals, nitrogen is detoxified in the liver and excreted as urea, a readily soluble and harmless product. The sequence leading to the formation of urea, commonly called the urea cycle, is summarized as follows: Ammonia, formed from glutamate and NAD^+ in the liver mitochondria, reacts with carbon dioxide and ATP to form carbamoyl phosphate, ADP, and inorganic phosphate, as shown in reaction.

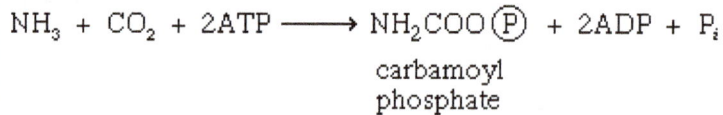

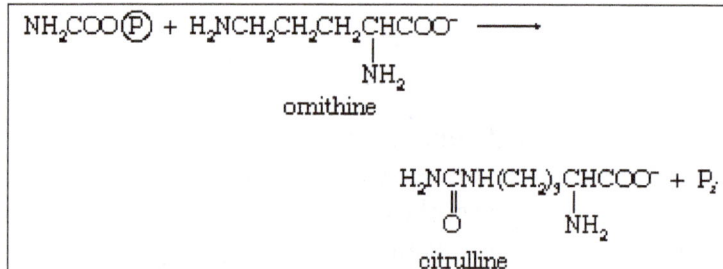

$$NH_3 + CO_2 + 2ATP \longrightarrow NH_2COO\,\textcircled{P} + 2ADP + P_i$$

carbamoyl
phosphate

$$NH_2COO\textcircled{P} + H_2NCH_2CH_2CH_2CHCOO^- \longrightarrow$$
$$\underset{\text{ornithine}}{\overset{|}{NH_2}}$$

$$H_2NCNH(CH_2)_3CHCOO^- + P_i$$
$$\underset{O}{\overset{\|}{}} \qquad \underset{NH_2}{\overset{|}{}}$$
citrulline

The reaction is catalyzed by carbamoyl phosphate synthetase. The carbamoyl moiety of carbamoyl phosphate (NH_2CO-) is transferred to ornithine, an amino acid, in a reaction catalyzed by ornithine transcarbamoylase; the products are citrulline and inorganic phosphate. Citrulline and aspartate formed from amino acids react to form argininosuccinate; argininosuccinic acid synthetase catalyzes the reaction. Argininosuccinate splits into fumarate and arginine during a reaction catalyzed by argininosuccinase.

In the final step of the urea cycle, arginine, in a reaction catalyzed by arginase, is hydrolyzed. Urea and ornithine are the products; ornithine thus is available to initiate another cycle.

Oxidation of the Carbon Skeleton

The carbon skeletons of amino acids (i.e., the portion of the molecule remaining after the removal of nitrogen) are fragmented to form only a few end products; all of them are intermediates of either glycolysis or the TCA cycle. The number and complexity of the catabolic steps by which each amino acid arrives at its catabolic end point reflect the chemical complexity of that amino acid. Thus, in the case of alanine, only the amino group must be removed to yield pyruvate; the amino acid threonine, on the other hand, must be transformed successively to the amino acids glycine and serine before pyruvate is formed. The fragmentation of leucine to acetyl coenzyme A involves seven steps; that of tryptophan to the same end product requires 11.

Combustion of Food Materials

Although the pathways for fragmentation of food materials effect the conversion of a large variety of relatively complex starting materials into only a few simpler intermediates of central metabolic routes—mainly pyruvate, acetyl coenzyme A, and a few intermediates of the TCA cycle—their operation releases but a fraction of the energy contained in the materials. The reason is that, in the fermentation process, catabolic intermediates serve also as the terminal acceptors of the reducing equivalents (hydrogen atoms or electrons) that are removed during the oxidation of food. The end products thus may be at the same oxidation level and may contain equivalent numbers of carbon, hydrogen, and oxygen atoms, as the material that was catabolized by a fermentative route. The necessity for pyruvate, for example, to act as the hydrogen acceptor in the fermentation of glucose to lactate results in the conservation of all the component atoms of the glucose molecule in the form of lactate. The consequent release of energy as ATP is thus small.

A more favourable situation arises if the reducing equivalents formed by oxidation of nutrients can be passed on to an inorganic acceptor such as oxygen. In this case, the products of fermentation need not act as "hydrogen sinks," in which the energy in the molecule is lost when they leave the cell; instead, the products of fermentation can be degraded further, during phase III of catabolism, and all the usable chemical energy of the nutrient can be transformed into ATP.

Oxidation of Molecular Fragments

Oxidation of Pyruvate

The oxidation of pyruvate involves the concerted action of several enzymes and coenzymes collectively called the pyruvate dehydrogenase complex; i.e., a multienzyme complex in which the substrates are passed consecutively from one enzyme to the next, and the product of the reaction catalyzed by the first enzyme immediately becomes the substrate for the second enzyme in the complex. The overall reaction is the formation of acetyl coenzyme A and carbon dioxide from pyruvate, with concomitant liberation of two reducing equivalents in the form of NADH + H+. The individual reactions that result in the formation of these end products are as follows.

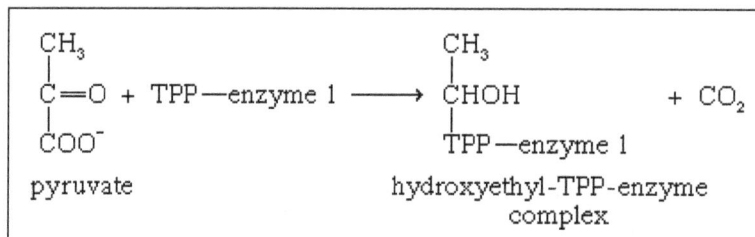

Pyruvate first reacts with the coenzyme of pyruvic acid decarboxylase (enzyme 1), thiamine pyrophosphate (TPP); in addition to carbon dioxide a hydroxyethyl–TPP–enzyme complex ("active acetaldehyde") is formed. Thiamine is vitamin B_1; the biological role of TPP was first revealed by the inability of vitamin B_1-deficient animals to oxidize pyruvate.

The hydroxyethyl moiety formed in the above reaction is immediately transferred to one of the two sulfur atoms (S) of the coenzyme (6,8-dithio-n-octanoate or $lipS_2$) of the second enzyme in the complex, dihydrolipoyl transacetylase (enzyme 2). The hydroxyethyl group attaches to $lipS_2$ at one of its sulfur atoms, as shown in the reaction given below; the result is that coenzyme $lipS_2$ is reduced and the hydroxyethyl moiety is oxidized.

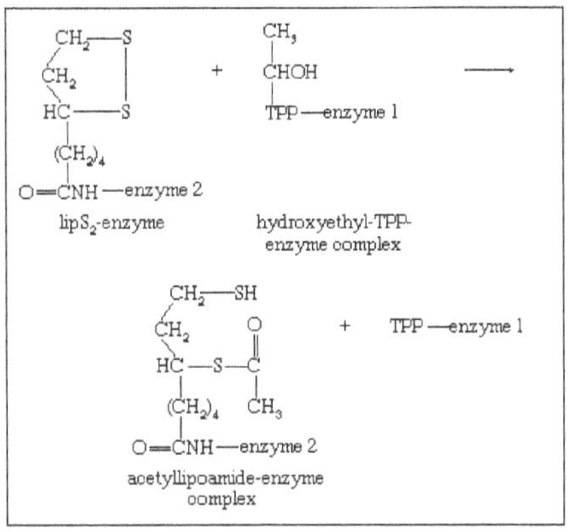

```
    CH2—S              CH3
   /      |            |
  CH2     |      +    CHOH                    ⟶
  HC——————S           |
  |                   TPP—enzyme 1
 (CH2)4
  |
O=CNH—enzyme 2
  lipS2-enzyme        hydroxyethyl-TPP-
                       enzyme complex

          CH2—SH
         /
        CH2      O        +    TPP—enzyme 1
        HC—S——C
        |      ‖
       (CH2)4  CH3
        |
      O=CNH—enzyme 2
      acetyllipoamide-enzyme
              complex
```

The acetyl group ($CH_3C|=O$) then is transferred to the sulfhydryl (−SH) group of coenzyme A, thereby completing the oxidation of pyruvate.

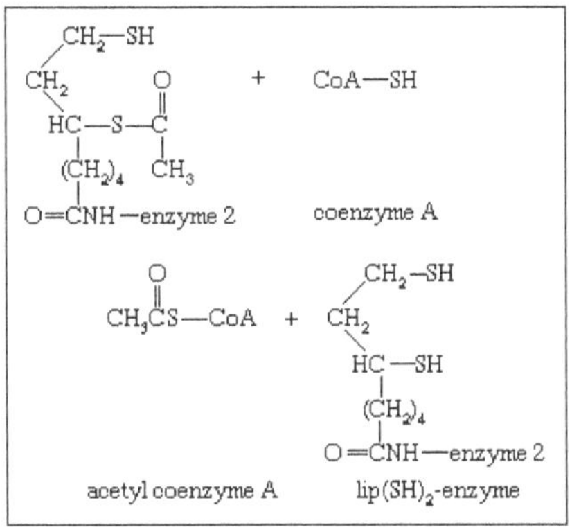

```
    CH2—SH
   /
  CH2      O         +    CoA—SH
  HC—S——C
  |      ‖
 (CH2)4  CH3
  |
O=CNH—enzyme 2           coenzyme A

          O                    CH2—SH
          ‖                   /
      CH3CS—CoA     +    CH2
                         HC—SH
                         |
                        (CH2)4
                         |
                       O=CNH—enzyme 2
    acetyl coenzyme A       lip(SH)2-enzyme
```

The coenzyme $lipS_2$ that accepted the hydroxyethyl moiety of the sequence, now reduced, must be reoxidized before another molecule of pyruvate can be oxidized. The reoxidation of the coenzyme is achieved by the enzyme-catalyzed transfer of two reducing equivalents initially to the coenzyme flavin adenine dinucleotide (FAD) and thence to the NAD^+ that is the first carrier in the so-called electron transport chain. The passage of two such reducing equivalents from reduced NAD^+ to oxygen is accompanied by the formation of three molecules of ATP.

The overall reaction may be written as shown in the below reaction, in which pyruvate reacts with coenzyme A in the presence of TPP and $lipS_2$ to form acetyl coenzyme A and carbon dioxide and to liberate two hydrogen atoms (in the form of $NADH + H^+$) that can subsequently yield energy by the reduction of oxygen to water. The $lipS_2$ reduced during this process is reoxidized in the presence of the enzyme lipoyl dehydrogenase, with the concomitant reduction of NAD^+.

$$\begin{array}{l} CH_3 \\ | \\ C{=}O \quad + \quad CoA{-}SH \quad + \quad NAD^+ \quad \longrightarrow \\ | \\ COO^- \end{array}$$

pyruvate   coenzyme A

$$CH_3\overset{O}{\overset{||}{C}}S{-}CoA \;+\; CO_2 \;+\; NADH \;+\; H^+$$

acetyl coenzyme A

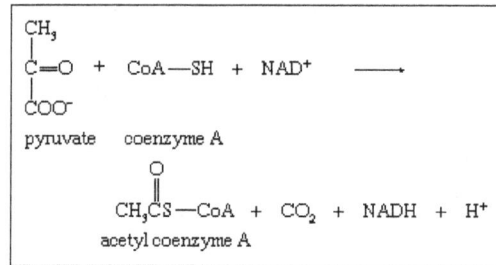

Tricarboxylic Acid (TCA) Cycle

Acetyl coenzyme A arises not only from the oxidation of pyruvate but also from that of fats and many of the amino acids constituting proteins. The sequence of enzyme-catalyzed steps that effects the total combustion of the acetyl moiety of the coenzyme represents the terminal oxidative pathway for virtually all food materials. The balance of the overall reaction of the TCA cycle is that three molecules of water react with acetyl coenzyme A to form carbon dioxide, coenzyme A, and reducing equivalents. The oxidation by oxygen of the reducing equivalents is accompanied by the conservation (as ATP) of most of the energy of the food ingested by aerobic organisms.

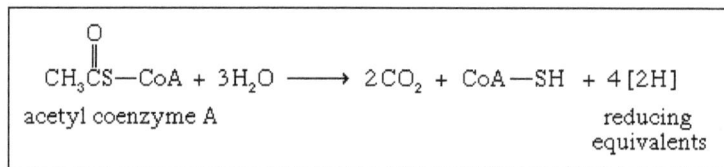

$$CH_3\overset{O}{\overset{||}{C}}S{-}CoA + 3H_2O \longrightarrow 2CO_2 + CoA{-}SH + 4\,[2H]$$

acetyl coenzyme A   reducing equivalents

Formation of coenzyme A, carbon dioxide, and reducing equivalent.

The relative complexity and number of chemical events that constitute the TCA cycle, and their location as components of spatially determined structures such as cell membranes in microorganisms and mitochondria in plants and higher animals, reflect the problems involved chemically in "dismembering" a compound having only two carbon atoms and releasing in a controlled and stepwise manner the reducing equivalents ultimately to be passed to oxygen. These problems have been overcome by the simple but effective device of initially combining the two-carbon compound with a four-carbon acceptor; it is much less difficult chemically to dismember and oxidize a compound having six carbon atoms.

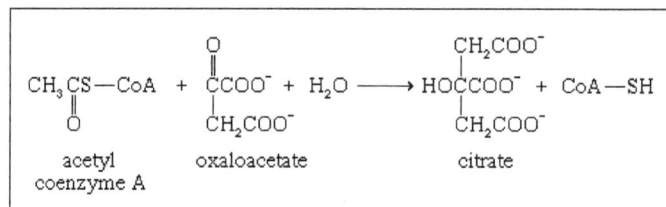

$$CH_3CS{-}CoA + \overset{O}{\overset{||}{C}}COO^- + H_2O \longrightarrow HO\overset{CH_2COO^-}{\underset{CH_2COO^-}{C}}COO^- + CoA{-}SH$$

acetyl coenzyme A   oxaloacetate   citrate

In the TCA cycle, acetyl coenzyme A initially reacts with oxaloacetate to yield citrate and to liberate coenzyme A. This above reaction is catalyzed by citrate synthase. Citrate undergoes isomerization (i.e., a rearrangement of certain atoms constituting the molecule) to form isocitrate. The reaction involves first the removal of the elements of water from citrate to form cis-aconitate and then the re-addition of water to cis-aconitate in such a way that isocitrate is formed. It is probable that all three reactants—citrate, cis-aconitate, and isocitrate—remain closely associated with aconitase, the enzyme that catalyzes the isomerization process, and that most of the cis-aconitate is not re-leased from the enzyme surface but is immediately converted to isocitrate.

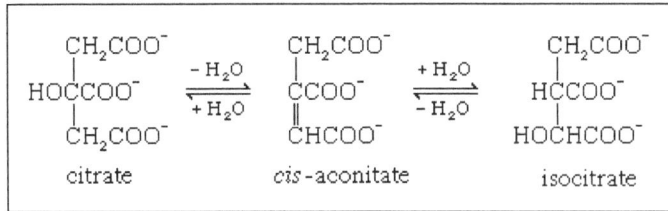

$$
\begin{array}{ccccc}
\text{CH}_2\text{COO}^- & & \text{CH}_2\text{COO}^- & & \text{CH}_2\text{COO}^- \\
| & -\text{H}_2\text{O} & | & +\text{H}_2\text{O} & | \\
\text{HOCCOO}^- & \rightleftharpoons & \text{CCOO}^- & \rightleftharpoons & \text{HCCOO}^- \\
| & +\text{H}_2\text{O} & \parallel & -\text{H}_2\text{O} & | \\
\text{CH}_2\text{COO}^- & & \text{CHCOO}^- & & \text{HOCHCOO}^- \\
\text{citrate} & & cis\text{-aconitate} & & \text{isocitrate}
\end{array}
$$

Isocitrate is oxidized—i.e., hydrogen is removed—to form oxalosuccinate. The two hydrogen atoms are usually transferred to NAD⁺, thus forming reduced NAD⁺ (shown in the following reaction).

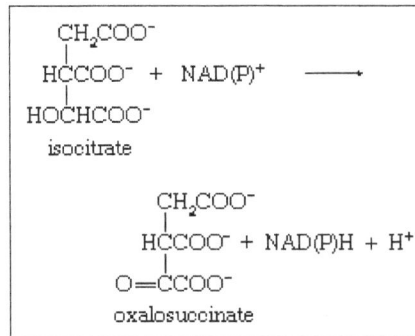

$$
\begin{array}{l}
\text{CH}_2\text{COO}^- \\
| \\
\text{HCCOO}^- \;+\; \text{NAD(P)}^+ \longrightarrow \\
| \\
\text{HOCHCOO}^- \\
\text{isocitrate}
\end{array}
$$

$$
\begin{array}{l}
\text{CH}_2\text{COO}^- \\
| \\
\text{HCCOO}^- \;+\; \text{NAD(P)H} \;+\; \text{H}^+ \\
| \\
\text{O}\!\!=\!\!\text{CCOO}^- \\
\text{oxalosuccinate}
\end{array}
$$

In some microorganisms, and during the biosynthesis of glutamate in the cytoplasm of animal cells, however, the hydrogen atoms may also be accepted by NADP⁺. Thus, the enzyme controlling this reaction, isocitrate dehydrogenase, differs in specificity for the coenzymes; various forms occur not only in different organisms but even within the same cell. In the above reaction, NAD(P)⁺ indicates that either NAD⁺ or NADP⁺ can act as a hydrogen acceptor.

The position of the carboxylate ($-$COO⁻) that is sandwiched in the middle of the oxalosuccinate molecule renders it very unstable, and, as a result, the carbon of this group is lost as carbon dioxide (note the dotted rectangle) in a reaction given below that can occur spontaneously but may be further accelerated by an enzyme.

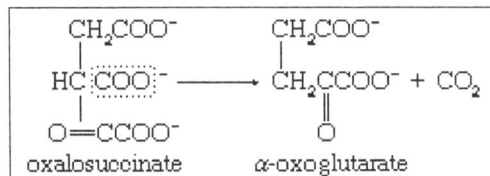

$$
\begin{array}{ccc}
\text{CH}_2\text{COO}^- & & \text{CH}_2\text{COO}^- \\
| & & | \\
\text{HC}\underline{\overline{\text{COO}}}^- & \longrightarrow & \text{CH}_2\text{CCOO}^- \;+\; \text{CO}_2 \\
| & & \parallel \\
\text{O}\!\!=\!\!\text{CCOO}^- & & \text{O} \\
\text{oxalosuccinate} & & \alpha\text{-oxoglutarate}
\end{array}
$$

The five-carbon product of the above reaction, α-oxoglutarate, has chemical properties similar to pyruvate (free-acid forms of both are so-called α-oxoacids), and the chemical events involved in the oxidation of α-oxoglutarate are analogous to those already described for the oxidation of pyruvate. The following reaction is effected by a multi-enzyme complex; TPP, lipS₂ (6,8-dithio-n-octanoate), and coenzyme A are required as coenzymes. The products are carbon dioxide and succinyl coenzyme A. As was noted with reaction (reduction of NAD⁺), this oxidation of α-oxoglutarate results in the reduction of lipS₂, which must be reoxidized. This is done by transfer of reducing equivalents to FAD and thence to NAD⁺. The resultant NADH + H⁺ is reoxidized by the passage of the electrons, ultimately, to oxygen, via the electron transport chain.

$$
\begin{array}{l}
CH_2COO^- \\
| \\
CH_2CCOO^- + CoA\!-\!SH + NAD^+ \longrightarrow \\
\quad \| \\
\quad O \\
\alpha\text{-oxoglutarate}
\end{array}
$$

$$
\begin{array}{l}
CH_2COO^- \\
| \\
CH_2CS\!-\!CoA + CO_2 + NADH + H^+ \\
\quad \| \\
\quad O \\
\text{succinyl} \\
\text{coenzyme A}
\end{array}
$$

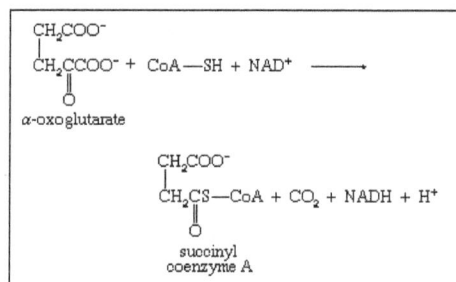

Unlike the acetyl coenzyme A produced from pyruvate in reaction (reduction of NAD^+), succinyl coenzyme A undergoes a phosphorolysis reaction—i.e., transfer of the succinyl moiety from coenzyme A to inorganic phosphate. The succinyl phosphate thus formed is not released from the enzyme surface; an unstable, high-energy compound called an acid anhydride, it transfers a high-energy phosphate to ADP, directly or via guanosine diphosphate (GDP).

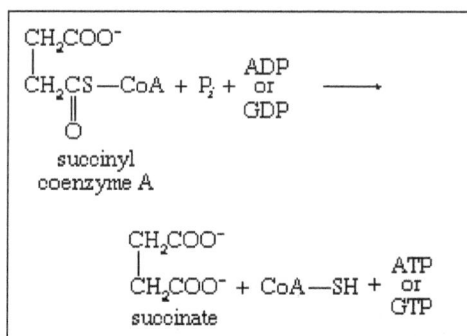

$$
\begin{array}{l}
CH_2COO^- \\
| \qquad\qquad\qquad\qquad ADP \\
CH_2CS\!-\!CoA + P_i + \quad\text{or} \quad \longrightarrow \\
\quad \| \qquad\qquad\qquad\quad GDP \\
\quad O \\
\quad \text{succinyl} \\
\quad \text{coenzyme A}
\end{array}
$$

$$
\begin{array}{l}
CH_2COO^- \\
| \qquad\qquad\qquad\qquad\qquad\quad ATP \\
CH_2COO^- + CoA\!-\!SH + \quad\text{or} \\
\text{succinate} \qquad\qquad\qquad\quad GTP
\end{array}
$$

If guanosine triphosphate (GTP) forms, ATP can readily arise from it in an exchange involving ADP:

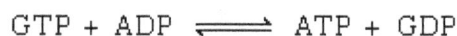

$$ GTP + ADP \rightleftharpoons ATP + GDP $$

Regeneration of Oxaloacetate

The remainder of the reactions of the TCA cycle serve to regenerate the initial four-carbon acceptor of acetyl coenzyme A (oxaloacetate) from succinate, the process requiring in effect the oxidation of a methylene group $(-CH_2-)$ to a carbonyl group $(-CO-)$, with concomitant release of $2 \times [2H]$ reducing equivalents. It is therefore similar to, and is affected in like manner to, the oxidation of fatty acids. As is the case with fatty acids, hydrogen atoms or electrons are initially removed from the succinate formed in the above reaction and are accepted by FAD; the reaction, catalyzed by succinate dehydrogenase, results in the formation of fumarate and reduced FAD.

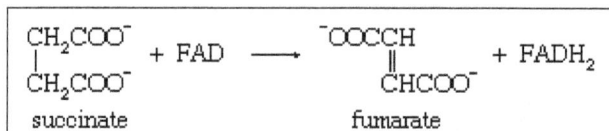

$$
\begin{array}{l}
CH_2COO^- \\
| \qquad\qquad + FAD \longrightarrow \\
CH_2COO^- \\
\text{succinate}
\end{array}
\qquad
\begin{array}{l}
^-OOCCH \\
\qquad \| \qquad\qquad + FADH_2 \\
\quad CHCOO^- \\
\text{fumarate}
\end{array}
$$

The elements of water are added across the double bond $(-CH=CH-)$ of fumarate in a reaction catalysed by fumarase. The product of the following reaction is malate.

$$\underset{\text{fumarate}}{\overset{\displaystyle{}^-OOCCH}{\underset{\displaystyle CHCOO^-}{\|}}} + H_2O \ \rightleftharpoons \ \underset{\text{malate}}{\overset{\displaystyle HOCHCOO^-}{\underset{\displaystyle CH_2COO^-}{|}}}$$

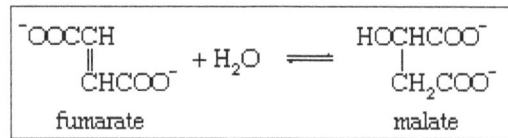

Malate can be oxidized to oxaloacetate by removal of two hydrogen atoms, which are accepted by NAD^+. This type of reaction is catalysed by malate dehydrogenase in the reaction given below. The formation of oxaloacetate completes the TCA cycle, which can now begin again with the formation of citrate.

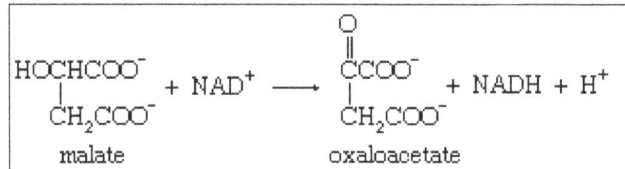

$$\underset{\text{malate}}{\overset{\displaystyle HOCHCOO^-}{\underset{\displaystyle CH_2COO^-}{|}}} + NAD^+ \ \longrightarrow \ \underset{\text{oxaloacetate}}{\overset{\displaystyle \overset{\displaystyle O}{\overset{\|}{C}}COO^-}{\underset{\displaystyle CH_2COO^-}{|}}} + NADH + H^+$$

ATP Yield of Aerobic Oxidation

The hydrogen ions and electrons that result in above four reactions are passed down the chain of respiratory carriers to oxygen, with the concomitant formation of three molecules of ATP per 2H as $NADH + H^+$. Similarly, the oxidation of the reduced FAD results in the formation of two ATP. Each turn of the cycle thus leads to the production of a total of 12 ATP. It will be recalled that the anaerobic fragmentation of glucose to two molecules of pyruvate yielded two ATP; the aerobic oxidation via the TCA cycle of two molecules of pyruvate thus makes available to the cell at least 15 times more ATP per molecule of glucose catabolized than is produced anaerobically. If, in addition, the $2 \times [NADH + H^+]$ generated per glucose in the second stage of glucose catabolism are passed on to oxygen, a further six ATP are generated. The advantage to living organisms is to be able to respire rather than merely to ferment.

Biological Energy Transduction

Adenosine Triphosphate as the Currency of Energy Exchange

When the terminal phosphate group is removed from ATP by hydrolysis, two negatively charged products are formed, ADP^{3-} and the phosphate group HPO_4^{2-}.

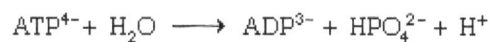

$$ATP^{4-} + H_2O \ \longrightarrow \ ADP^{3-} + HPO_4^{2-} + H^+$$

These products are electrically more stable than the parent molecule and do not readily recombine. The total free energy (G) of the products is much less than that of ATP; hence, energy is liberated (i.e., the reaction is exergonic). The amount of energy liberated under strictly defined conditions is called the standard free energy change ($\Delta G'$). This value for the hydrolysis of ATP is relatively high, at −8 kilocalories per mole. (One kilocalorie is the amount of heat required to raise the temperature of 1,000 grams of water one degree Celsius.) Conversely, the formation of ATP from ADP and inorganic phosphate (Pi) is an energy-requiring (i.e., endergonic) reaction with a standard free energy change of +8 kilocalories per mole.

The hydrolysis of the remaining phosphate-to-phosphate bond of ADP is also accompanied by a liberation of free energy (the standard free energy change is -6.5 kilocalories per mole); AMP hydrolysis liberates less energy (the standard free energy change is -2.2 kilocalories per mole).

The free energy of hydrolysis of a compound thus is a measure of the difference in energy content between the starting substances (reactants) and the final substances (products). ATP does not have the highest standard free energy of hydrolysis of all the naturally occurring phosphates but instead occupies a position at approximately the halfway point in a series of phosphate compounds with a wide range of standard free energies of hydrolysis. Compounds such as 1,3-diphosphoglycerate and phosphoenolpyruvate (PEP), which are above ATP on the scale, have large negative $\Delta G'$ values on hydrolysis and are often called high-energy phosphates. They are said to exhibit a high phosphate group transfer potential because they have a tendency to lose their phosphate groups. Compounds such as glucose 6-phosphate and fructose 6-phosphate, which are below ATP on the scale because they have smaller negative $\Delta G'$ values on hydrolysis, have a tendency to hold on to their phosphate groups and thus act as low-energy phosphate acceptors.

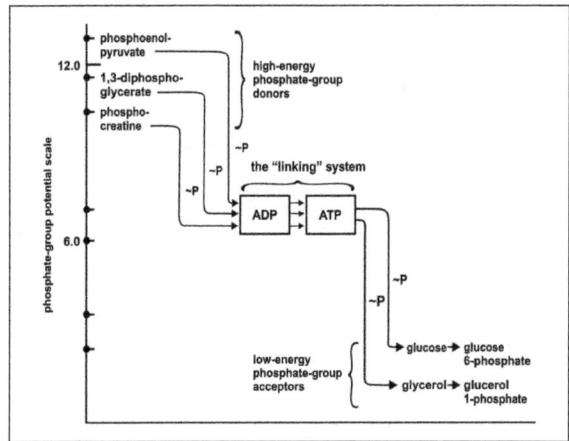

Transfer of phosphate groups from high-energy donors to low-energy acceptors.

The transfer of phosphate groups from high-energy donors to low-energy acceptors by way of the ATP-ADP system.

Both ATP and ADP act as intermediate carriers for the transfer of phosphate groups (which are more precisely called phosphoryl groups), and hence of energy, from compounds lying above ATP to those lying beneath it. Thus, in glycolysis, ADP acts as an acceptor of a phosphate group during the synthesis of ATP from PEP, and ATP functions as a donor of a phosphate group during the formation of fructose 1,6-diphosphate from fructose 6-phosphate.

The first step in glycolysis, the formation of glucose 6-phosphate (G6P), illustrates how an energetically unfavourable reaction may become feasible under intracellular conditions by coupling it to ATP.

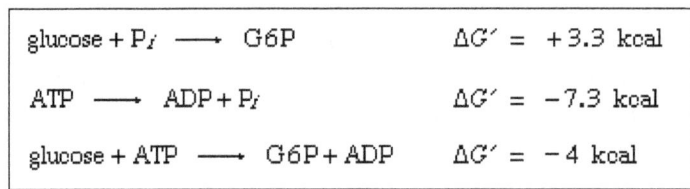

$$\text{glucose} + P_i \longrightarrow \text{G6P} \qquad \Delta G' = +3.3 \text{ kcal}$$

$$\text{ATP} \longrightarrow \text{ADP} + P_i \qquad \Delta G' = -7.3 \text{ kcal}$$

$$\text{glucose} + \text{ATP} \longrightarrow \text{G6P} + \text{ADP} \qquad \Delta G' = -4 \text{ kcal}$$

$$ATP \longrightarrow ADP + P_i \qquad\qquad \Delta G' = -7.3 \text{ kcal}$$

$$\text{glucose} + ATP \longrightarrow G6P + ADP \qquad \Delta G' = -4 \text{ kcal}$$

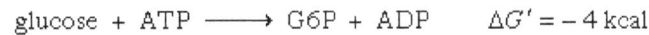

The above reaction has a positive $\Delta G'$ value, indicating that the reaction tends to proceed in the reverse direction. It is therefore necessary to use the standard free energy generated by the breaking of the first phosphate bond in ATP, which is −7.3 kilocalories per mole, to move the above reaction in the forward direction. Combining these reactions and their standard free energies gives reaction and a standard free energy value of −4 kilocalories per mole, indicating that the reaction will proceed in the forward direction. There are many intracellular reactions in which the formation of ADP or AMP from ATP provides energy for otherwise unfavourable biosyntheses. Some cellular reactions use equivalent phosphorylated analogues of ATP—for example, guanosine triphosphate (GTP) for protein synthesis.

The function of ATP as a common intermediate of energy transfer during anabolism is further dealt with below. In certain specialized cells or tissues, the chemical energy of ATP is used to perform work other than the chemical work of anabolism—for example, mechanical work, such as muscular contraction or the movement of contractile structures called cilia and flagella, which are responsible for the motility of many small organisms. The performance of osmotic work also requires ATP—e.g., the transport of ions or metabolites through membranes against a concentration gradient, a process that is basically responsible for many physiological functions, including nerve conduction, the secretion of hydrochloric acid in the stomach, and the removal of water from the kidneys.

Energy Conservation

The amount of ATP in a cell is limited, and it must be replaced continually to maintain repair and growth. This is achieved by using the energy liberated during the oxidative stages of catabolism to synthesize ATP from ADP and phosphate. The synthesis of ATP linked to catabolism occurs by two distinct mechanisms: substrate-level phosphorylation and oxidative, or respiratory-chain, phosphorylation. Oxidative phosphorylation is the major method of energy conservation under aerobic conditions in all nonphotosynthetic cells.

Substrate-level Phosphorylation

In substrate-level phosphorylation a phosphoryl group is transferred from an energy-rich donor (e.g., 1,3-diphosphoglycerate) to ADP to yield a molecule of ATP. This type of ATP synthesis does not require molecular oxygen (O_2), although it is frequently, but not always, preceded by an oxidation (i.e., dehydrogenation) reaction. Substrate-level phosphorylation is the major method of energy conservation in oxygen-depleted tissues and during fermentative growth of microorganisms.

Oxidative or Respiratory-chain Phosphorylation

In oxidative phosphorylation the oxidation of catabolic intermediates by molecular oxygen occurs via a highly ordered series of substances that act as hydrogen and electron carriers. They constitute the electron transfer system, or respiratory chain. In most animals, plants, and fungi, the electron transfer system is fixed in the membranes of mitochondria; in bacteria (which have no mitochondria) this system is incorporated into the plasma membrane. Sufficient free energy is released to allow the synthesis of ATP by a process described below. First, however, it is necessary to consider the nature of the respiratory chain.

Nature of the Respiratory Chain

Four types of hydrogen or electron carriers are known to participate in the respiratory chain, in which they serve to transfer two reducing equivalents (2H) from reduced substrate (AH_2) to molecular oxygen; the products are the oxidized substrate (A) and water (H_2O).

$$AH_2 + \tfrac{1}{2}O_2 \longrightarrow A + H_2O$$

The carriers are NAD^+ and, less frequently, $NADP^+$; the flavoproteins FAD and FMN (flavin mononucleotide); ubiquinone (or coenzyme Q); and several types of cytochromes. Each carrier has an oxidized and reduced form (e.g., FAD and $FADH_2$, respectively), the two forms constituting an oxidation-reduction, or redox, couple. Within the respiratory chain, each redox couple undergoes cyclic oxidation-reduction; i.e., the oxidized component of the couple accepts reducing equivalents from either a substrate or a reduced carrier preceding it in the series and in turn donates these reducing equivalents to the next oxidized carrier in the sequence. Reducing equivalents are thus transferred from substrates to molecular oxygen by a number of sequential redox reactions.

Most oxidizable catabolic intermediates initially undergo a dehydrogenation reaction, during which a dehydrogenase enzyme transfers the equivalent of a hydride ion ($H^+ + 2e^-$, with e^- representing an electron) to its coenzyme, either NAD^+ or $NADP^+$. The reduced NAD^+ (or $NADP^+$) thus produced (usually written as NADH + H^+ or NADPH + H^+) diffuses to the membrane-bound respiratory chain to be oxidized by an enzyme known as NADH dehydrogenase; the enzyme has as its coenzyme FMN. There is no corresponding NADPH dehydrogenase in mammalian mitochondria; instead, the reducing equivalents of NADPH + H^+ are transferred to NAD^+ in a reaction catalyzed by a transhydrogenase enzyme, with the products being reduced NADH + H^+ and $NADP^+$. A few substrates bypass this reaction and instead undergo immediate dehydrogenation by specific membrane-bound dehydrogenase enzymes. During the reaction, the coenzyme FAD accepts two hydrogen atoms and two electrons ($2H + 2e^-$). The reduced flavoproteins (i.e., $FMNH_2$ and $FADH_2$) donate their two hydrogen atoms to the lipid carrier ubiquinone, which is thus reduced.

The fourth type of carrier, the cytochromes, consists of hemoproteins—i.e., proteins with a nonprotein component, or prosthetic group, called heme (or a derivative of heme), which is an iron-containing pigment molecule. The iron atom in the prosthetic group is able to carry one electron and oscillates between the oxidized, or ferric (Fe^{3+}), and the reduced, or ferrous (Fe^{2+}), forms. The five cytochromes present in the mammalian respiratory chain, designated cytochromes b, c_1, c, a, and a_3, act in sequence between ubiquinone and molecular oxygen. The terminal cytochrome of this sequence (a_3, also known as cytochrome oxidase) is able to donate electrons to oxygen rather than to another electron carrier; a_3 is also the site of action of two substances that inhibit the respiratory chain, potassium cyanide and carbon monoxide. Special Fe-S complexes play a role in the activity of NADH dehydrogenase and succinate dehydrogenase.

In each redox couple, the reduced form has a tendency to lose reducing equivalents (i.e., to act as an electron or hydrogen donor); similarly, the oxidized form has a tendency to gain reducing equivalents (i.e., to act as an electron or hydrogen acceptor). The oxidation-reduction character-istics of each couple can be determined experimentally under well-defined standard conditions. The value thus obtained is the standard oxidation-reduction (redox) potential (E_6). Values for re-spiratory chain carriers range from $E_6 = -320$ millivolts (one millivolt = 0.001 volt) for NAD^+/re-duced NAD^+ to $E_6 = +820$ millivolts for $1/_2O_2/H_2O$; the values for intermediate carriers lie between. Reduced NAD^+ is the most electronegative carrier, oxygen the most electropositive acceptor. During respiration, reducing equivalents undergo stepwise transfer from the reduced form of the most electronegative carrier (reduced NAD^+) to the oxidized form of the most electropositive cou-ple (oxygen). Each step is accompanied by a decline in standard free energy ($\Delta G'$) proportional to the difference in the standard redox potentials (ΔE_0) of the two carriers involved.

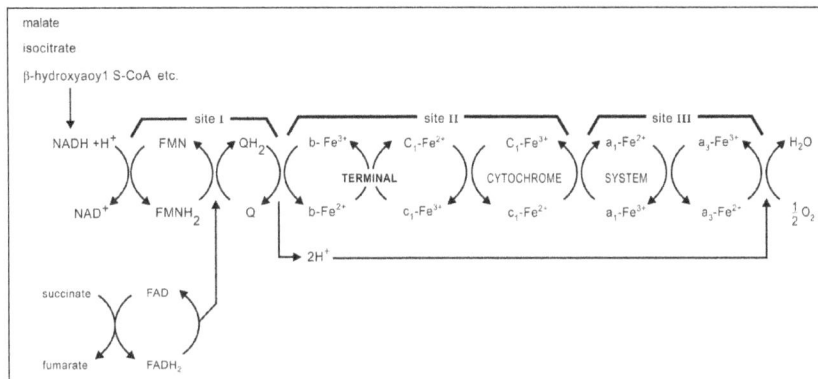

The respiratory chain

Overall oxidation of reduced NAD^+ by oxygen ($\Delta E_0 = +1,140$ millivolts) is accompanied by the liberation of free energy ($\Delta G' = -52.4$ kilocalories per mole). In theory, this energy is sufficient to allow the synthesis of six or seven molecules of ATP. In the cell, however, this synthesis of ATP, called oxidative phosphorylation, proceeds with an efficiency of about 46 percent. Thus, only three molecules of ATP are produced per atom of oxygen consumed—this being the so-called P/2e⁻, P/O, or ADP/O ratio. The energy that is not conserved as ATP is lost as heat. The oxidation of succinate by molecular oxygen ($\Delta E_0 = +790$ millivolts), which is accompanied by a smaller liberation of free energy ($\Delta G' = -36.5$ kilocalories per mole), yields only two molecules of ATP per atom of oxygen consumed (P/O = 2).

ATP Synthesis in Mitochondria

In order to understand the mechanism by which the energy released during respiration is conserved as ATP, it is necessary to appreciate the structural features of mitochondria. These are organelles in animal and plant cells in which oxidative phosphorylation takes place. There are many mitochondria in animal tissues—for example, in heart and skeletal muscle, which require large amounts of energy for mechanical work, and in the pancreas, where there is biosynthesis, and in the kidney, where the process of excretion begins. Mitochondria have an outer membrane, which allows the passage of most small molecules and ions, and a highly folded inner membrane (crista), which does not even allow the passage of small ions and so maintains a closed space within the cell. The electron-transferring molecules of the respiratory chain and the enzymes responsible for ATP synthesis are located in and on this inner membrane, while the space inside (matrix) contains the enzymes of the TCA cycle. The enzyme systems primarily responsible for the release and subsequent oxidation of reducing equivalents are thus closely related, so that the reduced coenzymes formed during catabolism (NADH + H$^+$ and FADH$_2$) are available as substrates for respiration. The movement of most charged metabolites into the matrix space is mediated by special carrier proteins in the crista that catalyze exchange-diffusion (i.e., a one-for-one exchange). The oxidative phosphorylation systems of bacteria are similar in principle but show a greater diversity in the composition of their respiratory carriers.

The mechanism of ATP synthesis appears to be as follows. During the transfer of hydrogen atoms from FMNH$_2$ or FADH$_2$ to oxygen, protons (H$^+$ ions) are pumped across the crista from the inside of the mitochondrion to the outside. Thus, respiration generates an electrical potential (and in mitochondria a small pH gradient) across the membrane corresponding to 200 to 300 millivolts, and the chemical energy in the substrate is converted into electrical energy. Attached to the crista is a complex enzyme (ATP synthetase) that binds ATP, ADP, and Pi. It has nine polypeptide chain subunits of five different kinds in a cluster and a unit of at least three more membrane proteins composing the attachment point of ADP and Pi. This complex forms a specific proton pore in the membrane. When ADP and Pi are bound to ATP synthetase, the excess of protons (H$^+$) that has formed outside of the mitochondria (an H$^+$ gradient) moves back into the mitochondrion through the enzyme complex. The energy released is used to convert ADP and Pi to ATP. In this process, electrical energy is converted to chemical energy, and it is the supply of ADP that limits the rate of this process. The precise mechanism by which the ATP synthetase complex converts the energy stored in the electrical H$^+$ gradient to the chemical bond energy in ATP is not well understood. The H$^+$ gradient may power other endergonic (energy-requiring) processes besides ATP synthesis, such as the movement of bacterial cells and the transport of carbon substrates or ions.

ATP Formation during Photosynthesis

Photosynthesis generates ATP by a mechanism that is similar in principle. The organelles responsible are different from mitochondria, but they also form membrane-bounded closed sacs (thylakoids) often arranged in stacks (grana). Solar energy splits two molecules of H$_2$O into molecular oxygen (O$_2$), four protons (H$^+$), and four electrons.

This is the source of oxygen evolution, clearly visible as bubbles from underwater plants in bright sunshine. The process involves a chlorophyll molecule, P$_{680}$, that changes its redox potential from +820 millivolts (in which there is a tendency to accept electrons) to about −680 millivolts (in which there is a tendency to lose electrons) upon excitation with light and acquisition of electrons. The electrons are subsequently passed along a series of carriers (plastoquinone, cytochromes b and f, and plastocyanin), analogous to the mitochondrial respiratory chain. This process pumps protons across the membrane from the outside of the thylakoid membrane to the inside. Protons (H$^+$) do not move freely across the membrane although chloride ions (Cl$^-$) do, creating a pH gradient. An ATP synthetase enzyme similar to that of the mitochondria is present, but on the outside of the thylakoid membrane. Passage of protons (H$^+$) through it from inside to outside generates ATP.

Hence, a gradient of protons (H$^+$) across the membrane is the high-energy intermediate for forming ATP in plant photosynthesis and in the respiration of all cells capable of passing reducing equivalents (hydrogen atoms or electrons) to electron acceptors.

Biosynthesis of Cell Components

Stages of Biosynthesis

The biosynthesis of cell components (anabolism) may be regarded as occurring in two main stages. In the first, intermediate compounds of the central routes of metabolism are diverted from further catabolism and are channeled into pathways that usually lead to the formation of the relatively small molecules that serve as the building blocks, or precursors, of macromolecules.

In the second stage of biosynthesis, the building blocks are combined to yield the macromolecules—proteins, nucleic acids, lipids, and polysaccharides—that make up the bulk of tissues and cellular components. In organisms with the appropriate genetic capability, for example, all of the amino acids can be synthesized from ammonia and intermediates of the main routes of carbohydrate fragmentation and oxidation. Such intermediates act also as precursors for the purines, the pyrimidines, and the pentose sugars that constitute DNA and for a number of types of RNA. The assembly of proteins necessitates the precise combination of specific amino acids in a highly ordered and controlled manner; this in turn involves the copying, or transcription, into RNA of specific parts of DNA. The first stage of biosynthesis thus requires the specificity normally required for the efficient functioning of sequences of enzyme-catalyzed reactions. The second stage also involves—directly for protein and nucleic acid synthesis, less directly for the synthesis of other macromolecules—the maintenance and expression of the biological information that specifies the identity of the cell, the tissue, and the organism.

Utilization of ATP

The two stages of biosynthesis—the formation of building blocks and their specific assembly into macromolecules—are energy-consuming processes and thus require ATP. Although the ATP is derived from catabolism, catabolism does not "drive" biosynthesis. The occurrence of chemical reactions in the living cell is accompanied by a net decrease in free energy. Although biological growth and development result in the creation of ordered systems from less ordered ones and of complex systems from simpler ones, these events must occur at the expense of energy-yielding reactions. The overall coupled reactions are, on balance, still accompanied by a decrease in free energy and are thus essentially irreversible in the direction of biosynthesis. The total energy released from ATP, for example, is usually much greater than is needed for a particular biosynthetic step; thus, many of the reactions involved in biosynthesis release inorganic pyrophosphate (PPi) rather than phosphate (Pi) from ATP, and hence yield AMP rather than ADP. Since inorganic pyrophosphate readily undergoes virtually irreversible hydrolysis to two equivalents of inorganic phosphate, the creation of a new bond in the product of synthesis may be accompanied by the breaking of two high-energy bonds of ATP—although, in theory, one might have sufficed.

The efficient utilization for anabolic processes of ATP and some intermediate compound formed during a catabolic reaction requires the cell to have simultaneously a milieu favourable for both ATP generation and consumption. Catabolism occurs readily only if sufficient ADP is available; hence, the concentration of ATP is low. On the other hand, biosynthesis requires a high level of ATP and consequently low levels of ADP and AMP. Suitable conditions for the simultaneous function of both processes are met in two ways. Biosynthetic reactions often take place in compartments within the cell different from those in which catabolism occurs; there is thus a physical separation of energy-requiring and energy-yielding processes. Furthermore, biosynthetic reactions are regulated independently of the mechanisms by which catabolism is controlled. Such independent control is made possible by the fact that catabolic and anabolic pathways are not identical; the pacemaker, or key, enzyme that controls the overall rate of a catabolic route usually does not play any role in the biosynthetic pathway of a compound. Similarly, the pacemaker enzymes of biosynthesis are not involved in catabolism. Catabolic pathways are often regulated by the relative amounts of ATP, ADP, and AMP in the cellular compartment in which the pacemaker enzymes are located. In general, ATP inhibits and ADP (or AMP) stimulates such enzymes. In contrast, many biosynthetic routes are regulated by the concentration of the end products of particular anabolic processes, so that the cell synthesizes only as much of these building blocks as it needs.

Supply of Biosynthetic Precursors

When higher animals consume a mixed diet, sufficient quantities of compounds for both biosynthesis and energy supply are available. Carbohydrates yield intermediates of glycolysis and of the phosphogluconate pathway, which in turn yield acetyl coenzyme A (or acetyl-CoA); lipids yield glycolytic intermediates and acetyl coenzyme A; and many amino acids form intermediates of both the TCA cycle and glycolysis. Any intermediate withdrawn for biosynthesis can thus be readily replenished by the catabolism of further nutrients. This situation does not always hold, however. Microorganisms in particular can derive all of their carbon and energy requirements by utilizing a single carbon source. The sole carbon source may be a substance such as a carbohydrate or a fatty acid, or an intermediate of the TCA cycle (or a substance readily converted to one).

Anaplerotic Routes

Although the catabolism of carbohydrates can occur via a variety of routes, all give rise to pyruvate. During the catabolism of pyruvate, one carbon atom is lost as carbon dioxide and the remaining two form acetyl coenzyme A; these two are involved in the TCA cycle. Because the TCA cycle is initiated by the condensation of acetyl coenzyme A with oxaloacetate, which is regenerated in each turn of the cycle, the removal of any intermediate from the cycle would cause the cycle to stop. Yet, various essential cell components are derived from α-oxoglutarate, succinyl coenzyme A, and oxaloacetate, so that these compounds are, in fact, removed from the cycle. Microbial growth with a carbohydrate as the sole carbon source is thus possible only if a cellular process occurs that effects the net formation of some TCA cycle intermediate from an intermediate of carbohydrate catabolism. Such a process, which replenishes the TCA cycle, has been described as an anaplerotic reaction.

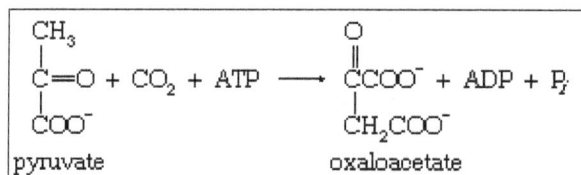

The anaplerotic function may be carried out by either of two enzymes that catalyze the fixation of carbon dioxide onto a three-carbon compound, either pyruvate or phosphoenolpyruvate to form oxaloacetate, which has four carbon atoms. Both reactions require energy. In the above reaction it is supplied by the cleavage of ATP to ADP and inorganic phosphate (Pi), and in the below mentioned reaction, it is supplied by the release of the high-energy phosphate of PEP as inorganic phosphate. Pyruvate serves as a carbon dioxide acceptor not only in many bacteria and fungi but also in the livers and kidneys of higher organisms, including humans; PEP serves as the carbon dioxide acceptor in many bacteria, such as those that inhabit the gut.

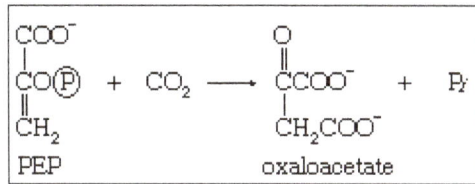

$$\begin{array}{c} COO^- \\ | \\ CO\text{\textcircled{P}} \\ || \\ CH_2 \end{array} + CO_2 \longrightarrow \begin{array}{c} O \\ || \\ CCOO^- \\ | \\ CH_2COO^- \end{array} + P_i$$

PEP   oxaloacetate

Unlike higher organisms, many bacteria and fungi can grow on acetate or compounds such as ethanol or a fatty acid that can be catabolized to acetyl coenzyme A. Under these conditions, the net formation of TCA cycle intermediates can proceed via different ways. For example, in obligate anaerobic bacteria, pyruvate can be formed from acetyl coenzyme A and carbon dioxide; reducing equivalents [2H] are necessary for the reaction. The pyruvate so formed can then react via either of the above two reactions.

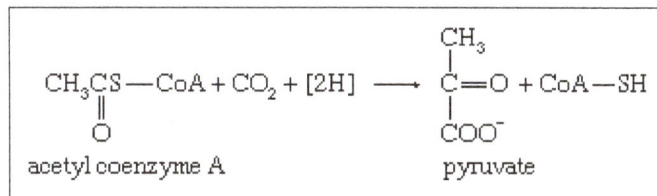

$$CH_3CS\!-\!CoA + CO_2 + [2H] \longrightarrow \begin{array}{c} CH_3 \\ | \\ C\!=\!O + CoA\!-\!SH \\ | \\ COO^- \end{array}$$

acetyl coenzyme A   pyruvate

The above reaction does not occur in facultative anaerobic organisms or in strict aerobes, however. Instead, in these organisms two molecules of acetyl coenzyme A give rise to the net synthesis of a four-carbon intermediate of the TCA cycle via a route known as the glyoxylate cycle. In this route, the steps of the TCA cycle that lead to the loss of carbon dioxide are bypassed. Instead of being oxidized to oxalosuccinate, isocitrate is split by isocitrate lyase. The dotted line in the below mentioned reaction indicates the way in which isocitrate is split. The products are succinate and glyoxylate.

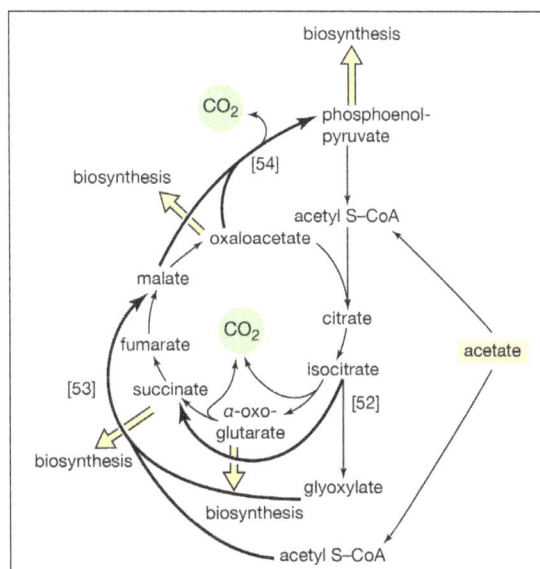

The glyoxylate cycle.

$$\begin{array}{c} CH_2COO^- \\ | \\ HCCOO^- \\ | \\ HOCHCOO^- \end{array} \longrightarrow \begin{array}{c} CH_2COO^- \\ | \\ CH_2COO^- \end{array} + \begin{array}{c} CHO \\ | \\ COO^- \end{array}$$

isocitrate   succinate   glyoxylate

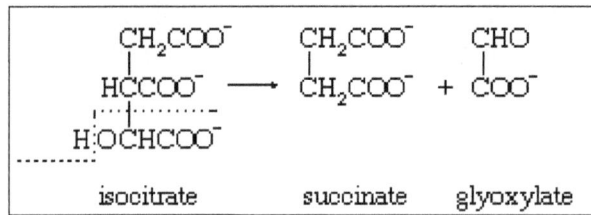

Glyoxylate, like oxaloacetate, is the anion of an α-oxoacid and thus can condense, in a reaction catalyzed by malate synthase, with acetyl coenzyme A; the products of this reaction are coenzyme A and malate.

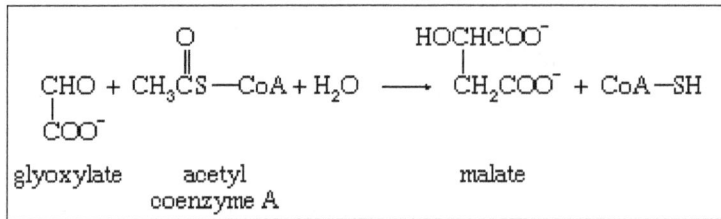

$$\begin{array}{c} O \\ || \\ CHO + CH_3CS-CoA + H_2O \\ | \\ COO^- \end{array} \longrightarrow \begin{array}{c} HOCHCOO^- \\ | \\ CH_2COO^- \end{array} + CoA-SH$$

glyoxylate   acetyl   malate
                  coenzyme A

In conjunction with the reactions of the TCA cycle that effect the re-formation of isocitrate from malate lead to the net production of a four-carbon compound (malate) from two two-carbon units (glyoxylate and acetyl coenzyme A). The sequence thus complements the TCA cycle, enabling the cycle to fulfill the dual roles of providing both energy and biosynthetic building blocks when the sole carbon source is a two-carbon compound such as acetate.

Other examples of anaplerotic pathways used to form cellular building blocks include the ethylmalonyl-CoA pathway and the methylaspartate pathway. The ethylmalonyl-CoA pathway is used by organisms lacking the isocitrate lyase enzyme, such as the bacterium Rhodobacter sphaeroides. In this pathway two acetyl-CoA molecules are combined to produce acetoactyl-CoA, which subsequently reacts to form the intermediate ethylmalonyl-CoA. Ethylmalonyl-CoA is acted upon to form methylmalonyl-CoA, which is cleaved to produce glyoxylate and propionyl-CoA, leading to the formation of malate and succinyl-CoA, respectively. In the methylaspartate pathway the intermediate compound methylaspartate is formed from acetyl-CoA and undergoes a series of reactions to produce glyoxylate. Glyoxylate then reacts with acetyl-CoA, ultimately forming malate. The methylaspartate pathway of acetyl-CoA assimilation was discovered in a primitive single-celled prokaryotic organism known as Haloarcula marismortui, which lacks several of the genes that encode enzymes needed for the glyoxylate and ethylmalonyl-CoA pathways.

Growth of Microorganisms on TCA Cycle Intermediates

Most aerobic microorganisms grow readily on substances such as succinate or malate as their sole source of carbon. Under these circumstances, the formation of the intermediates of carbohydrate metabolism requires an enzymatic step ancillary to the central pathways. In most cases this step is catalyzed by phosphoenolpyruvate (PEP) carboxykinase. Oxaloacetate is decarboxylated (i.e., carbon dioxide is removed) during this energy-requiring reaction. The energy may be supplied by ATP or a similar substance (e.g., GTP) that can readily be derived from. The products are PEP, carbon dioxide, and ADP.

$$
\begin{array}{c}
\underset{\substack{\text{O}\\||\\\text{CCOO}^-\\|\\\text{CH}_2\text{COO}^-}}{} + \text{ATP} \longrightarrow \underset{\substack{\text{COO}^-\\|\\\text{CO}\textcircled{P}\\||\\\text{CH}_2}}{} + \text{CO}_2 + \text{ADP}\\
\text{oxaloacetate} \qquad\qquad\qquad \text{PEP}
\end{array}
$$

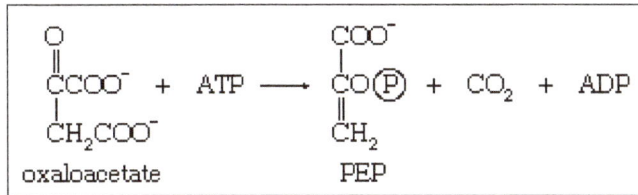

Another reaction that can yield an intermediate of carbohydrate catabolism is catalyzed by the so-called malic enzyme; in reaction given below, malate is decarboxylated to pyruvate, with concomitant reduction of $NADP^+$. The primary role of malic enzyme, however, may be to generate reduced $NADP^+$ for biosynthesis rather than to form an intermediate of carbohydrate catabolism.

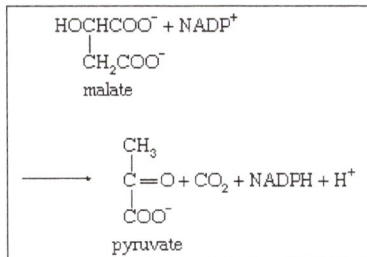

$$
\begin{array}{l}
\underset{\substack{\text{HOCHCOO}^- + \text{NADP}^+\\|\\\text{CH}_2\text{COO}^-}}{}\\
\text{malate}\\
\\
\longrightarrow \underset{\substack{\text{CH}_3\\|\\\text{C}=\text{O} + \text{CO}_2 + \text{NADPH} + \text{H}^+\\|\\\text{COO}^-}}{}\\
\qquad\quad \text{pyruvate}
\end{array}
$$

Synthesis of Building Blocks

Gluconeogenesis

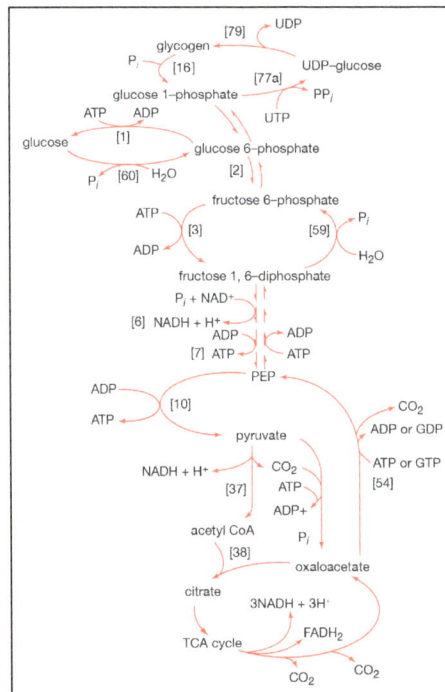

Catabolism and biosynthesis of glucose and glycogen: Shown at left are reactions peculiar to catabolism. At right are reactions peculiar to anabolism. Numbers in brackets refer to reactions explained in text.

The formation of sugars from noncarbohydrate precursors, gluconeogenesis, is of major importance in all living organisms. In the light, photosynthetic plants and microorganisms incorporate, or fix, carbon dioxide onto a five-carbon sugar and, via a sequence of transfer reactions, re-form the same sugar while also effecting the net synthesis of the glycolytic intermediate, 3-phosphoglycerate. Phosphoglycerate is the precursor of starch, cell-wall carbohydrates, and other plant polysaccharides. A situation similar in principle applies to the growth of microorganisms on precursors of acetyl coenzyme A or on intermediates of the TCA cycle—that is, a large variety of cell components are derived from carbohydrates that, in turn, are synthesized from these noncarbohydrate precursors. Higher organisms also readily convert glucogenic amino acids (i.e., those that do not yield acetyl coenzyme A as a catabolic product) into TCA cycle intermediates, which are then converted into glucose. The amounts of glucose thus transformed depend on the needs of the organism for protein synthesis and on the availability of fuels other than glucose. The synthesis of blood glucose from lactate, which occurs largely in liver, is a particularly active process during recovery from intense muscular activity.

Most of the steps in the pathway for the biosynthesis of glucose from pyruvate are catalyzed by the enzymes of glycolysis; the direction of the reactions is reversed. Three virtually irreversible steps in glucose catabolism that cannot be utilized in gluconeogenesis, however, are bypassed by alternative reactions that tend to proceed in the direction of glucose synthesis.

Formation of PEP from Pyruvate

The first alternative reaction is the conversion of pyruvate to PEP. Three mechanisms for overcoming the energy barrier associated with the direct reversal of the pyruvate kinase reaction are known. In some bacteria, PEP is formed from pyruvate by the utilization of two of the high-energy bonds of ATP; the products include, in addition to PEP, AMP and inorganic phosphate. A variant of this reaction occurs in some bacteria, in which ATP and inorganic phosphate are reactants and AMP and inorganic pyrophosphate are products; as mentioned above, inorganic pyrophosphate is likely to be hydrolyzed to two equivalents of inorganic phosphate, so that the net balance of the reaction is identical with the reaction given below:

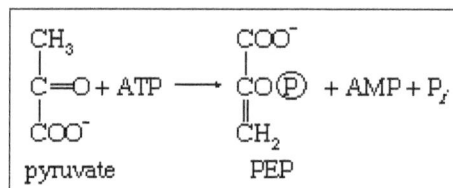

The enzyme adenylate kinase catalyzes the interconversion of the various adenine nucleotides.

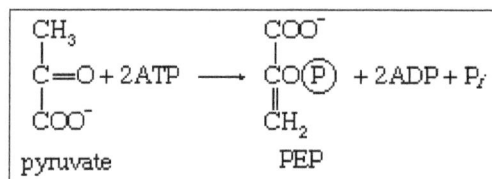

The combination of the above and below reactions yields the same energy balance as does the direct conversion of pyruvate to PEP.

Hydrolysis of fructose 1,6-diphosphate and glucose 6-phosphate.

The second step of glycolysis bypassed in gluconeogenesis is that catalyzed by phosphofructoki-nase (reaction Above). Instead, the fructose 1,6-diphosphate synthesized from dihydroxyaceto-nephosphate and glyceraldehyde 3-phosphate in the reaction catalyzed by aldolase is hydrolyzed, with the loss of the phosphate group linked to the first carbon atom.

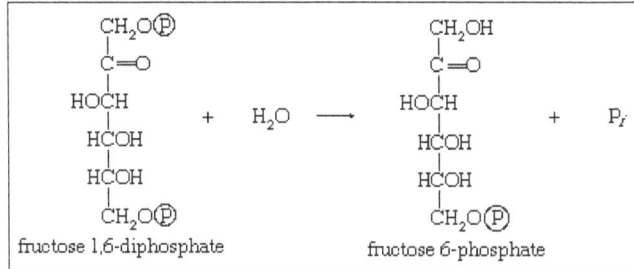

The enzyme fructose diphosphatase catalyzes reaction, in which the products are fructose 6-phos-phate and inorganic phosphate. The fructose 6-phosphate thus formed is a precursor of mucopoly-saccharides (polysaccharides with nitrogen-containing components). In addition, its conversion to glucose 6-phosphate provides the starting material for the formation of storage polysaccharides such as starch and glycogen, of monosaccharides other than glucose, of disaccharides (carbohydrates with two sugar components), and of some structural polysaccharides (e.g., cellulose). The maintenance of the glucose content of vertebrate blood requires glucose 6-phosphate to be converted to glucose. This process occurs in the kidney, in the lining of the intestine, and most importantly in the liver. The reaction does not occur by reversal of the hexokinase or glucokinase reactions that effect the forma-tion of glucose 6-phosphate from glucose and ATP; rather, glucose 6-phosphate is hydrolyzed in a reaction catalyzed by glucose 6-phosphatase, and the phosphate is released as inorganic phosphate.

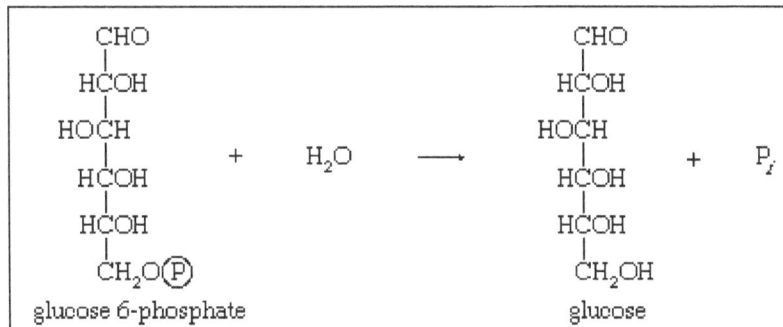

Lipid Components

The component building blocks of the lipids found in storage fats, in lipoproteins (combinations of lipid and protein), and in the membranes of cells and organelles are glycerol, the fatty acids, and a number of other compounds (e.g., serine, inositol).

Glycerol

Glycerol is readily derived from dihydroxyacetone phosphate, an intermediate of glycolysis. The reaction given below, catalyzed by glycerol 1-phosphate dehydrogenase, dihydroxyacetone phos-phate is reduced to glycerol 1-phosphate. Reduced NAD^+ provides the reducing equivalents for the reaction and is oxidized. This compound reacts further.

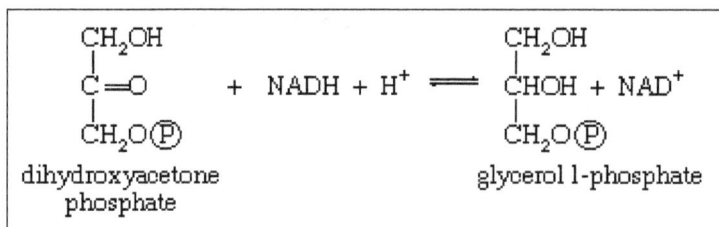

$$\begin{array}{ccc}
\text{CH}_2\text{OH} & & \text{CH}_2\text{OH} \\
| & & | \\
\text{C}=\text{O} \quad + \text{ NADH} + \text{H}^+ \rightleftharpoons & \text{CHOH} + \text{NAD}^+ \\
| & & | \\
\text{CH}_2\text{O}\textcircled{P} & & \text{CH}_2\text{O}\textcircled{P} \\
\text{dihydroxyacetone} & & \text{glycerol 1-phosphate} \\
\text{phosphate} & &
\end{array}$$

Fatty Acids

Although all the carbon atoms of the fatty acids found in lipids are derived from the acetyl coenzyme A produced by the catabolism of carbohydrates and fatty acids, the molecule first undergoes a carboxylation, forming malonyl coenzyme A, before participating in fatty acid synthesis. The carboxylation reaction is catalyzed by acetyl CoA carboxylase, an enzyme whose prosthetic group is the vitamin biotin. The biotin–enzyme first undergoes a reaction that results in the attachment of carbon dioxide to biotin; ATP is required and forms ADP and inorganic phosphate.

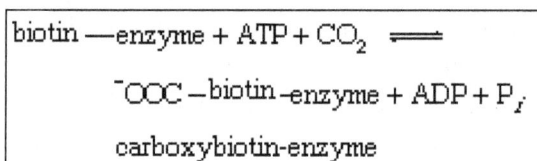

$$\text{biotin}-\text{enzyme} + \text{ATP} + \text{CO}_2 \rightleftharpoons$$
$$^-\text{OOC}-\text{biotin}-\text{enzyme} + \text{ADP} + \text{P}_i$$
$$\text{carboxybiotin-enzyme}$$

The complex product, called carboxybiotin–enzyme, releases the carboxy moiety to acetyl coenzyme A, forming malonyl coenzyme A and restoring the biotin–enzyme.

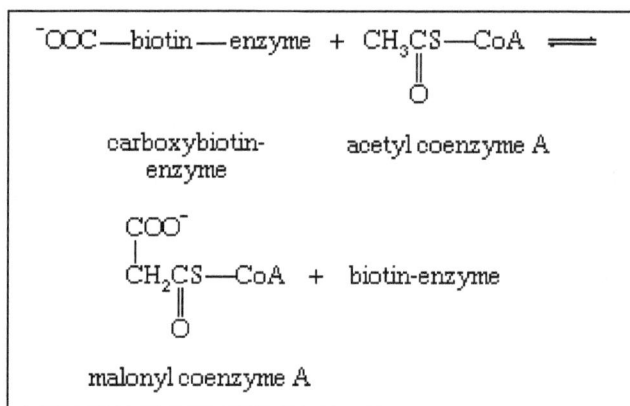

$$^-\text{OOC}-\text{biotin}-\text{enzyme} + \text{CH}_3\overset{\text{O}}{\underset{\|}{\text{C}}}\text{S}-\text{CoA} \rightleftharpoons$$

carboxybiotin-enzyme   acetyl coenzyme A

$$\overset{\text{COO}^-}{\underset{}{|}} \text{CH}_2\overset{\text{O}}{\underset{\|}{\text{C}}}\text{S}-\text{CoA} + \text{biotin-enzyme}$$

malonyl coenzyme A

The above two reactions, catalyzed by acetyl coenzyme A carboxylase thus involves the expenditure of one molecule of ATP for the formation of each molecule of malonyl coenzyme A from acetyl coenzyme A and carbon dioxide.

Malonyl coenzyme A and a molecule of acetyl coenzyme A react (in bacteria) with the sulfhydryl group of a relatively small molecule known as acyl-carrier protein (ACP–SH); in higher organisms ACP–SH is part of a multienzyme complex called fatty acid synthetase. ACP–SH is involved in all of the reactions leading to the synthesis of a fatty acid such as palmitic acid from acetyl coenzyme A and malonyl coenzyme A. The products of the two reactions given below are acetyl-S-ACP, malonyl-S-ACP, and coenzyme A. The enzymes catalyzing the two reactions given below are known as acetyl transacylase and malonyl transacylase, respectively. Acetyl-ACP and malonyl-ACP react in a reaction catalyzed by β-ketoacyl-ACP synthetase so that the acetyl moiety (CH_3CO-) is transferred to the malonyl moiety ($^-OOCH_2CO-$). Simultaneously, the carbon dioxide fixed in the above reaction is lost, leaving as a product a four-carbon moiety attached to ACP and called acetoacetyl-S-ACP.

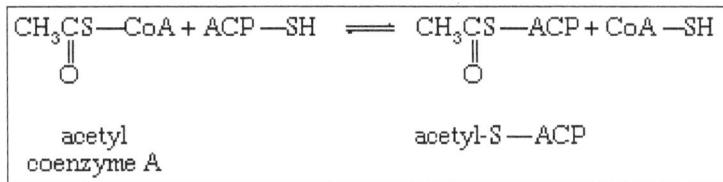

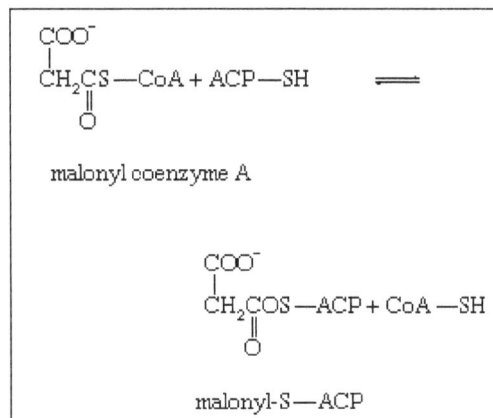

$$CH_3\overset{\|}{\underset{O}{C}}S{-}CoA + ACP{-}SH \rightleftharpoons CH_3\overset{\|}{\underset{O}{C}}S{-}ACP + CoA{-}SH$$

acetyl   acetyl-S—ACP
coenzyme A

$$\overset{COO^-}{\underset{\|}{\underset{O}{|}}}\ \ CH_2\overset{\|}{\underset{O}{C}}S{-}CoA + ACP{-}SH \rightleftharpoons$$

malonyl coenzyme A

$$\overset{COO^-}{|}\ CH_2\overset{\|}{\underset{O}{C}}OS{-}ACP + CoA{-}SH$$

malonyl-S—ACP

It should be noted that the carbon atoms of acetyl-S-ACP occur at the end of acetoacetyl-S-ACP and that carbon dioxide plays an essentially catalytic role; the decarboxylation of the malonyl-S-ACP in the below reaction provides a strong thermodynamic pull toward fatty acid synthesis.

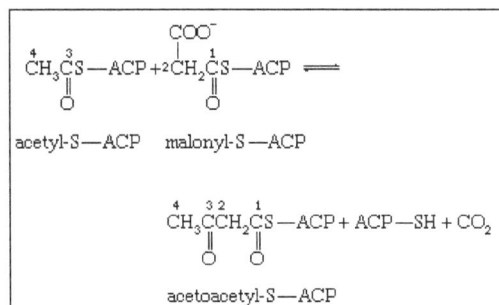

$$\overset{4}{C}H_3\overset{3}{\underset{\|}{\underset{O}{C}}}S{-}ACP + {}^2\overset{COO^-}{\underset{\|}{\underset{O}{C}}}H_2\overset{1}{C}S{-}ACP \rightleftharpoons$$

acetyl-S—ACP   malonyl-S—ACP

$$\overset{4}{C}H_3\overset{3\ 2}{\underset{\|}{\underset{O}{C}}}CH_2\overset{1}{\underset{\|}{\underset{O}{C}}}S{-}ACP + ACP{-}SH + CO_2$$

acetoacetyl-S—ACP

The analogy between the above reaction of fatty acid synthesis and the cleavage reaction of fatty acid catabolism is apparent in the other reactions of fatty acid synthesis. The acetoacetyl-S-ACP, for example, undergoes reduction to β-hydroxybutyryl-S-ACP; the reaction is catalyzed by β-ketoacyl-ACP reductase. Reduced NADP⁺ is the electron donor, however, and not reduced NAD⁺ (which would participate in the reversal of reaction. NADP⁻ is thus a product in the following reaction.

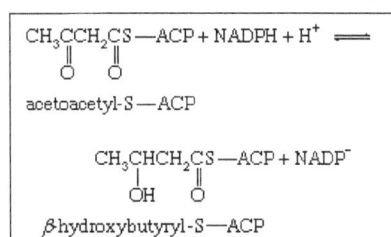

$$CH_3\overset{\|}{\underset{O}{C}}CH_2\overset{\|}{\underset{O}{C}}S{-}ACP + NADPH + H^+ \rightleftharpoons$$

acetoacetyl-S—ACP

$$CH_3\overset{}{\underset{OH}{C}}HCH_2\overset{\|}{\underset{O}{C}}S{-}ACP + NADP^-$$

β-hydroxybutyryl-S—ACP

In the below reaction, β-hydroxybutyryl-S-ACP is dehydrated (i.e., one molecule of water is removed), in a reaction catalyzed by enoyl-ACP-hydrase, and then undergoes a second reduction, in which reduced NADP$^+$ again acts as the electron donor. The products of the reaction given below are crotonyl-S-ACP and water.

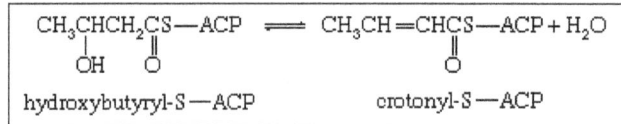

$$CH_3CHCH_2CS\!-\!ACP \rightleftharpoons CH_3CH\!=\!CHCS\!-\!ACP + H_2O$$

hydroxybutyryl-S —ACP   crotonyl-S —ACP

The formation of butyryl-S-ACP in the reaction given below completes the first of several cycles, in each of which one molecule of malonyl coenzyme. In the cycle following the one ending with the butyryl moiety is transferred to malonyl-S-ACP, and a molecule of carbon dioxide is again lost; a six-carbon compound results. In subsequent cycles, each of which adds two carbon atoms to the molecule via reaction above, successively longer β-oxoacyl-S-ACP derivatives are produced.

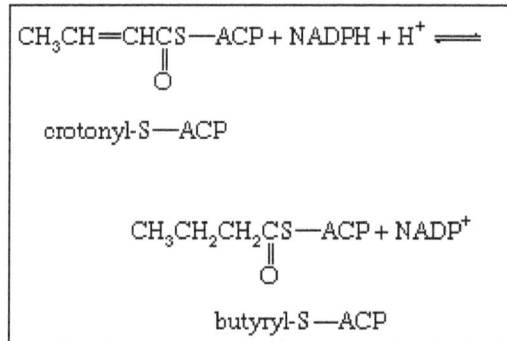

$$CH_3CH\!=\!CHCS\!-\!ACP + NADPH + H^+ \rightleftharpoons$$

crotonyl-S—ACP

$$CH_3CH_2CH_2CS\!-\!ACP + NADP^+$$

butyryl-S—ACP

Ultimately, a molecule with 16 carbon atoms, palmityl-S-ACP, is formed. In most organisms a deacylase catalyzes the release of free palmitic acid; in a few, synthesis continues, and an acid with 18 carbon atoms is formed. The fatty acids can then react with coenzyme A to form fatty acyl coenzyme A, which can condense with the glycerol 1-phosphate; the product is a phosphatidic acid. The overall formation of each molecule of palmitic acid from acetyl coenzyme A and repeated cycles of the above five reactions requires the investment of seven molecules of ATP and 14 of reduced NADP$^+$. The process is thus an energy-requiring one (endergonic) and represents a major way by which the reducing power generated in NADP-linked dehydrogenation reactions of carbohydrate catabolism is utilized.

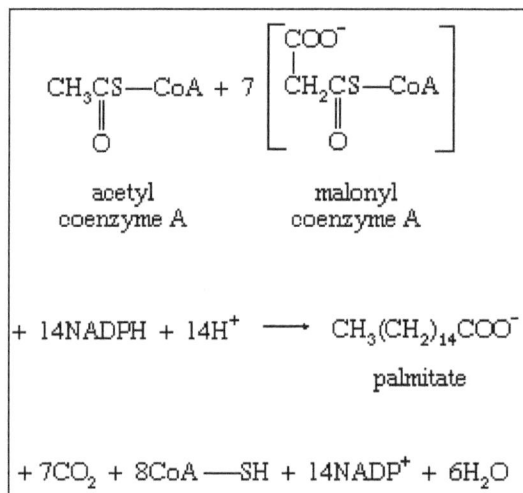

$$CH_3CS\!-\!CoA + 7 \left[\begin{array}{c} COO^- \\ | \\ CH_2CS\!-\!CoA \end{array} \right]$$

acetyl   malonyl
coenzyme A   coenzyme A

$$+ \; 14NADPH + 14H^+ \longrightarrow CH_3(CH_2)_{14}COO^-$$

palmitate

$$+ \; 7CO_2 + 8CoA\!-\!SH + 14NADP^+ + 6H_2O$$

Other Components

The major lipids that serve as components of membranes, called phospholipids, as well as lipoproteins, contain, in addition to two molecules of fatty acid, one molecule of a variety of different compounds. The precursors of these compounds include serine, inositol, and glycerol 1-phosphate. They are derived from intermediates of the central metabolic pathways.

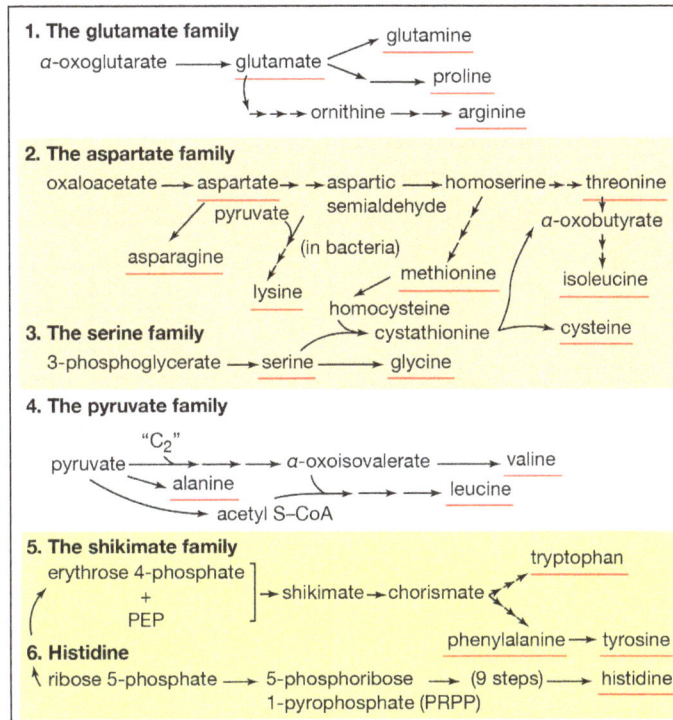

Family relationships in amino acid biosynthesis:Components of proteins are underlined. Not all of the intermediates formed are named.

Amino Acids

Organisms differ considerably in their ability to synthesize amino acids from the intermediates of central metabolic pathways. Most vertebrates can form only the chemically most simple amino acids; the others must be supplied in the diet. Humans, for example, synthesize about 10 of the 20 commonly encountered amino acids; these are known as nonessential amino acids. The essential amino acids must be supplied in food.

Higher plants are more versatile than animals; they can make all of the amino acids required for protein synthesis, with either ammonia (NH_3) or nitrate (NO_3^-) as the nitrogen source. Some bacteria, and leguminous plants (e.g., peas) that harbour such bacteria in their root nodules, are able to utilize nitrogen from the air to form ammonia and use the latter for amino acid synthesis.

Bacteria differ widely in their ability to synthesize amino acids. Some species, such as Escherichia coli, which can grow in media supplied with only a single carbon source and ammonium salts, can make all of their amino acids from these starting materials. Other bacteria may require as many as 16 different amino acids.

Each of the 20 common amino acids is synthesized by a different pathway, the complexity of which reflects the chemical complexity of the amino acid formed. As with other compounds, the pathway for the synthesis of an amino acid is for the most part different from that by which it is catabolized.

First, ammonia is incorporated into the intermediates of metabolic pathways mainly via the glutamate dehydrogenase reaction, which proceeds from right to left in biosynthetic reactions. Similarly, the transaminase enzymes enable the amino group (NH_2^-) to be transferred to other amino acids.

Second, a group of several amino acids may be synthesized from one amino acid, which acts as a "parent" of an amino acid "family." The families are also interrelated in several instances. Bacteria can synthesize 20 amino acids, all derived from intermediates of pathways already considered. Alpha-oxoglutarate and oxaloacetate are intermediates of the TCA cycle; pyruvate, 3-phosphoglycerate, and PEP are intermediates of glycolysis; and ribose 5-phosphate and erythrose 4-phosphate are formed in the phosphogluconate pathway.

Mononucleotides

Most organisms can synthesize the purine and pyrimidine nucleotides that serve as the building blocks of RNA (containing nucleotides in which the pentose sugar is ribose, called ribonucleotides) and DNA (containing nucleotides in which the pentose sugar is deoxyribose, called deoxyribonucleotides) as well as the agents of energy exchange.

Purine Ribonucleotides

The purine ribonucleotides (AMP and GMP) are derived from ribose 5-phosphate. The overall sequence that leads to the parent purine ribonucleotide, which is inosinic acid, involves 10 enzymatic steps. Inosinic acid can be converted to AMP and GMP; these in turn yield the triphosphates (i.e., ATP and GTP) via reactions catalyzed by adenylate kinase and nucleoside diphosphate kinase.

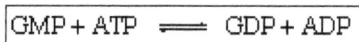

$$\text{GMP} + \text{ATP} \rightleftharpoons \text{GDP} + \text{ADP}$$

Pyrimidine Ribonucleotides

The biosynthetic pathway for the pyrimidine nucleotides is somewhat simpler than that for the purine nucleotides.

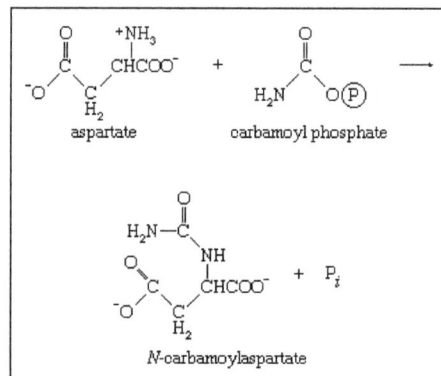

aspartate + carbamoyl phosphate ⟶ N-carbamoylaspartate + P_i

Aspartate (derived from the TCA cycle intermediate, oxaloacetate) and carbamoyl phosphate condense to form N-carbamoylaspartate, which loses water in a reaction given below catalyzed by dihydroorotase.

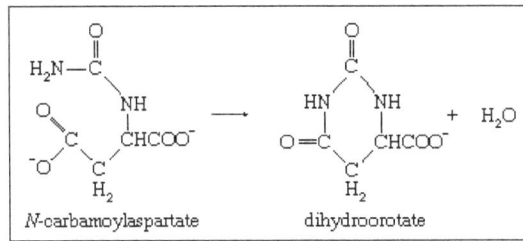

The product, dihydroorotate, is then oxidized to orotate in a reaction catalyzed by dihydroorotic acid dehydrogenase, in which NAD^+ is reduced.

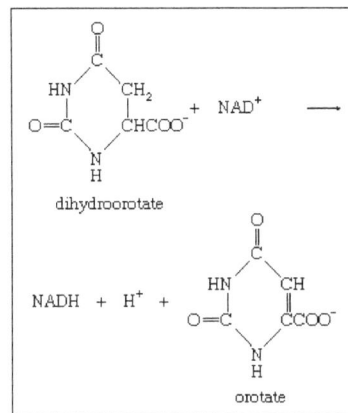

The orotate accepts a pentose phosphate moiety from 5-phosphoribose 1-pyrophosphate (PRPP); PRPP, which is formed from ribose 5-phosphate and ATP, also initiates the pathways for biosynthesis of purine nucleotides and of histidine. The product loses carbon dioxide to yield the parent pyrimidine nucleotide, uridylic acid.

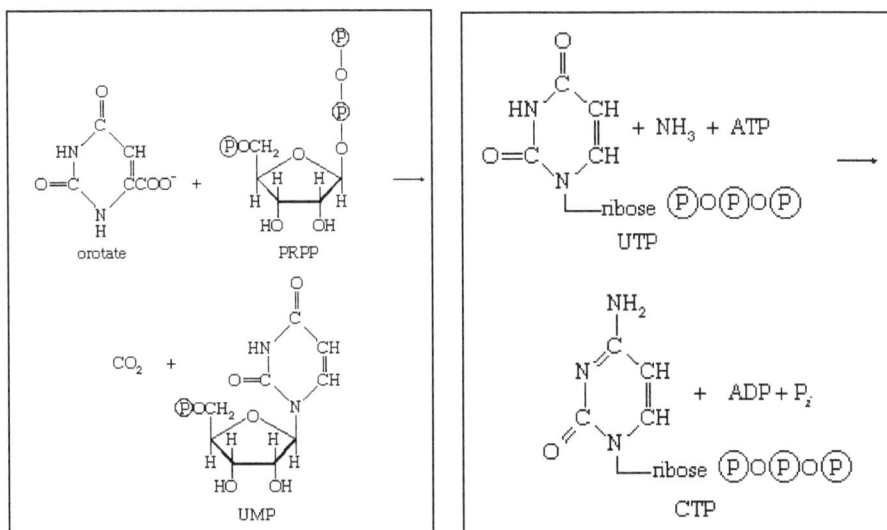

Analogous to the phosphorylation of purine nucleotides is the phosphorylation of UMP to UDP and thence to UTP by interaction with two molecules of ATP. Uridine triphosphate (UTP) can be converted to the other pyrimidine building block of RNA, cytidine triphosphate (CTP). In bacteria, the nitrogen for this in the reaction given below is derived from ammonia; in higher animals, glutamine is the nitrogen donor.

Deoxyribonucleotides

The building blocks for the synthesis of DNA differ from those for the synthesis of RNA in two respects. In DNA the purine and pyrimidine nucleotides contain the pentose sugar 2-deoxyribose instead of ribose. In addition, the pyrimidine base uracil, found in RNA, is replaced in DNA by thymine. The deoxyribonucleoside diphosphate can be derived directly from the corresponding ribonucleoside diphosphate by a process involving the two sulfhydryl groups of the protein, thioredoxin, and a flavoprotein, thioredoxin reductase that can in turn be reduced by reduced $NADP^+$. Thus, for the reduction of XDP, in which X represents a purine base or cytosine, the reaction may be written as shown in the two reactions given below. In the following reaction oxidized thioredoxin-S_2 is reduced to thioredoxin-$(SH)_2$ by NADPH, which is oxidized in the process. Thioredoxin-$(SH)_2$ then reduces XDP to deoxyXDP in reaction, in which thioredoxin is re-formed.

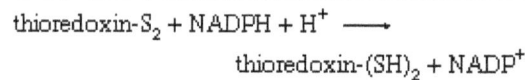

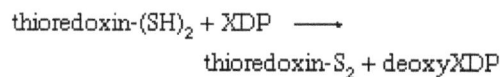

$$\text{thioredoxin-}S_2 + \text{NADPH} + H^+ \longrightarrow$$
$$\text{thioredoxin-}(SH)_2 + \text{NADP}^+$$

$$\text{thioredoxin-}(SH)_2 + \text{XDP} \longrightarrow$$
$$\text{thioredoxin-}S_2 + \text{deoxyXDP}$$

Deoxythymidylic acid (dTMP) is derived from deoxyuridylic acid (dUMP).

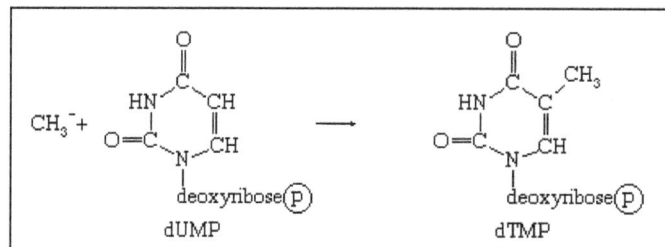

Deoxyuridine diphosphate (dUDP) is first converted to dUMP, by reaction proceeding from right to left. Deoxyuridylic acid then accepts a methyl group (CH_3-) in a reaction catalyzed by an enzyme (thymidylate synthetase) with the vitamin folic acid as a coenzyme; the product is dTMP.

Synthesis of Macromolecules

Carbohydrates and Lipids

The formation of polysaccharides and of phospholipids from their component building blocks not only requires the investment of the energy of nucleoside triphosphates but uses these molecules in a novel manner. The biosynthetic reactions described thus far have mainly been accompanied by the formation of energy-rich intermediates with the formation of either AMP or ADP; however, nucleotides serve as intermediate carriers in the formation of glycogen, starch, and a variety of lipids. This unique process necessitates reactions by which ATP, or another nucleoside triphosphate, which can be readily derived from ATP, combines with a phosphorylated reactant to form a nucleoside-diphosphate product. Although the change in standard free energy is small in this reaction, the subsequent hydrolysis of the inorganic pyrophosphate also released effectively makes the reaction irreversible in the direction of synthesis. The nucleoside triphosphate is represented as NTP in the reaction given below, and the phosphorylated reactant as $R-\textcircled{P}$.

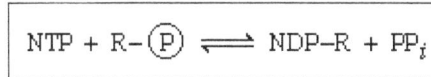

$$\text{NTP} + \text{R}-\textcircled{P} \rightleftharpoons \text{NDP--R} + \text{PP}_i$$

Such types of reactions are catalyzed by pyrophosphorylases.

Formation of Storage Polysaccharides

In the formation of storage polysaccharides—i.e., glycogen in animals, starch in plants is preceded by the conversion of glucose 6-phosphate to glucose 1-phosphate, in a reaction catalyzed by phosphoglucomutase. Glucose 1-phosphate functions as $R-\textcircled{P}$ in reaction.

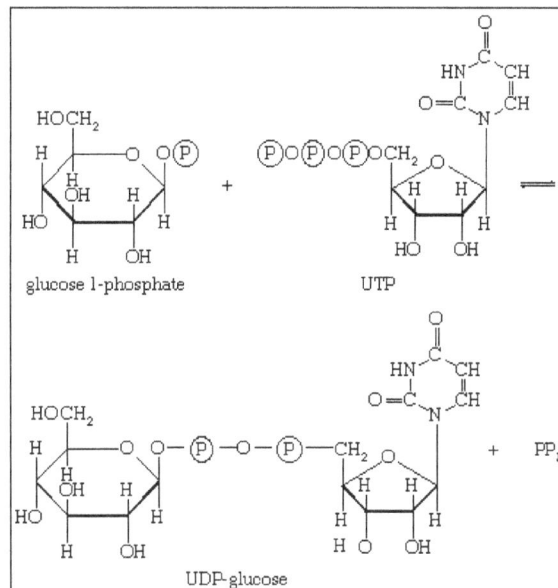

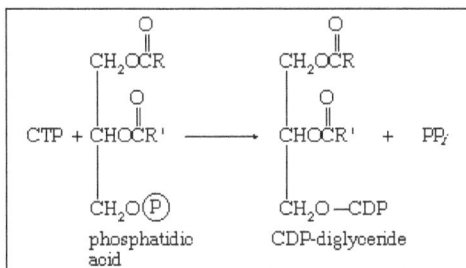

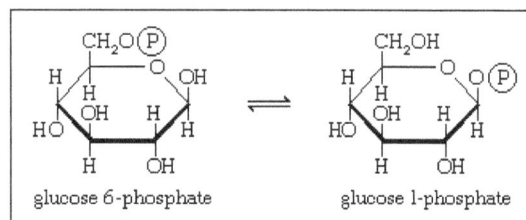

UTP is the specific NTP for glycogen synthesis in animals; the products are UDP-glucose and pyrophosphate. In bacteria, fungi, and plants, ATP, CTP, or GTP serves instead of UTP. In all cases the nucleoside diphosphate glucose (NDP-glucose) thus synthesized can donate glucose to the terminal glucose of a polysaccharide chain, thereby increasing the number (n) of glucose molecules by one to n + 1. UDP is released in this process, which is catalyzed by glycogen synthetase. Starch synthesis in plants occurs by an analogous pathway catalyzed by amylose synthetase; ADP-glucose rather than UDP-glucose is the preferred glucose donor. Similarly, cellulose, the major structural polysaccharide in plant cell walls, is synthesized in some plants by reaction; other plants undergo analogous reactions in which GDP-glucose or CDP-glucose acts as the glucose donor.

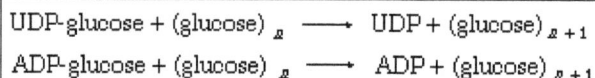

$$\text{UDP-glucose} + (\text{glucose})_n \longrightarrow \text{UDP} + (\text{glucose})_{n+1}$$
$$\text{ADP-glucose} + (\text{glucose})_n \longrightarrow \text{ADP} + (\text{glucose})_{n+1}$$

Nucleoside diphosphate sugars also participate in the synthesis of disaccharides; for example, common table sugar, sucrose (consisting of glucose and fructose), is formed in sugarcane by the two reactions given below; UDP-glucose and fructose 6-phosphate first form a phosphorylated derivative of sucrose, sucrose 6′-phosphate, which is hydrolyzed to sucrose and inorganic phosphate.

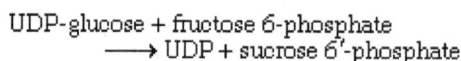

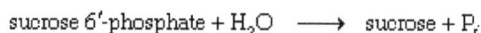

$$\text{UDP-glucose} + \text{fructose 6-phosphate} \longrightarrow \text{UDP} + \text{sucrose 6′-phosphate}$$

$$\text{sucrose 6′-phosphate} + H_2O \longrightarrow \text{sucrose} + P_i$$

Lactose, which consists of galactose and glucose, is the principal sugar of milk. It is synthesized in the mammary gland as shown in the reaction given below; UDP-galactose and glucose react to form lactose; UDP is also a product.

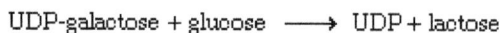

$$\text{UDP-galactose} + \text{glucose} \longrightarrow \text{UDP} + \text{lactose}$$

Formation of Lipids

The neutral fats, or triglycerides, that constitute storage lipids, and the phospholipid components of lipoproteins and membranes, are synthesized from their building blocks by a route that branches after the first biosynthetic reaction. Initially, one molecule of glycerol 1-phosphate, the intermediate derived from carbohydrate catabolism, and two molecules of the appropriate fatty acyl coenzyme A combine, yielding phosphatidic acid.

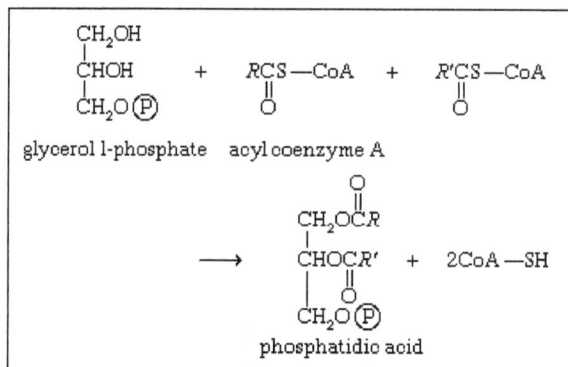

This reaction occurs preferentially with acyl coenzyme A derivatives of fatty acids containing 16 or 18 carbon atoms. In the above reaction, R and R′ represent the hydrocarbon moieties ($Ch_3(CH_2$)

n−) of two fatty acid molecules. A triglyceride molecule (neutral fat) is formed from phosphatidic acid in a reaction catalyzed by a phosphatase that results in loss of the phosphate group; the diglyceride thus formed can then accept a third molecule of fatty acyl coenzyme A (represented as R″C ∥ OS−CoA.

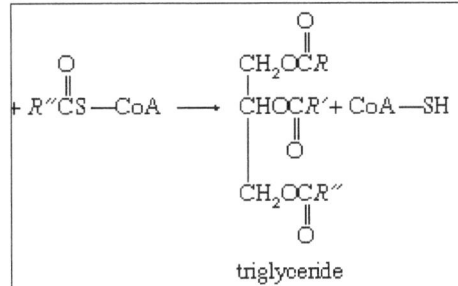

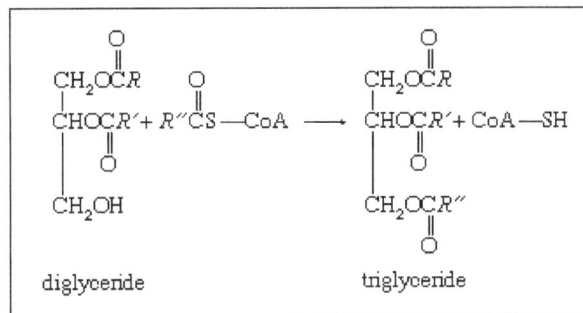

triglyceride

diglyceride   triglyceride

In the biosynthesis of phospholipids, however, phosphatidic acid is not hydrolyzed; rather, it acts as the R−Ⓟ, the NTP here being cytidine triphosphate (CTP). A CDP-diglyceride is produced, and inorganic pyrophosphate is released. CDP-diglyceride is the common precursor of a variety of phospholipids. In subsequent reactions, each catalyzed by a specific enzyme, CMP is displaced from CDP-diglyceride by one of three compounds—serine, inositol, or glycerol 1-phosphate—to form CMP and, respectively, phosphatidylserine, phosphatidylinositol, or 3-phosphatidyl-glycerol 1′-phosphate. These reactions differ from those of polysaccharide biosynthesis in that phosphate is retained in the phospholipid, and the nucleotide product (CMP) is therefore a nucleoside monophosphate rather than the diphosphate. These compounds can react further: phosphatidylserine to give, sequentially, phosphatidylethanolamine and phosphatidylcholine; phosphatidylinositol to yield mono- and diphosphate derivatives that are components of brain tissue and of mitochondrial membranes; and PGP to yield the phosphatidylglycerol abundant in many bacterial membranes and the diphosphatidylglycerol that is also a major component of mitochondrial and bacterial membranes.

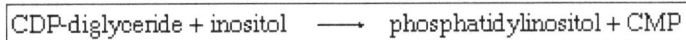

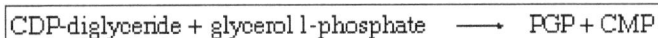

CDP-diglyceride + inositol $\longrightarrow$ phosphatidylinositol + CMP

CDP-diglyceride + glycerol 1-phosphate $\longrightarrow$ PGP + CMP

Nucleic Acids and Proteins

As with the synthesis of polysaccharides and lipids, the formation of the nucleic acids and proteins from their building blocks requires the input of energy. Nucleic acids are formed from nucleoside triphosphates, with concomitant elimination of inorganic pyrophosphate, which is subsequently hydrolyzed. Amino acids also are activated, forming, at the expense of ATP, aminoacyl-complexes. This activation process is also accompanied by loss of inorganic pyrophosphate. But, although these biochemical processes are basically similar to those involved in the biosynthesis of other macromolecules, their occurrence is specifically subservient to the genetic information in DNA. DNA contains within its structure the blueprint both for its own exact duplication and for the synthesis of a number of types of RNA, among which is a class termed messenger RNA (mRNA). A complementary relationship exists between the sequence of purines (i.e., adenine and guanosine) and pyrimidines (cytosine and thymine) in the DNA comprising a gene and the sequence in mRNA into which this genetic information is transcribed. This information is then translated into the sequence of amino acids in a protein, a process that involves the functioning of a variety of other classes of ribonucleic acids.

Synthesis of DNA

The maintenance of genetic integrity demands not only that enzymes exist for the synthesis of DNA but that they function so as to ensure the replication of the genetic information (encoded in the DNA to be copied) with absolute fidelity. This implies that the assembly of new regions of a DNA molecule must occur on a template of DNA already present in the cell. The synthetic processes must also be capable of repairing limited regions of DNA, which may have been damaged, for example, as a consequence of exposure to ultraviolet irradiation. The physical structure of DNA is ideally adapted to its biological roles. Two strands of nucleotides are wound around each other in the form of a double helix. The helix is stabilized by hydrogen bonds that occur between the purine and pyrimidine bases of the strands. Thus, the adenine of one strand pairs with the thymine of the other, and the guanine of one strand with the cytosine of the other. The base pairs may be visualized as the treads of a spiral staircase, in which the two chains of repeating units (i.e., ribose-phosphate-ribose) form the sides.

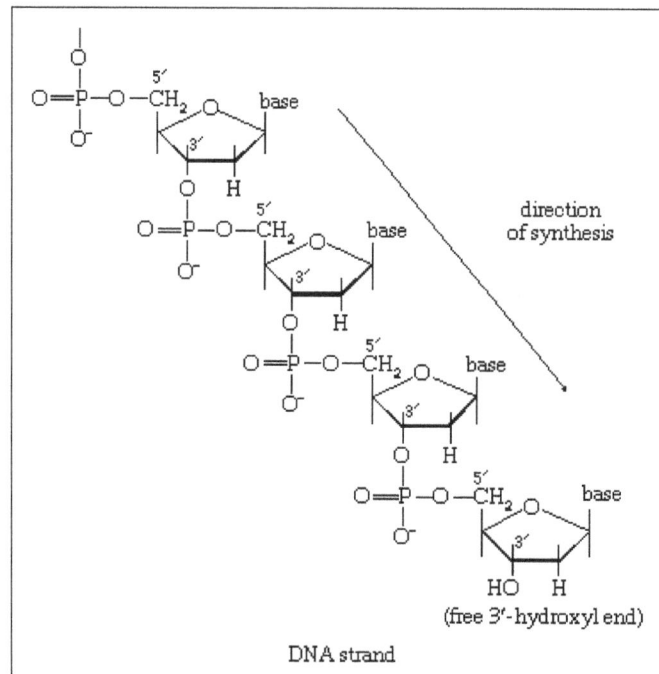

DNA strand

During the biosynthesis of DNA, the two strands unwind, and each serves as a template for the synthesis of a new, complementary strand, in which the bases pair in exactly the same manner as occurred in the parent double helix. The process is catalyzed by a DNA polymerase enzyme, which catalyzes the addition of the appropriate deoxyribonucleoside triphosphate (NTP) in the reaction given below onto one end, specifically, the free 3′-hydroxyl end (−OH) of the growing DNA chain. In the reaction given below, the addition of a deoxyribonucleoside monophosphate (dNMP) moiety onto a growing DNA chain (5′-DNA-polymer-3′-OH) is shown; the other product is inorganic pyrophosphate. The specific nucleotide inserted in the growing chain is dictated by the base in the complementary (template) strand of DNA with which it pairs. The functioning of DNA polymerase thus requires the presence of all four deoxyribonucleoside triphosphates (i.e., dATP, dTPP, dGTP, and dCTP) as well as preformed DNA to act as a template. Although a number of DNA polymerase enzymes have been purified from different organisms, it is not yet certain whether those that have been most extensively studied are necessarily involved in the formation of new DNA molecules, or whether they are primarily concerned with the repair of damaged regions of molecules. A polynucleotide ligase that effects the formation of the phosphate bond between adjacent sugar molecules is concerned with the repair function but may also have a role in synthesis.

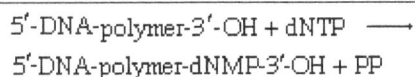

$$5'\text{-DNA-polymer-}3'\text{-OH} + \text{dNTP} \longrightarrow$$
$$5'\text{-DNA-polymer-dNMP-}3'\text{-OH} + \text{PP}$$

Synthesis of RNA

Various types of RNA are found in living organisms: messenger RNA (mRNA) is involved in the immediate transcription of regions of DNA; transfer RNA (tRNA) is concerned with the incorporation of amino acids into proteins; and structural RNA is found in the ribosomes that form the protein-synthesizing machinery of the cell. In cells of organisms with well-defined nuclei (i.e., eukaryotes), a heterogenous RNA fraction of unknown function is constantly broken down and resynthesized in the nucleus of the cell but does not leave it. The different types of RNA are synthesized via RNA polymerases, the action of which is analogous to that of the DNA polymerases that catalyze reaction. The growing RNA chain is represented by 5′-RNA-polymer-3′-OH, and the ribonucleoside triphosphate by NTP. One product (5′-RNA-polymer-NMP-3′-OH) reflects the incorporation of ribonucleoside monophosphate; the other product is inorganic pyrophosphate. Synthesis of RNA requires DNA as a template, thus ensuring that the base composition of the RNA faithfully reflects that of the DNA; in addition, as in DNA synthesis, all four nucleoside triphosphates must be present. The major differences between reactions above and below are that, in the latter, the nucleotides contain ribose instead of deoxyribose, and that, in RNA, uracil replaces the thymine of DNA.

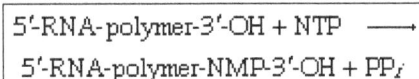

$$5'\text{-RNA-polymer-}3'\text{-OH} + \text{NTP} \longrightarrow$$
$$5'\text{-RNA-polymer-NMP-}3'\text{-OH} + \text{PP}_i$$

It appears that, although only one strand of the DNA double helix serves as template during the formation of RNA, some regions are transcribed from one strand, some from the other.

An important constraint on RNA synthesis is that the accurate copying of the appropriate DNA strand by RNA polymerase must start at the beginning of a gene—and not somewhere along it—and must stop as soon as the genetic information has been transcribed. The way in which this selectivity is achieved is not yet fully understood, although it has been established that E. coli contains a protein, the sigma factor, that is not required for the incorporation of the nucleoside triphosphates into the growing RNA chain but apparently is essential for binding RNA polymerase to the proper DNA sites to initiate RNA synthesis. After the initiation step, the sigma factor is released; the role of the sigma factor in transcription suggests that the DNA at the initiation sites must be unique in some way so as to ensure that the correct strand is used as the template. Evidence indicates further that other protein factors are involved in the termination of transcription.

Synthesis of Proteins

Approximately 120 macromolecules are involved directly or indirectly in the process of the translation of the base sequence of a messenger RNA molecule into the amino acid sequence of a protein. The relationship between the base sequence and the amino acid sequence constitutes the genetic code. The basic properties of the code are: it is triplet—i.e., a linear sequence of three bases in mRNA specifies one amino acid in a protein; it is nonoverlapping—i.e., each triplet is discrete and does not overlap either neighbour; it is degenerate—i.e., many of the 20 amino acids are specified by more than one of the 64 possible triplets of bases; and it appears to apply universally to all living organisms.

The main sequence of events associated with the expression of this genetic code, as elucidated for E. coli, may be summarized as follows:

1. Messenger RNA binds to the smaller of two subunits of large particles termed ribosomes.

2. The amino acid that begins the assembly of the protein chain is activated and transferred to a specific transfer RNA (tRNA). The activation step, catalyzed by an aminoacyl–tRNA synthetase specific for a particular amino acid, effects the formation of an aminoacyl–AMP complex; ATP is required, and inorganic pyrophosphate is a product. The aminoacyl–AMP, which remains bound to the enzyme, is transferred to a specific molecule of tRNA in a reaction catalyzed by the same enzyme. AMP is released, and the other product is called aminoacyl–tRNA. In E. coli the amino acid that begins the assembly of the protein is always formylmethionine (f-Met). There is no evidence that f-Met is involved in protein synthesis in eukaryotic cells.

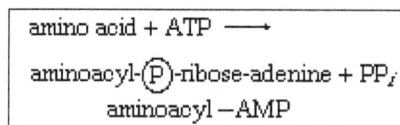

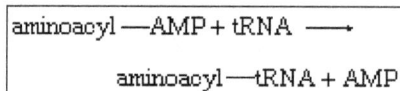

amino acid + ATP ⟶
aminoacyl-(P)-ribose-adenine + PP$_i$
aminoacyl –AMP

aminoacyl —AMP + tRNA ⟶
aminoacyl—tRNA + AMP

3. Aminoacyl–tRNA binds to the mRNA-ribosomal complex in a reaction in which energy is provided by the hydrolysis of GTP to GDP and inorganic phosphate. In this step and in 5 below, the genetic code is translated. All of the different tRNAs contain triplets of bases that pair specifically with the complementary base triplets in mRNA; the base triplets in mRNA specify the amino acids to be added to the protein chain. During or shortly after the

pairing occurs the aminoacyl–tRNA moves from the aminoacyl-acceptor (A) site on the ribosome to another site, called a peptidyl-donor (P) site.

4. The larger subunit of the ribosome then joins the mRNA–f-Met–tRNA–smaller ribosomal subunit complex.

5. The second amino acid to be added to the protein chain is specified by the triplet of bases adjacent to the initiator triplet in mRNA. The amino acid is activated and transferred to its tRNA by a repetition of the above two reactions. This newly formed aminoacyl–tRNA now binds to the A site of the mRNA–ribosome complex, with concomitant hydrolysis of GTP.

6. The enzyme peptidyl transferase, which is part of the larger of the two ribosomal subunits, catalyzes the transfer of formylmethionine from the tRNA to which it is attached (designated tRNA$^{f\text{-Met}}$) to the second amino acid; for example, if the second amino acid were leucine, the fifth reaction would have achieved the binding of leucyl–tRNA (Leu–tRNA^{Leu}) next to f-Met–tRNA$^{f\text{-Met}}$ on the ribosome–mRNA complex. Step 6 catalyzes the transfer reaction that is shown in the reaction given below, in which tRNA$^{f\text{-Met}}$ is released from formyl-methionine (f-Met), and Leu–tRNA^{Leu} is bound to formyl-methionine.

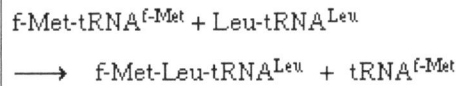

$$\text{f-Met-tRNA}^{f\text{-Met}} + \text{Leu-tRNA}^{Leu}$$
$$\longrightarrow \quad \text{f-Met-Leu-tRNA}^{Leu} + \text{tRNA}^{f\text{-Met}}$$

7. In the next step three results are achieved. The dipeptide f-Met–Leu (a dipeptide consists of two amino acids) moves from the A (aminoacyl-acceptor) site to the P (peptidyl-donor) site on the ribosome; the tRNA$^{f\text{-Met}}$ is thereby displaced from the P site, and the ribosome moves the length of one triplet (three bases) along the mRNA molecule. The occurrence of these events is accompanied by the hydrolysis of a second molecule of GTP and leaves the system ready to receive the next aminoacyl–tRNA (by repetition of step 5). The cycle of events in 5, 6, and 7 is repeated until the ribosome moves to a triplet on the mRNA that does not specify an amino acid but provides the signal for termination of the amino acid chain. Triplets of this type are represented by one uracil (U) preceding and adjacent to, two adenines (UAA) or preceding one adenine and one guanosine in either order (UGA, or UAG).

8. At the termination of synthesis the completed protein is released from the tRNA to which it had remained linked. Two further events then occur in E. coli. First, the formyl constituent of the f-methionyl moiety is hydrolyzed by the catalytic action of a formylase, producing a protein with methionine at the end. If the required protein does not contain methionine in this position (and the majority of proteins in E. coli appear to), the methionine and possibly other amino acids that follow it are removed by enzymatic reactions. Second, the ribosome–mRNA complex dissociates, and the ribosomal subunits become available for a new round of translation by binding another mRNA molecule step 1.

For the sake of brevity, other ancillary protein factors that participate in this sequence of events 1 to 8 have been omitted. The role of many of these factors is as yet poorly understood.

Regulation of Metabolism

Fine Control

The flux of nutrients along each metabolic pathway is governed chiefly by two factors: (1) the availability of substrates on which pacemaker, or key, enzymes of the pathway can act and (2) the intracellular levels of specific metabolites that affect the reaction rates of pacemaker enzymes. Key enzymes are usually complex proteins that, in addition to the site at which the catalytic process occurs (i.e., the active site), contain sites to which the regulatory metabolites bind. Interactions with the appropriate molecules at these regulatory sites cause changes in the shape of the enzyme molecule. Such changes may either facilitate or hinder the changes that occur at the active site. The rate of the enzymatic reaction is thus speeded up or slowed down by the presence of a regulatory metabolite.

In many cases, the specific small molecules that bind to the regulatory sites have no obvious structural similarity to the substrates of the enzymes; these small molecules are therefore termed allosteric effectors, and the regulatory sites are termed allosteric sites. Allosteric effectors may be formed by enzyme-catalyzed reactions in the same pathway in which the enzyme regulated by the effectors functions. In this case a rise in the level of the allosteric effector would affect the flux of nutrients along that pathway in a manner analogous to the feedback phenomena of homeostatic processes. Such effectors may also be formed by enzymatic reactions in apparently unrelated pathways. In this instance the rate at which one metabolic pathway operates would be profoundly affected by the rate of nutrient flux along another. It is this situation that, to a large extent, governs the sensitive and immediately responsive coordination of the many metabolic routes in the cell.

End-product Inhibition

A biosynthetic pathway is usually controlled by an allosteric effector produced as the end product of that pathway, and the pacemaker enzyme on which the effector acts usually catalyzes the first step that uniquely leads to the end product. This phenomenon, called end-product inhibition, is illustrated by the multienzyme, branched pathway for the formation from oxaloacetate of the aspartate family of amino acids. Only plants and microorganisms can synthesize many of these amino acids, most animals requiring such amino acids to be supplied preformed in their diets.

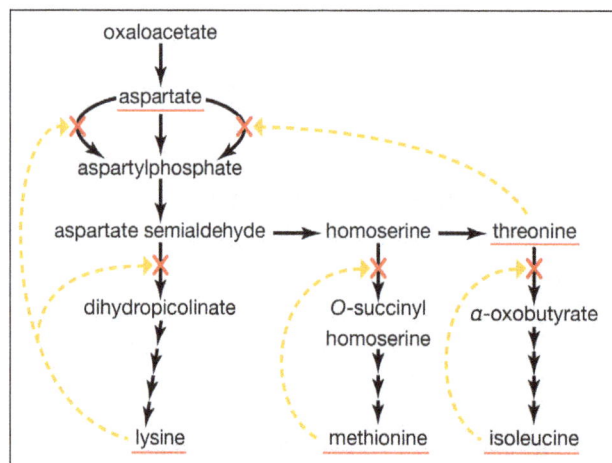

"Fine control" of the enzymes of the aspartate family in *E. coli.*

There are a number of pacemaker enzymes in the biosynthetic route for the aspartate family of amino acids, most of which are uniquely involved in the formation of one product. Each of the enzymes functions after a branch point in the pathway, and all are inhibited specifically by the end product that emerges from the branch point. Thus, the supplies of lysine, methionine, and isoleucine required by a cell can be independently regulated. Threonine, however, is both an amino acid essential for protein synthesis and a precursor of isoleucine. If the rate of synthesis of threonine from aspartate were regulated as are the rates of lysine, methionine, and isoleucine, an imbalance in the supply of isoleucine might result. This risk is overcome in E. coli by the existence of three different aspartokinase enzymes, all of which catalyze the first step common to the production of all the products derived from aspartate. Each has a different regulatory effector molecule. Thus, one type of aspartokinase is inhibited by lysine, a second by threonine. The third kinase is not inhibited by any naturally occurring amino acid, but its rate of synthesis is controlled by the concentration of methionine within the cell. The triple control mechanism resulting from the three different aspartokinases ensures that the accumulation of one amino acid does not shut off the supply of aspartyl phosphate necessary for the synthesis of the others.

Another example of control through end-product inhibition also illustrates the manner in which the operation of two biosynthetic pathways may be coordinated. Both DNA and the various types of RNA are assembled from purine and pyrimidine nucleotides; these in turn are built up from intermediates of central metabolic pathways. The first step in the synthesis of pyrimidine nucleotides is that catalyzed by aspartate carbamoyltransferase. This step initiates a sequence of reactions that leads to the formation of pyrimidine nucleotides such as UTP and CTP. Studies of aspartate carbamoyltransferase have revealed that the affinity of this enzyme for its substrate (aspartate) is markedly decreased by the presence of CTP. This effect can be overcome by the addition of ATP, a purine nucleotide. The enzyme can be dissociated into two subunits: one contains the enzymatic activity and (in the dissociated form) does not bind CTP; the other binds CTP but has no catalytic activity. Apart from providing physical evidence that pacemaker enzymes contain distinct catalytic and regulatory sites, the interaction of aspartate carbamoyltransferase with the different nucleotides provides an explanation for the control of the supply of nucleic acid precursors. If a cell contains sufficient pyrimidine nucleotides (e.g., UTP), aspartate carbamoyltransferase, the first enzyme of pyrimidine biosynthesis, is inhibited. If, however, the cell contains high levels of purine nucleotides (e.g., ATP), as required for the formation of nucleic acids, the inhibition of aspartate carbamoyltransferase is relieved, and pyrimidines are formed.

Positive Modulation

Not all pacemaker enzymes are controlled by inhibition of their activity. Instead, some are subject to positive modulation—i.e., the effector is required for the efficient functioning of the enzyme. Such enzymes exhibit little activity in the absence of the appropriate allosteric effector. One instance of positive modulation is the anaplerotic fixation of carbon dioxide onto pyruvate and phosphoenolpyruvate (PEP); this example also illustrates how a metabolic product of one route controls the rate of nutrient flow of another.

The carboxylation of pyruvate in higher organisms and the carboxylation of phosphoenolpyruvate in gut bacteria ccurs at a significant rate only if acetyl coenzyme A is present. Acetyl coenzyme A acts as a positive allosteric effector and is not broken down in the course of the reaction. Moreover, some pyruvate carboxylases and the PEP carboxylase of gut bacteria are inhibited by four-carbon compounds (e.g., aspartate). These substances inhibit because they interfere with the binding of the positive effector, acetyl coenzyme A. Such enzymatic controls are reasonable in a physiological sense: it will be recalled that anaplerotic formation of oxaloacetate from pyruvate or PEP is required to provide the acceptor for the entry of acetyl coenzyme A into the TCA cycle. The reaction need occur only if acetyl coenzyme A is present in sufficient amounts. On the other hand, an abundance of four-carbon intermediates obviates the necessity for forming more through carboxylation reactions.

Similar reasoning, though in the opposite sense, can be applied to the control of another anaplerotic sequence, the glyoxylate cycle. The biosynthesis of cell materials from the two-carbon compound acetate is, in principle, akin to biosynthesis from TCA cycle intermediates. In both processes, it is the availability of intermediates such as PEP and pyruvate that determines the rate at which a cell forms the many components produced through gluconeogenesis. Although in the strictest sense the glyoxylate cycle has no defined end product, PEP and pyruvate are, for these physiological reasons, best fitted to regulate the rate at which the glyoxylate cycle is required to operate. It is thus not unexpected that the pacemaker enzyme of the glyoxylate cycle, isocitrate lyase, is allosterically inhibited by PEP and by pyruvate.

Energy State of the Cell

It is characteristic of catabolic routes that they do not lead to uniquely identifiable end products. The major products of glycolysis and the TCA cycle, for example, are carbon dioxide and water. Within the cell, the concentrations of both are unlikely to vary sufficiently to allow them to serve as effective regulatory metabolites. The processes by which water is produced initially involve, however, the reduction of coenzymes, the reoxidation of which is accompanied by the synthesis of ATP from ADP. The utilization of ATP in energy-consuming reactions yields ADP and AMP. At any given moment, therefore, a living cell contains ATP, ADP, and AMP; the relative proportion of the three nucleotides provides an index of the energy state of the cell. It is thus reasonable that the flux of nutrients through catabolic routes is, in general, impeded by high intracellular levels of both reduced coenzymes (e.g., $FADH_2$, reduced NAD^+) and ATP, and that these inhibitory effects are often overcome by AMP.

The control exerted by the levels of ATP, ADP, and AMP within the cell is illustrated by the regulatory mechanisms of glycolysis and the TCA cycle; these nucleotides also serve to govern the occurrence of the opposite pathway, gluconeogenesis, and to avoid mutual interference of the catabolic and anabolic sequences. Although not all of the controls mentioned below have been found to operate in all living organisms examined, it has been observed that, in general:

1. Glucose 6-phosphate stimulates glycogen synthesis from glucose 1-phosphate and inhibits both glycogen breakdown and its own formation from glucose.

2. Phosphofructokinase, the most important pacemaker enzyme of glycolysis, is inhibited by high levels of its own substrates (fructose 6-phosphate and ATP); this inhibition is overcome by AMP. In tissues, such as heart muscle, which use fatty acids as a major fuel, inhibition of glycolysis by citrate may be physiologically the more important means of control. Control by citrate, the first intermediate of the TCA cycle, which produces the bulk of the cellular ATP, is thus the same, in principle, as control through ATP.

3. Fructose 1,6-diphosphatase, which catalyzes the reaction opposite to phosphofructokinase, is strongly inhibited by AMP.

4. Rapid catabolism of carbohydrate requires the efficient conversion of PEP to pyruvate. In the liver and in some bacteria, the activity of the pyruvate kinase that catalyzes this process is greatly stimulated by the presence of fructose 1,6-diphosphate, which thus acts as a potentiator of a reaction required for its ultimate catabolism.

5. The oxidation of pyruvate to acetyl coenzyme A is inhibited by acetyl coenzyme A. Because acetyl coenzyme A also acts as a positive modulator of pyruvate carboxylation, this control reinforces the partition between pyruvate catabolism and its conversion to four-carbon intermediates for anaplerosis and gluconeogenesis.

6. Citrate synthase, the first enzyme of the TCA cycle, is inhibited by ATP in higher organisms and by reduced NAD^+ in many microorganisms. In some strictly aerobic bacteria, the inhibition by reduced NAD^+ is overcome by AMP.

7. Citrate acts as a positive effector for the first enzyme of fatty acid biosynthesis. A high level of citrate, which also indicates a sufficient energy supply, thus inhibits carbohydrate fragmentation and diverts the carbohydrate that has been fragmented from combustion to the formation of lipids.

8. Some forms of isocitrate dehydrogenase are maximally active only in the presence of ADP or AMP and are inhibited by ATP. This is an example of regulation by covalent modification of an enzyme since the action of ATP here is to phosphorylate, and consequently to inactivate, the isocitrate dehydrogenase. A specific phosphatase, which is a different enzymatic activity of the protein that effects the phosphorylation by ATP, catalyzes the splitting-off by water of the phosphate moiety on the inactive isocitrate dehydrogenase and thus restricts activity. Again, the energy state of the cell serves as the signal regulating an enzyme involved in energy transduction.

Coarse Control

Although fine control mechanisms allow the sensitive adjustment of the flux of nutrients along metabolic pathways relative to the needs of cells under relatively constant environmental conditions, these processes may not be adequate to cope with severe changes in the chemical milieu.

Such severe changes may arise in higher organisms with a change in diet or when, in response to other stimuli, the hormonal balance is altered. In starvation, for example, the overriding need to maintain blood glucose levels may require the liver to synthesize glucose from noncarbohydrate products of tissue breakdown at rates greater than can be achieved by the enzymes normally present in the liver. Under such circumstances, cellular concentrations of key enzymes of gluconeogenesis, such as pyruvate carboxylase and PEP carboxykinase, may rise by as much as 10-fold, while the concentration of glucokinase and of the enzymes of fatty acid synthesis decreases to a similar extent. Conversely, high carbohydrate diets and administration of the hormone insulin to diabetic animals elicit a preferential synthesis of glucokinase and pyruvate kinase. These changes in the relative proportions and absolute amounts of key enzymes are the net result of increases in the rate of their synthesis and decreases in the rate of their destruction. Although such changes reflect changes in the rates of either transcription, translation, or both of specific regions of the genome, the mechanisms by which the changes are effected have not yet been clarified.

Microorganisms sometimes encounter changes in environment much more severe than those encountered by the cells of tissues and organs, and their responses are correspondingly greater. Mention has already been made of the ability of E. coli to form β-galactosidase when transferred to a medium containing lactose as the sole carbon source; such a transfer may result in an increase of 1,000-fold or more in the cellular concentration of the enzyme. Because this preferential enzyme synthesis is elicited by exposure of the cells to lactose, or to non-metabolizable but chemically similar analogues, and because synthesis ceases as soon as the eliciting agents (inducers) are removed, β-galactosidase is termed an inducible enzyme. It has been established that a regulator gene exists that specifies the amino-acid sequence of a so-called repressor protein, and that the repressor protein binds to a unique portion of the region of DNA concerned with β-galactosidase formation. Under these circumstances the DNA is not transcribed to mRNA, and virtually no enzyme is made. The repressor, however, is an allosteric protein and readily combines with inducers. Such a combination prevents the repressor from binding to DNA and allows transcription and translation of β-galactosidase to proceed.

Although this mechanism for the specific control of gene activity may not apply to the regulation of all inducible enzymes—for example, those concerned with the utilization of the sugar arabinose—and is not universally applicable to all coarse control processes in all microorganisms, it can explain the manner in which the presence in growth media of at least some cell components represses (i.e., inhibits the synthesis of) enzymes normally involved in the formation of such components by gut bacteria such as E. coli. Although, for example, the bacteria must obviously make amino acids from ammonia if that is the sole source of nitrogen available to them, it would not be necessary for the bacteria to synthesize enzymes required for the formation of amino acids supplied preformed in the medium. Thus, of the three aspartokinases formed by E. coli, two are repressed by their end products, methionine and lysine. On the other hand, the third aspartokinase, which is inhibited by threonine, is repressed by threonine only if isoleucine is also present. This example of so-called multivalent repression is of obvious physiological utility. It is likely that the amino acids that thus specifically inhibit the synthesis of aspartokinases do so by combining with specific protein repressor molecules; however, whereas the combination of the inducer with the repressor of β-galactosidase inactivates the repressor protein and hence permits synthesis of the enzyme, the repressor proteins for biosynthetic enzymes would not bind to DNA unless they were also combined with the appropriate amino acid. Aspartokinase synthesis would thus occur in the absence of the end-product effectors and not in their presence.

This explanation applies also to the coarse control of the anaplerotic glyoxylate cycle. The synthesis of both of the enzymes unique to that cycle, isocitrate lyase and malate synthase, is controlled by a regulator gene that presumably specifies a repressor protein unable to bind to DNA unless combined with pyruvate or PEP. Cells growing on acetate do not contain high levels of these intermediates because they are continuously being removed for biosynthesis. The enzymes of the glyoxylate cycle are therefore formed at high rates. If pyruvate or substances catabolized to PEP or pyruvate are added to the medium, however, further synthesis of the two enzymes is speedily repressed.

Metabolic Rate

The metabolic rate of the body is the overall rate of tissue oxidation of fuels by all the body's organs. The dietary fuels are the carbohydrate, fat, protein, alcohol, and minor dietary components that are oxidized in the tissues, oxygen being taken up by the lungs and the combusted end products (carbon dioxide, water, and urea) being excreted by the lungs, urine, and skin. The total rate of body metabolism is assessed by monitoring the rate of oxygen uptake by the lungs. The sources of fuel can then be estimated from the proportion of carbon dioxide produced and the rate of urea production. The equations for calculating these are set out below. The rates of utilization of body stores of carbohydrate (c, expressed in terms of monosaccharide units) and fat (f), in g h^{-1}, were calculated from the VO$_2$ and VCO$_2$ (1 h^{-1}) and the rate of leucine oxidation (L, mmol h^{-1}) using formulae derived by Garlick (1987). C and F are the rates of dietary intake of carbohydrate and fat. In the fasted state, the rates were as follows:

$$c = (4.574 \times V_{co_2}) - (3.260 \times V_{o_2}) - 0.864L$$

$$f = (1.673 \times V_{o_2}) - (1.682 \times V_{co_2}) - 0.434L.$$

In the fed state, the rates were as follows:

$$c = (4.574 \times V_{co_2}) - (3.260 \times V_{o_2}) - 0.850L - 0.077F - C$$

$$f = (1.673 \times V_{o_2}) - (1.682 \times V_{co_2}) - 0.383L - 0.947F.$$

The energy equivalence of oxygen varies, depending on the precise nature of the fuels being oxidized, but a value of 20 kJ per liter of oxygen is taken as an appropriate average.

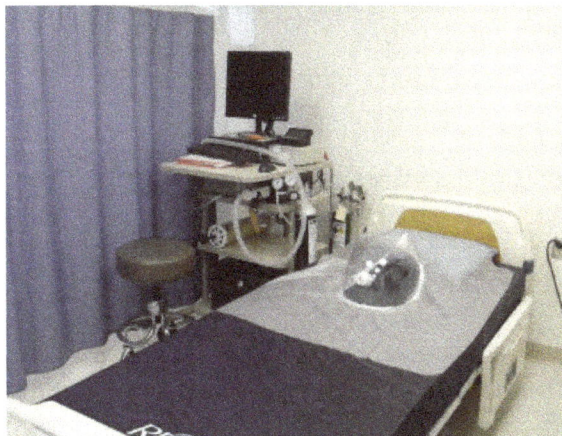

Metabolic rate has been measured using direct calorimeters and closed-circuit indirect calorimetry systems, but it is now generally measured with an open-flow indirect calorimetry system. Room air is drawn through a clear plastic hood covering the individual's face, and the flow and concentration of oxygen and carbon dioxide in the intake and expired air are accurately measured for calculation of RMR. This technique is known as indirect calorimetry because it does not directly measure heat but, rather, measures O$_2$ consumption and CO$_2$ production, which are then used to calculate energy expenditure. The pretesting environment impacts the measurement of RMR. Food, ethanol, caffeine, nicotine, and physical activity impact RMR and should be controlled before measurements are taken. A number of commercial indirect calorimetry systems are available, with some being more reliable than others. Smaller, portable indirect calorimeters are also available, allowing investigators more mobility for field measurement of metabolic rate.

Metabolic rate (estimated by O_2 consumption) is more closely related to body surface area than bodyweight so it has been suggested that small animals within a species may require a higher dose per kg than larger animals, when scaling is more closely linked to metabolic rate. This is particularly relevant to dogs where the body size within the species covers such a large range. Where there is a narrow therapeutic range for the drug, this factor can become very important. The dose of a drug with a narrow therapeutic ratio (e.g. digoxin, cytotoxic drugs) is usually calculated on body surface area rather than bodyweight. There can be a large difference in the calculated dose for dogs of extreme size (small or large) when weight or body surface areas are used. For drugs with a wide margin of safety such accurate dosing may not be clinically important. However, for drugs with a narrow margin of safety, failure to calculate the dose appropriately can result in toxicity or reduced therapeutic efficacy.

Another consideration when adjusting dosages for body size is the fat component of the bodyweight. Drug dosages are usually expressed per unit weight within a particular species. One should attempt to estimate the appropriate lean bodyweight and use this to calculate an appropriate dosage for nonlipid-soluble drugs even if using body surface area. Drugs which have a narrow margin of safety and are not lipid soluble include digoxin and the aminoglycoside antibiotics. For lipid-soluble drugs, increased body fat can act as a sink and reservoir, leading to protracted drug elimination if metabolism to a more water-soluble form is not involved.

Metabolic Fuel

Metabolic fuel is a well-known parameter which measures the body's fuel preference in energy production.

Our body primarily relies on three sources of fuel for energy: carbs, fats, and proteins. Proteins aren't a major source of energy as the body uses them primarily as building blocks. Fats and carbs, our body's main energy sources, are partnered up to fuel us in varying situations. However, in every given situation, the ratio of fat to carb usage shifts.

In order to live our bodies must regulate the fluxes of multiple fuel sources to support changing metabolic rates that result from variations in physiological circumstances. The aim of fuel selection strategies is to exploit the advantages of individual substrates while minimizing the impact of disadvantages from years of torpor to seconds of sprinting. The regulation of energy metabolism is a complex challenge because the fuels available vary greatly in stored quantity, energy density, speed of conversion to ATP and water solubility.

RQ (respiratory quotient) is the gold standard measurement for directly determining metabolic fuel usage. However, it is an invasive, challenging and unavailable technique for most. RER (respiratory exchange ratio) is currently the preferred method for determining metabolic fuel. RER estimates the relative contribution of carbohydrate and lipids to overall energy expenditure, via CO_2 production and O_2 uptake, in an indirect manner.

Metabolic States of the Body

You eat periodically throughout the day; however, your organs, especially the brain, need a continuous supply of glucose. How does the body meet this constant demand for energy? Your body processes the food you eat both to use immediately and, importantly, to store as energy for later demands. If there were no method in place to store excess energy, you would need to eat constantly in order to meet energy demands. Distinct mechanisms are in place to facilitate energy storage, and to make stored energy available during times of fasting and starvation.

Absorptive State

The absorptive state, or the fed state, occurs after a meal when your body is digesting the food and absorbing the nutrients (anabolism exceeds catabolism). Digestion begins the moment you put food into your mouth, as the food is broken down into its constituent parts to be absorbed through the intestine. The digestion of carbohydrates begins in the mouth, whereas the digestion of proteins and fats begins in the stomach and small intestine. The constituent parts of these carbohydrates, fats, and proteins are transported across the intestinal wall and enter the bloodstream (sugars and amino acids) or the lymphatic system (fats). From the intestines, these systems transport them to the liver, adipose tissue, or muscle cells that will process and use, or store, the energy.

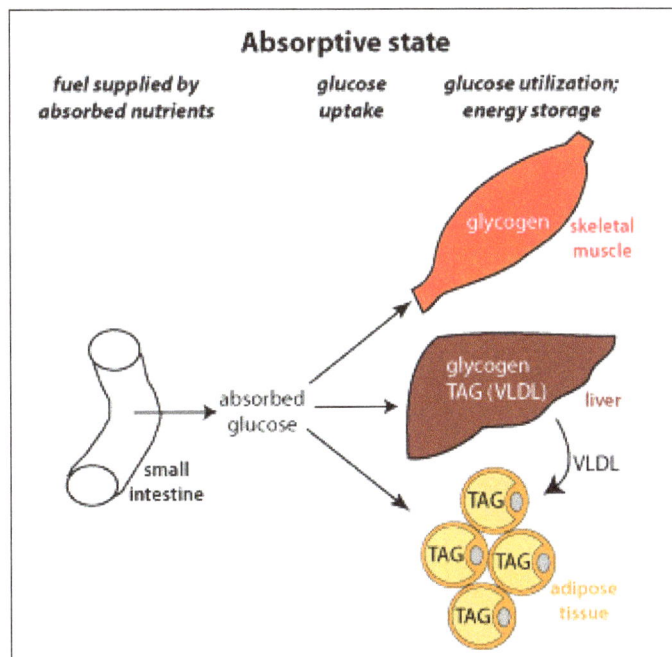

Absorptive State: During the absorptive state, the body digests food and absorbs the nutrients.

Depending on the amounts and types of nutrients ingested, the absorptive state can linger for up to 4 hours. The ingestion of food and the rise of glucose concentrations in the bloodstream stimulate pancreatic beta cells to release insulin into the bloodstream, where it initiates the absorption of blood glucose by liver hepatocytes, and by adipose and muscle cells. Once inside these cells, glucose is immediately converted into glucose-6-phosphate. By doing this, a concentration gradient is established where glucose levels are higher in the blood than in the cells. This allows for glucose to continue moving from the blood to the cells where it is needed. Insulin also stimulates the storage of glucose as glycogen in the liver and muscle cells where it can be used for later energy needs of the body. Insulin also promotes the synthesis of protein in muscle.

If energy is exerted shortly after eating, the dietary fats and sugars that were just ingested will be processed and used immediately for energy. If not, the excess glucose is stored as glycogen in the liver and muscle cells, or as fat in adipose tissue; excess dietary fat is also stored as triglycerides in adipose tissues. Figure below summarizes the metabolic processes occurring in the body during the absorptive state.

Postabsorptive State

The postabsorptive state, or the fasting state, occurs when the food has been digested, absorbed, and stored. You commonly fast overnight, but skipping meals during the day puts your body in the postabsorptive state as well. During this state, the body must rely initially on stored glycogen. Glucose levels in the blood begin to drop as it is absorbed and used by the cells. In response to the decrease in glucose, insulin levels also drop. Glycogen and triglyceride storage slows. However, due to the demands of the tissues and organs, blood glucose levels must be maintained in the normal range of 80–120 mg/dL. In response to a drop in blood glucose concentration, the hormone glucagon is released from the alpha cells of the pancreas. Glucagon acts upon the liver cells, where it inhibits the synthesis of glycogen and stimulates the breakdown of stored glycogen back into glucose. This glucose is released from the liver to be used by the peripheral tissues and the brain. As a result, blood glucose levels begin to rise. Gluconeogenesis will also begin in the liver to replace the glucose that has been used by the peripheral tissues.

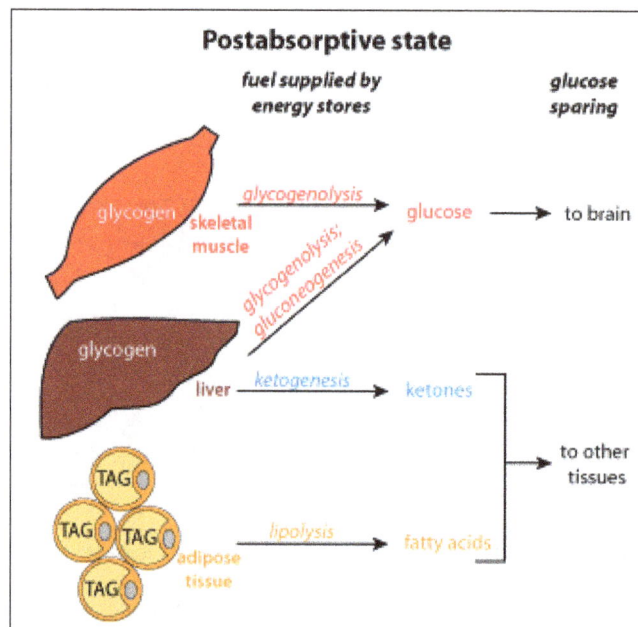

Postabsorptive State: During the postabsorptive state, the body must rely on stored glycogen for energy.

After ingestion of food, fats and proteins are processed as described previously; however, the glucose processing changes a bit. The peripheral tissues preferentially absorb glucose. The liver, which normally absorbs and processes glucose, will not do so after a prolonged fast. The gluconeogenesis that has been ongoing in the liver will continue after fasting to replace the glycogen stores that were depleted in the liver. After these stores have been replenished, excess glucose that is absorbed by the liver will be converted into triglycerides and fatty acids for long-term storage. Figure summarizes the metabolic processes occurring in the body during the postabsorptive state.

Starvation

When the body is deprived of nourishment for an extended period of time, it goes into "survival mode." The first priority for survival is to provide enough glucose or fuel for the brain. The second priority is the conservation of amino acids for proteins. Therefore, the body uses ketones to satisfy the energy needs of the brain and other glucose-dependent organs, and to maintain proteins in the cells. Because glucose levels are very low during starvation, glycolysis will shut off in cells that can use alternative fuels. For example, muscles will switch from using glucose to fatty acids as fuel. As previously explained, fatty acids can be converted into acetyl CoA and processed through the Krebs cycle to make ATP. Pyruvate, lactate, and alanine from muscle cells are not converted into acetyl CoA and used in the Krebs cycle, but are exported to the liver to be used in the synthesis of glucose. As starvation continues, and more glucose is needed, glycerol from fatty acids can be liberated and used as a source for gluconeogenesis.

After several days of starvation, ketone bodies become the major source of fuel for the heart and other organs. As starvation continues, fatty acids and triglyceride stores are used to create ketones for the body. This prevents the continued breakdown of proteins that serve as carbon sources for gluconeogenesis. Once these stores are fully depleted, proteins from muscles are released and broken down for glucose synthesis. Overall survival is dependent on the amount of fat and protein stored in the body.

Energy and Heat Balance

The body tightly regulates the body temperature through a process called thermoregulation, in which the body can maintain its temperature within certain boundaries, even when the surrounding temperature is very different. The core temperature of the body remains steady at around 36.5–37.5 °C (or 97.7–99.5 °F). In the process of ATP production by cells throughout the body, approximately 60 percent of the energy produced is in the form of heat used to maintain body temperature. Thermoregulation is an example of negative feedback.

The hypothalamus in the brain is the master switch that works as a thermostat to regulate the body's core temperature. If the temperature is too high, the hypothalamus can initiate several processes to lower it. These include increasing the circulation of the blood to the surface of the body to allow for the dissipation of heat through the skin and initiation of sweating to allow evaporation of water on the skin to cool its surface. Conversely, if the temperature falls below the set core temperature, the hypothalamus can initiate shivering to generate heat. The body uses more energy and generates more heat. In addition, thyroid hormone will stimulate more energy use and heat production by cells throughout the body. An environment is said to be thermoneutral when the body does not expend or release energy to maintain its core temperature. For a naked human, this is an ambient air temperature of around 84 °F. If the temperature is higher, for example, when wearing clothes, the body compensates with cooling mechanisms. The body loses heat through the mechanisms of heat exchange.

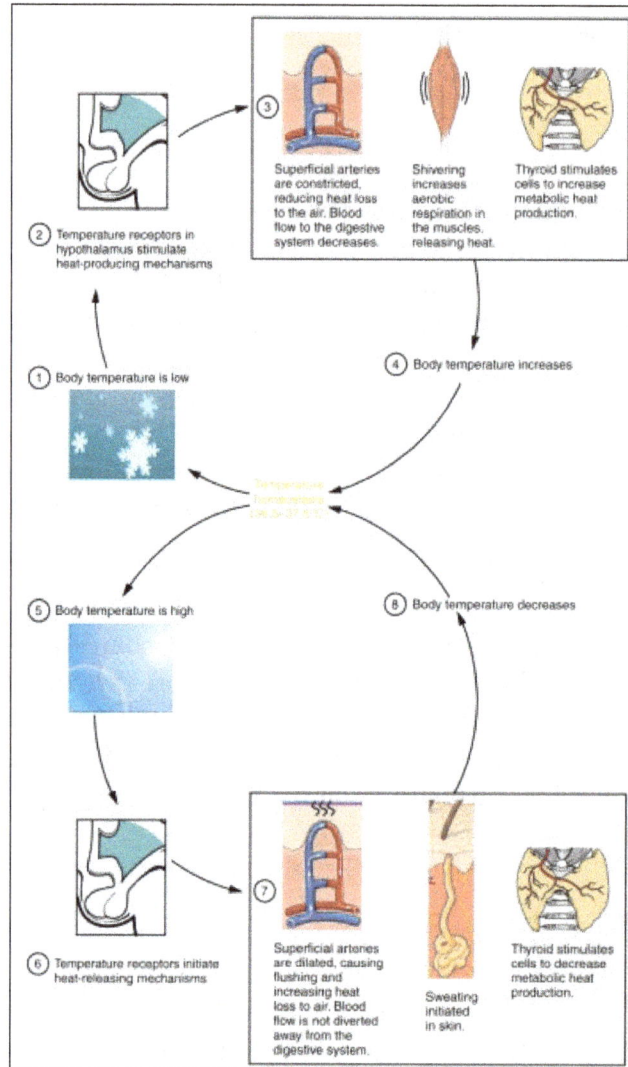

Hypothalamus Controls Thermoregulation: The hypothalamus controls thermoregulation.

Mechanisms of Heat Exchange

When the environment is not thermoneutral, the body uses four mechanisms of heat exchange to maintain homeostasis: conduction, convection, radiation, and evaporation. Each of these mechanisms relies on the property of heat to flow from a higher concentration to a lower concentration; therefore, each of the mechanisms of heat exchange varies in rate according to the temperature and conditions of the environment.

Conduction is the transfer of heat by two objects that are in direct contact with one another. It occurs when the skin comes in contact with a cold or warm object. For example, when holding a glass of ice water, the heat from your skin will warm the glass and in turn melt the ice. Alternatively, on a cold day, you might warm up by wrapping your cold hands around a hot mug of coffee. Only about 3 percent of the body's heat is lost through conduction.

Convection is the transfer of heat to the air surrounding the skin. The warmed air rises away from the body and is replaced by cooler air that is subsequently heated. Convection can also occur in water. When the water temperature is lower than the body's temperature, the body loses heat by warming the water closest to the skin, which moves away to be replaced by cooler water. The convection currents created by the temperature changes continue to draw heat away from the body more quickly than the body can replace it, resulting in hyperthermia. About 15 percent of the body's heat is lost through convection.

Radiation is the transfer of heat via infrared waves. This occurs between any two objects when their temperatures differ. A radiator can warm a room via radiant heat. On a sunny day, the radiation from the sun warms the skin. The same principle works from the body to the environment. About 60 percent of the heat lost by the body is lost through radiation.

Evaporation is the transfer of heat by the evaporation of water. Because it takes a great deal of energy for a water molecule to change from a liquid to a gas, evaporating water (in the form of sweat) takes with it a great deal of energy from the skin. However, the rate at which evaporation occurs depends on relative humidity—more sweat evaporates in lower humidity environments. Sweating is the primary means of cooling the body during exercise, whereas at rest, about 20 percent of the heat lost by the body occurs through evaporation.

References

- Biological-energy-transduction, science: britannica.com, Retrieved 14 February, 2019

- Metabolic-rate, medicine-and-dentistry: sciencedirect.com, Retrieved 17 April, 2019

- What-is-metabolic-fuel: lumen.me, Retrieved 7 June, 2019

- Metabolic-states-of-the-body, anatomyandphysiology: opentextbc.ca, Retrieved 12 January, 2019

- Energy-and-heat-balance, anatomyandphysiology: opentextbc.ca, Retrieved 20 March, 2019

Chapter 3
Nutrients: An Integrated Study

The different types of nutrients include minerals, carbohydrates, proteins, lipids and vitamins. Some of the major minerals are sodium, potassium, chloride, calcium, phosphorus, magnesium and sulfur. The topics elaborated in this chapter will help in gaining a better perspective about these different nutrients.

Carbohydrate

Carbohydrate is the class of naturally occurring compounds and derivatives formed from them. Carbohydrates are probably the most abundant and widespread organic substances in nature, and they are essential constituents of all living things. Carbohydrates are formed by green plants from carbon dioxide and water during the process of photosynthesis. Carbohydrates serve as energy sources and as essential structural components in organisms; in addition, part of the structure of nucleic acids, which contain genetic information, consists of carbohydrate.

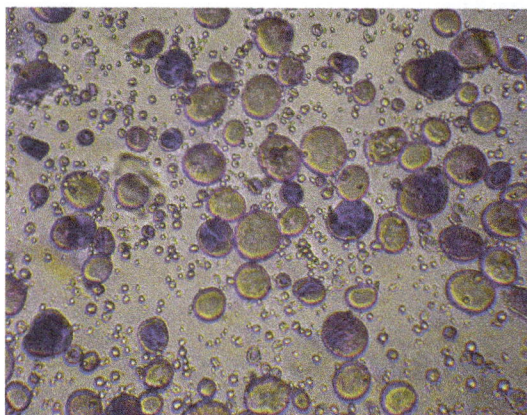

Wheat starch granules stained with iodine.

Classification and Nomenclature

Although a number of classification schemes have been devised for carbohydrates, the division into four major groups—monosaccharides, disaccharides, oligosaccharides, and polysaccharides—used here is among the most common. Most monosaccharides, or simple sugars, are found in grapes, other fruits, and honey. Although they can contain from three to nine carbon atoms, the most common representatives consist of five or six joined together to form a chainlike molecule. Three of the most important simple sugars—glucose (also known as dextrose, grape sugar, and corn sugar), fructose (fruit sugar), and galactose—have the same molecular formula, $(C_6H_{12}O_6)$, but, because their atoms have different structural arrangements, the sugars have different characteristics; i.e., they are isomers.

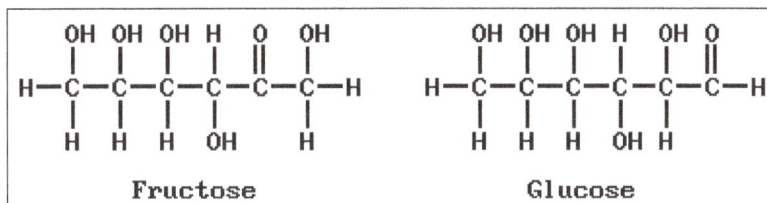

Slight changes in structural arrangements are detectable by living things and influence the biological significance of isomeric compounds. It is known, for example, that the degree of sweetness of various sugars differs according to the arrangement of the hydroxyl groups (−OH) that compose part of the molecular structure. A direct correlation that may exist between taste and any specific structural arrangement, however, has not yet been established; that is, it is not yet possible to predict the taste of a sugar by knowing its specific structural arrangement. The energy in the chemical bonds of glucose indirectly supplies most living things with a major part of the energy that is necessary for them to carry on their activities. Galactose, which is rarely found as a simple sugar, is usually combined with other simple sugars in order to form larger molecules.

Two molecules of a simple sugar that are linked to each other form a disaccharide, or double sugar. The disaccharide sucrose, or table sugar, consists of one molecule of glucose and one molecule of fructose; the most familiar sources of sucrose are sugar beets and cane sugar. Milk sugar, or lactose, and maltose are also disaccharides. Before the energy in disaccharides can be utilized by living things, the molecules must be broken down into their respective monosaccharides. Oligosaccharides, which consist of three to six monosaccharide units, are rather infrequently found in natural sources, although a few plant derivatives have been identified.

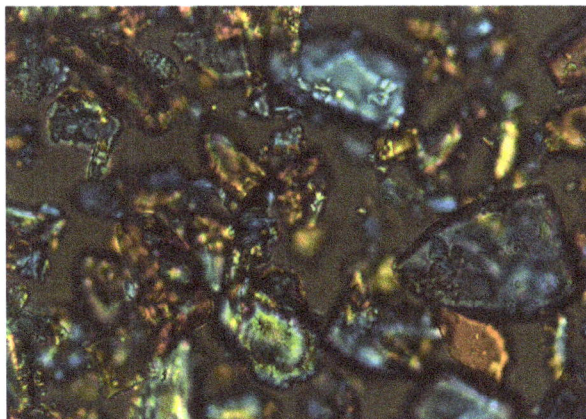

Lactose crystals are shown suspended in oil: Their distinct shape allows them to be identified in foods examined for research.

Polysaccharides (the term means many sugars) represent most of the structural and energy-reserve carbohydrates found in nature. Large molecules that may consist of as many as 10,000 monosaccharide units linked together, polysaccharides vary considerably in size, in structural complexity, and in sugar content; several hundred distinct types have thus far been identified. Cellulose, the principal structural component of plants, is a complex polysaccharide comprising many glucose units linked together; it is the most common polysaccharide. The starch found in plants and the glycogen found in animals also are complex glucose polysaccharides.

Starch is found mostly in seeds, roots, and stems, where it is stored as an available energy source for plants. Plant starch may be processed into foods such as bread, or it may be consumed directly—as in potatoes, for instance. Glycogen, which consists of branching chains of glucose molecules, is formed in the liver and muscles of higher animals and is stored as an energy source.

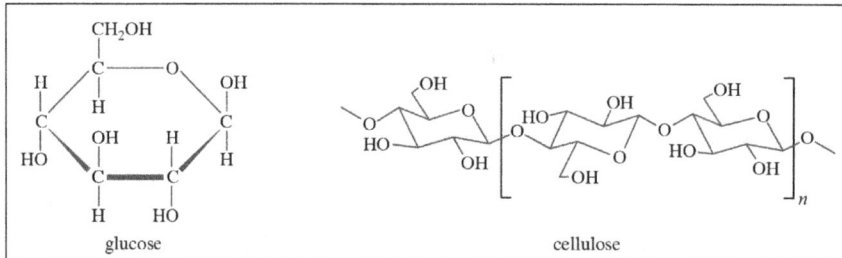

Composition of cellulose and glucose: Cellulose and glucose are examples of carbohydrates.

The generic nomenclature ending for the monosaccharides is -ose; thus, the term pentose (pent = five) is used for monosaccharides containing five carbon atoms, and hexose (hex = six) is used for those containing six. In addition, because the monosaccharides contain a chemically reactive group that is either an aldehyde group or a keto group, they are frequently referred to as aldopentoses or ketopentoses or aldohexoses or ketohexoses. The aldehyde group can occur at position 1 of an aldopentose, and the keto group can occur at a further position (e.g., 2) within a ketohexose. Glucose is an aldohexose—i.e., it contains six carbon atoms, and the chemically reactive group is an aldehyde group.

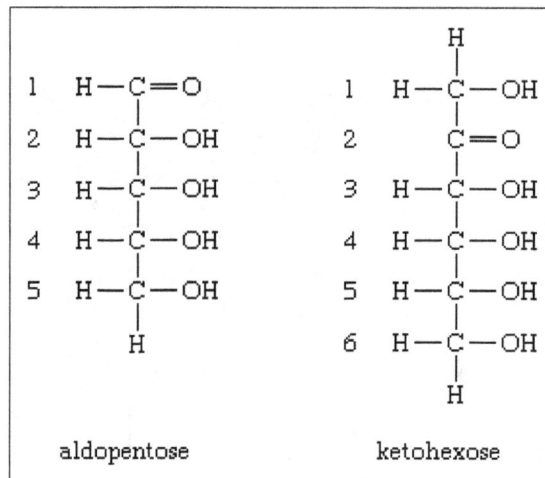

The total caloric, or energy, requirement for an individual depends on age, occupation, and other factors but generally ranges between 2,000 and 4,000 calories per 24-hour period (one calorie, as this term is used in nutrition, is the amount of heat necessary to raise the temperature of 1,000 grams of water from 15 to 16 °C [59 to 61 °F]; in other contexts this amount of heat is called the kilocalorie). Carbohydrate that can be used by humans produces four calories per gram as opposed to nine calories per gram of fat and four per gram of protein. In areas of the world where nutrition is marginal, a high proportion (approximately one to two pounds) of an individual's

Role in Human Nutrition

daily energy requirement may be supplied by carbohydrate, with most of the remainder coming from a variety of fat sources.

Although carbohydrates may compose as much as 80 percent of the total caloric intake in the human diet, for a given diet, the proportion of starch to total carbohydrate is quite variable, depending upon the prevailing customs. In East Asia and in areas of Africa, for example, where rice or tubers such as manioc provide a major food source, starch may account for as much as 80 percent of the total carbohydrate intake. In a typical Western diet, 33 to 50 percent of the caloric intake is in the form of carbohydrate. Approximately half (i.e., 17 to 25 percent) is represented by starch; another third by table sugar (sucrose) and milk sugar (lactose); and smaller percentages by monosaccharides such as glucose and fructose, which are common in fruits, honey, syrups, and certain vegetables such as artichokes, onions, and sugar beets. The small remainder consists of bulk, or indigestible carbohydrate, which comprises primarily the cellulosic outer covering of seeds and the stalks and leaves of vegetables.

Classes of Carbohydrates

Monosaccharides

The most common naturally occurring monosaccharides are D-glucose, D-mannose, D-fructose, and D-galactose among the hexoses and D-xylose and L-arabinose among the pentoses. In a special sense, D-ribose and 2-deoxy-D-ribose are ubiquitous because they form the carbohydrate component of ribonucleic acid (RNA) and deoxyribonucleic acid (DNA), respectively; these sugars are present in all cells as components of nucleic acids.

Some naturally occurring monosaccharides	
sugar	sources
L-arabinose	Mesquite gum, wheat bran
D-ribose	All living cells; as component of ribonucleic acid
D-xylose	Corncobs, seed hulls, straw
D-ribulose	As an intermediate in photosynthesis
2-deoxy-D-ribose	As constituent of deoxyribonucleic acid
D-galactose	Lactose, agar, gum arabic, brain glycolipids
D-glucose	Sucrose, cellulose, starch, glycogen
D-mannose	Seeds, ivory nut
D-fructose	Sucrose, artichokes, honey
L-fucose	Marine algae, seaweed
L-rhamnose	Poison-ivy blossom, oak bark
D-mannoheptulose	Avocado
D-altroheptulose	Numerous plants

D-Xylose, found in most plants in the form of a polysaccharide called xylan, is prepared from corncobs, cottonseed hulls, or straw by chemical breakdown of xylan. D-Galactose, a common constituent of both oligosaccharides and polysaccharides, also occurs in carbohydrate-containing lipids, called glycolipids, which are found in the brain and other nervous tissues of most animals. Galactose is generally prepared by acid hydrolysis (breakdown involving water) of lactose, which is composed of galactose and glucose. Since the biosynthesis of galactose in animals occurs through intermediate compounds derived directly from glucose, animals do not require galactose in the diet. In fact, in most human populations the majority of people do not retain the ability to manufacture the enzyme necessary to metabolize galactose after they reach the age of four, and many individuals possess a hereditary defect known as galactosemia and never have the ability to metabolize galactose.

D-Glucose is, the naturally occurring form, is found in fruits, honey, blood, and, under abnormal conditions, in urine. It is also a constituent of the two most common naturally found disaccharides, sucrose and lactose, as well as the exclusive structural unit of the polysaccharides cellulose, starch, and glycogen. Generally, D-glucose is prepared from either potato starch or cornstarch.

D-Fructose, a ketohexose, is one of the constituents of the disaccharide sucrose and is also found in uncombined form in honey, apples, and tomatoes. Fructose, generally considered the sweetest monosaccharide, is prepared by sucrose hydrolysis and is metabolized by humans.

Chemical Reactions

The reactions of the monosaccharides can be conveniently subdivided into those associated with the aldehyde or keto group and those associated with the hydroxyl groups.

The relative ease with which sugars containing a free or potentially free aldehyde or keto group can be oxidized to form products has been known for a considerable time and once was the basis for the detection of these so-called reducing sugars in a variety of sources. For many years, analyses of blood glucose and urinary glucose were carried out by a procedure involving the use of an alkaline copper compound. Because the reaction has undesirable features—extensive destruction of carbohydrate structure occurs, and the reaction is not very specific (i.e., sugars other than glucose give similar results) and does not result in the formation of readily identifiable products—blood and urinary glucose now are analyzed by using the enzyme glucose oxidase, which catalyzes the oxidation of glucose to products that include hydrogen peroxide. The hydrogen peroxide then is used to oxidize a dye present in the reaction mixture; the intensity of the colour is directly proportional to the amount of glucose initially present. The enzyme, glucose oxidase, is highly specific for β-D-glucose.

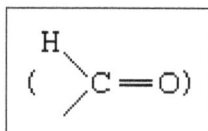

$$\left(\overset{H}{\diagdown}_{\diagup} C = O \right)$$

In another reaction, the aldehyde group of glucose reacts with alkaline iodine to form a class of compounds called aldonic acids. One important aldonic acid is ascorbic acid (vitamin C), an essential dietary component for humans and guinea pigs. The formation of similar acid derivatives does not occur with the keto sugars.

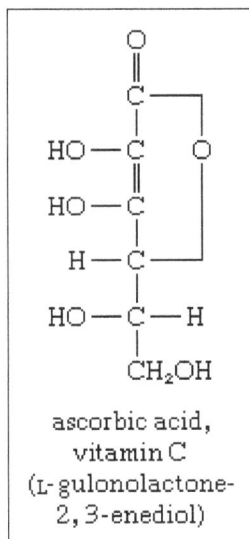

ascorbic acid,
vitamin C
(L-gulonolactone-
2,3-enediol)

Either the aldehyde or the keto group of a sugar may be reduced (i.e., hydrogen added) to form an alcohol; compounds formed in this way are called alditols, or sugar alcohols. The product formed as a result of the reduction of the aldehyde carbon of D-glucose is called sorbitol (D-glucitol). D-Glucitol also is formed when L-sorbose is reduced. The reduction of mannose results in mannitol, that of galactose in dulcitol.

Sugar alcohols that are of commercial importance include sorbitol (D-glucitol), which is commonly used as a sweetening agent, and D-mannitol, which is also used as a sweetener, particularly in chewing gums, because it has a limited water solubility and remains powdery and granular on long storage.

Formation of Glycosides

The hydroxyl group that is attached to the anomeric carbon atom (i.e., the carbon containing the aldehyde or keto group) of carbohydrates in solution has unusual reactivity, and derivatives, called glycosides, can be formed; glycosides formed from glucose are called glucosides. It is not possible for equilibration between the α- and β-anomers of a glycoside in solution (i.e., mutarotation) to occur. The reaction by which a glycoside is formed involves the hydroxyl group (−OH) of the anomeric carbon atom (numbered 1) of both α and β forms of D-glucose—α and β forms of D-glucose are shown in equilibrium in the reaction sequence—and the hydroxyl group of an alcohol (methyl alcohol in the reaction sequence); methyl α-D-glucosides and β-D-glucosides are formed as products, as is water.

Among the wide variety of naturally occurring glycosides are a number of plant pigments, particularly those red, violet, and blue in colour; these pigments are found in flowers and consist of a pigment molecule attached to a sugar molecule, frequently glucose. Plant indican (from Indigofera species), composed of glucose and the pigment indoxyl, was important in the preparation of indigo dye before synthetic dyes became prevalent. Of a number of heart muscle stimulants that occur as glycosides, digitalis is still used. Other naturally occurring glycosides include vanillin, which is found in the vanilla bean, and amygdalin (oil of bitter almonds); a variety of glycosides found in mustard have a sulfur atom at position 1 rather than oxygen.

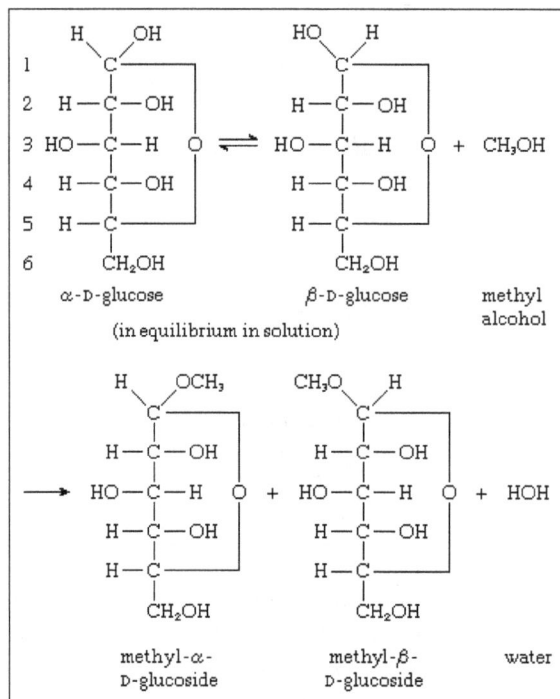

α-D-glucose and β-D-glucose (in equilibrium in solution) + methyl alcohol $\rightleftharpoons$ methyl-α-D-glucoside and methyl-β-D-glucoside + water

A number of important antibiotics are glycosides; among the best known are streptomycin and erythromycin. Glucosides—i.e., glycosides formed from glucose—in which the anomeric carbon atom (at position 1) has phosphoric acid linked to it, are extremely important biological compounds. For example, α-D-glucose-1-phosphate is an intermediate product in the biosynthesis of cellulose, starch, and glycogen; similar glycosidic phosphate derivatives of other monosaccharides participate in the formation of naturally occurring glycosides and polysaccharides.

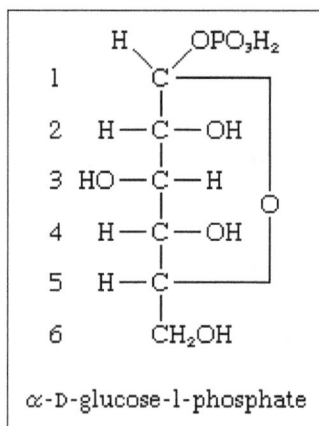

α-D-glucose-1-phosphate

The hydroxyl groups other than the one at the anomeric carbon atom can undergo a variety of reactions. Esterification, which consists of reacting the hydroxyl groups with an appropriate acidic compound, results in the formation of a class of compounds called sugar esters. Among the common ones are the sugar acetates, in which the acid is acetic acid. Esters of phosphoric acid and sulfuric acid are important biological compounds; glucose-6-phosphate, for example, plays a central role in the energy metabolism of most living cells, and D-ribulose 1,5-diphosphate is important in photosynthesis.

Formation of Methyl Ethers

Treatment of a carbohydrate with methyl iodide or similar agents under appropriate conditions results in the formation of compounds in which the hydroxyl groups are converted to methyl groups ($-CH_3$). Called methyl ethers, these compounds are employed in structural studies of oligosaccharides and polysaccharides because their formation does not break the bonds, called glycosidic bonds, that link adjacent monosaccharide units. An example is the etherification of a starch molecule carried out using methyl iodide, in which methyl groups become attached to the glucose molecules, forming a methylated segment in the starch molecule; note that the glycosidic bonds are not broken by the reaction with methyl iodide. When the methylated starch molecule then is broken down (hydrolyzed), hydroxyl groups are located at the positions in the molecule previously involved in linking one sugar molecule to another, and a methylated glucose, in this case named 2,3,6 tri-O-methyl-D-glucose, forms. The linkage positions (which are not methylated) in a complex carbohydrate can be established by analyzing the locations of the methyl groups in the monosaccharides. This technique is useful in determining the structural details of polysaccharides, particularly since the various methylated sugars are easily separated by techniques involving gas chromatography, in which a moving gas stream carries a mixture through a column of a stationary liquid or solid, the components thus being resolved.

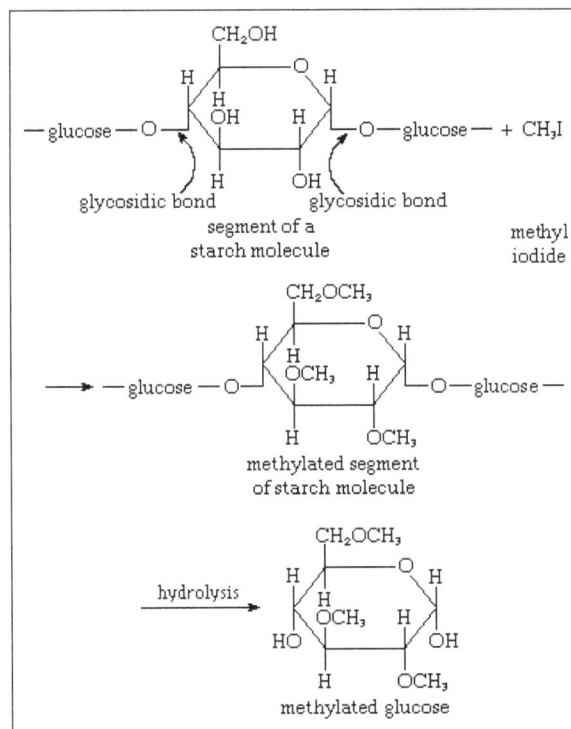

When the terminal group (CH_2OH) of a monosaccharide is oxidized chemically or biologically, a product called a uronic acid is formed. Glycosides that are derived from D-glucuronic acid (the uronic acid formed from D-glucose) and fatty substances called steroids appear in the urine of animals as normal metabolic products; in addition, foreign toxic substances are frequently converted in the liver to glucuronides before excretion in the urine. D-Glucuronic acid also is a major component of connective tissue polysaccharides, and D-galacturonic acid and D-mannuronic acid, formed from D-galactose and D-mannose, respectively, are found in several plant sources.

Other compounds formed from monosaccharides include those in which one hydroxyl group, usually at the carbon at position 2, is replaced by an amino group ($-NH_2$); these compounds, called amino sugars, are widely distributed in nature. The two most important ones are glucosamine (2-amino-2-deoxy-D-glucose) and galactosamine (2-amino-2-deoxy-D-galactose).

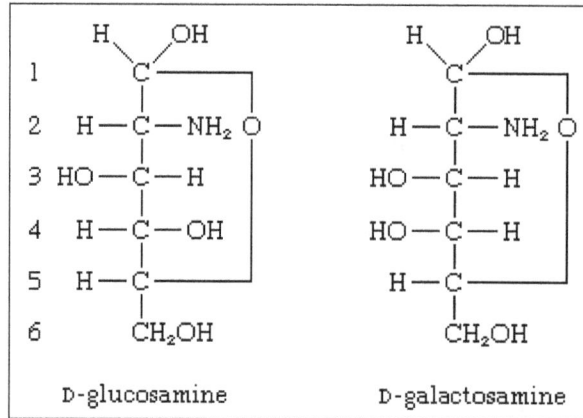

D-glucosamine   D-galactosamine

Neither amino sugar is found in the uncombined form. Both occur in animals as components of glycolipids or polysaccharides; e.g., the primary structural polysaccharide (chitin) of insect outer skeletons and various blood group substances.

In a number of naturally occurring sugars, known as deoxy sugars, the hydroxyl group at a particular position is replaced by a hydrogen atom. By far the most important representative is 2-deoxy-D-ribose, the pentose sugar found in deoxyribonucleic acid (DNA); the hydroxyl group at the carbon atom at position 2 has been replaced by a hydrogen atom.

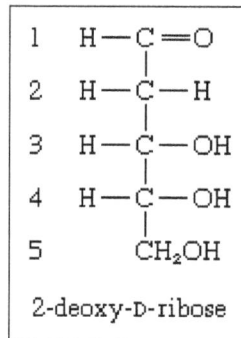

2-deoxy-D-ribose

Other naturally occurring deoxy sugars are hexoses, of which L-rhamnose (6-deoxy-L-mannose) and L-fucose (6-deoxy-L-galactose) are the most common; the latter, for example, is present in the carbohydrate portion of blood group substances and on the outer surface of red blood cells.

Disaccharides and Oligosaccharides

Disaccharides are a specialized type of glycoside in which the anomeric hydroxyl group of one sugar has combined with the hydroxyl group of a second sugar with the elimination of the elements of water. Although an enormous number of disaccharide structures are possible, only a limited number are of commercial or biological significance.

Sucrose and Trehalose

Sucrose, or common table sugar, is a major commodity worldwide. By the second decade of the 21st century, its world production had amounted to more than 170 million tons annually. The unusual type of linkage between the two anomeric hydroxyl groups of glucose and fructose means that neither a free aldehyde group (on the glucose moiety) nor a free keto group (on the fructose moiety) is available to react unless the linkage between the monosaccharides is destroyed; for this reason, sucrose is known as a nonreducing sugar. Sucrose solutions do not exhibit mutarotation, which involves formation of an asymmetrical centre at the aldehyde or keto group. If the linkage between the monosaccharides composing sucrose is broken, the optical rotation value of sucrose changes from positive to negative; the new value reflects the composite rotation values for D-glucose, which is dextrorotatory (+52°), and D-fructose, which is levorotatory (−92°). The change in the sign of optical rotation from positive to negative is the reason sucrose is sometimes called invert sugar.

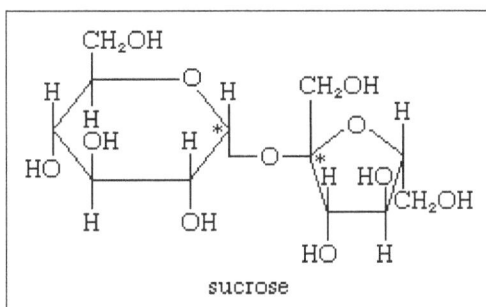

sucrose

The commercial preparation of sucrose takes advantage of the alkaline stability of the sugar, and a variety of impurities are removed from crude sugarcane extracts by treatment with alkali. After this step, syrup preparations are crystallized to form table sugar. Successive "crops" of sucrose crystals are "harvested," and the later ones are known as brown sugar. The residual syrupy material is called either cane final molasses or blackstrap molasses; both are used in the preparation of antibiotics, as sweetening agents, and in the production of alcohol by yeast fermentation. Sucrose is formed following photosynthesis in plants by a reaction in which sucrose phosphate first is formed.

The disaccharide trehalose is similar in many respects to sucrose but is much less widely distributed. It is composed of two molecules of α-D-glucose and is also a nonreducing sugar. Trehalose is present in young mushrooms and in the resurrection plant (Selaginella); it is of considerable biological interest because it is also found in the circulating fluid (hemolymph) of many insects. Since trehalose can be converted to a glucose phosphate compound by an enzyme-catalyzed reaction that does not require energy, its function in hemolymph may be to provide an immediate energy source, a role similar to that of the carbohydrate storage forms (i.e., glycogen) found in higher animals.

Lactose and Maltose

Lactose is one of the sugars (sucrose is another) found most commonly in human diets throughout the world; it constitutes about 7 percent of human milk and about 4–5 percent of the milk of mammals such as cows, goats, and sheep. Lactose consists of two aldohexoses—β-D-galactose and glucose—linked so that the aldehyde group at the anomeric carbon of glucose is free to react; i.e., lactose is a reducing sugar.

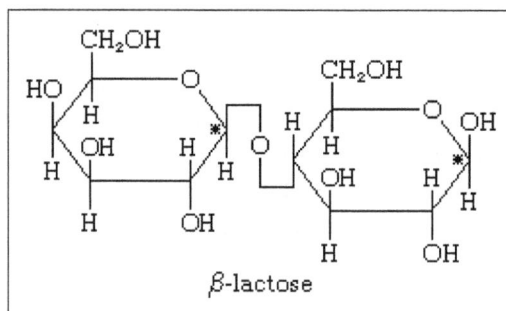

β-lactose

A variety of metabolic disorders related to lactose may occur in infants; in some cases, they are the result of a failure to metabolize properly the galactose portion of the molecule.

Although not found in uncombined form in nature, the disaccharide maltose is biologically important because it is a product of the enzymatic breakdown of starches during digestion. Maltose consists of α-D-glucose linked to a second glucose unit in such a way that maltose is a reducing sugar. Maltose, which is readily hydrolyzed to glucose and can be metabolized by animals, is employed as a sweetening agent and as a food for infants whose tolerance for lactose is limited.

Polysaccharides

Polysaccharides, or glycans, may be classified in a number of ways; the following scheme is frequently used. Homopolysaccharides are defined as polysaccharides formed from only one type of monosaccharide. Homopolysaccharides may be further subdivided into straight-chain and branched-chain representatives, depending upon the arrangement of the monosaccharide units. Heteropolysaccharides are defined as polysaccharides containing two or more different types of monosaccharides; they may also occur in both straight-chain and branched-chain forms. In general, extensive variation of linkage types does not occur within a polysaccharide structure, nor are there many polysaccharides composed of more than three or four different monosaccharides; most contain one or two.

Representative homopolysaccharides				
Homopolysaccharide	Sugar component	Linkage	Function	Sources
Cellulose	Glucose	$\beta, 1 \rightarrow 4$	Structural	Throughout plant kingdom
Amylose	Glucose	$\alpha, 1 \rightarrow 4$	Food storage	Starches, especially corn, potatoes, rice
Chitin	N-acetylglucosamine	$\beta, 1 \rightarrow 4$	Structural	Insect and crustacean skeleton
Inulin	Fructose	$\beta, 2 \rightarrow 1$	Food storage	Artichokes, chicory
Xylan	Xylose	$\beta, 1 \rightarrow 4$	Structural	All land plants
Glycogen	Glucose	$\alpha, 1 \rightarrow 4,$ $6 \leftarrow 1, \alpha$	Food storage	Liver and muscle cells of all animals
Amylopectin	Glucose	$\alpha, 1 \rightarrow 4,$ $6 \leftarrow 1, \alpha$	Food storage	Starches, especially corn, potatoes, rice
Dextran	Glucose	$\alpha, 1 \rightarrow 6,$ $4 \leftarrow 1, \alpha$	Unknown	Primarily bacterial
Agar	Galactose	$\alpha, 1 \rightarrow 3$	Structural	Seaweeds

Homopolysaccharides

In general, homopolysaccharides have a well-defined chemical structure, although the molecular weight of an individual amylose or xylan molecule may vary within a particular range, depending on the source; molecules from a single source also may vary in size, because most polysaccharides are formed biologically by an enzyme-catalyzed process lacking genetic information regarding size.

The basic structural component of most plants, cellulose, is widely distributed in nature. It has been estimated that 50 billion to 100 billion tons of cellulose are synthesized yearly as a result of photosynthesis by higher plants. The proportion of cellulose to total carbohydrate found in plants may vary in various types of woods from 30 to 40 percent, and to more than 98 percent in the seed hair of the cotton plant. Cellulose, a large, linear molecule composed of 3,000 or more β-D-glucose molecules, is insoluble in water.

The chains of glucose units composing cellulose molecules are frequently aligned within the cell-wall structure of a plant to form fibre-like or crystalline arrangements. This alignment permits very tight packing of the chains and promotes their structural stability but also makes structural analysis difficult. The relationships between cellulose and other polysaccharides present in the cell wall are not well established; in addition, the presence of unusual chemical linkages or nonglucose units within the cellulose structure has not yet been established with certainty.

During the preparation of cellulose, raw plant material is treated with hot alkali; this treatment removes most of the lignin, the hemicelluloses, and the mucilaginous components. The cellulose then is processed to produce papers and fibres. The high resistance of cellulose to chemical or enzymatic breakdown is important in the manufacture of paper and cloth. Cellulose also is modified chemically for other purposes; e.g., compounds such as cellulose acetate are used in the plastics industry, in the production of photographic film, and in the rayon-fibre industry. Cellulose nitrate (nitrocellulose) is employed in the lacquer and explosives industries.

The noteworthy biological stability of cellulose is dramatically illustrated by trees, the life-span of which may be several thousand years. Enzymes capable of breaking down cellulose are generally found only among several species of bacteria and molds. The apparent ability of termites to utilize cellulose as an energy source depends on the presence in their intestinal tracts of protozoans that can break it down. Similarly, the single-celled organisms present in the rumina of sheep and cattle are responsible for the ability of these animals to utilize the cellulose present in typical grasses and other feeds.

Xylans are almost as ubiquitous as cellulose in plant cell walls and contain predominantly β-D-xylose units linked as in cellulose. Some xylans contain other sugars, such as L-arabinose, but they form branches and are not part of the main chain. Xylans are of little commercial importance.

The term starch refers to a group of plant reserve polysaccharides consisting almost exclusively of a linear component (amylose) and a branched component (amylopectin). The use of starch as an energy source by humans depends on the ability to convert it completely to individual glucose units; the process is initiated by the action of enzymes called amylases, synthesized by the salivary glands in the mouth, and continues in the intestinal tract. The primary product of amylase action is maltose, which is hydrolyzed to two component glucose units as it is absorbed through the walls of the intestine.

A characteristic reaction of the amylose component of starch is the formation with iodine of a complex compound with a characteristic blue colour. About one iodine molecule is bound for each seven or eight glucose units, and at least five times that many glucose units are needed in an amylose chain to permit the effective development of the colour.

The amylopectin component of starch is structurally similar to glycogen in that both are composed of glucose units linked together in the same way, but the distance between branch points is greater in amylopectin than in glycogen, and the former may be thought of as occupying more space per unit weight.

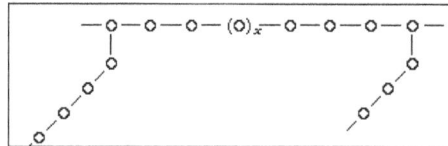
Schematic amylopectin structure.

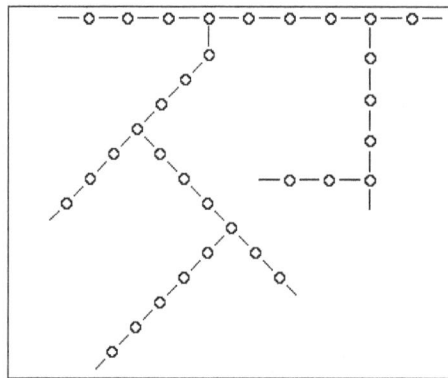
Schematic Glycogen structure

The applications of starches other than as foods are limited. Starches are employed in adhesive manufacture, and starch nitrate has some utility as an explosive.

Glycogen, which is found in all animal tissues, is the primary animal storage form of carbohydrate and, indirectly, of rapidly available energy. The distance between branch points in a glycogen molecule is only five or six units, which results in a compact treelike structure. The ability of higher animals to form and break down this extensively branched structure is essential to their well-being; in conditions known as glycogen storage diseases, these activities are abnormal, and the asymmetrical glycogen molecules that are formed have severe, often fatal, consequences. Glycogen synthesis and breakdown are controlled by substances called hormones.

Large molecules—e.g., pectins and agars—composed of galactose or its uronic-acid derivative (galacturonic acid) are important because they can form gels. Pectins, which are predominantly galacturonans, are produced from citrus fruit rinds; they are used commercially in the preparation of jellies and jams. Agar is widely employed in biological laboratories as a solidifying agent for growth media for microorganisms and in the bakery industry as a gelling agent; it forms a part of the diet of people in several areas of East Asia.

Dextrans, a group of polysaccharides composed of glucose, are secreted by certain strains of bacteria as slimes. The structure of an individual dextran varies with the strain of microorganism.

Dextrans can be used as plasma expanders (substitutes for whole blood) in cases of severe shock. In addition, a dextran derivative compound is employed medically as an anticoagulant for blood.

Chitin is structurally similar to cellulose, but the repeating sugar is 2-deoxy-2-acetamido-D-glucose (N-acetyl-D-glucosamine) rather than glucose.

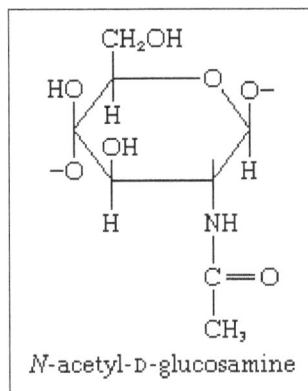

N-acetyl-D-glucosamine

Sometimes referred to as animal cellulose, chitin is the major component of the outer skeletons of insects, crustaceans, and other arthropods, as well as annelid and nematode worms, mollusks, and coelenterates. The cell walls of most fungi also are predominantly chitin, which comprises nearly 50 percent of the dry weight of some species. Since chitin is nearly as chemically inactive as cellulose and easily obtained, numerous attempts, none of which has thus far been successful, have been made to develop it commercially. The nitrogen content of the biosphere, however, is stabilized by the ability of soil microorganisms to degrade nitrogen-containing compounds such as those found in insect skeletons; these microorganisms convert the nitrogen in complex molecules to a form usable by plants. If such microorganisms did not exist, much of the organic nitrogen present in natural materials would be unavailable to plants.

Heteropolysaccharides

In general, heteropolysaccharides (heteroglycans) contain two or more different monosaccharide units. Although a few representatives contain three or more different monosaccharides, most naturally occurring heteroglycans contain only two different ones and are closely associated with lipid or protein. The complex nature of these substances has made detailed structural studies extremely difficult. The major heteropolysaccharides include the connective-tissue polysaccharides, the blood group substances, glycoproteins (combinations of carbohydrates and proteins) such as gamma globulin, and glycolipids (combinations of carbohydrates and lipids), particularly those found in the central nervous system of animals and in a wide variety of plant gums.

Representative heteropolysaccharides			
Heteropolysaccharide	Component sugars	Functions	Distribution
Hyaluronic acid	D-glucuronic acid and n-acetyl-d-glucosamine	Lubricant, shock absorber, water binding	Connective tissue, skin
Chondroitin-4-sulfate*	D-glucuronic acid and n-acetyl-d-galactosamine-4-o-sulfate	Calcium accumulation, cartilage and bone formation	Cartilage
Heparin*	D-glucuronic acid, l-iduronic acid, n-sulfo-d-glucosamine	Anticoagulant	Mast cells, blood

Gamma globulin*	N-acetyl-hexosamine, d-mannose, d-galactose	Antibody	Blood
Blood group substance*	D-glucosamine, d-galactosamine, l-fucose, d-galactose	Blood group specificity	Cell surfaces, especially red blood cells
*Covalently linked to protein; the proportion of protein to carbohydrate in such complex molecules varies from about 10% protein in the case of chondroitin-4-sulfate to better than 95% for gamma globulin			

The most important heteropolysaccharides are found in the connective tissues of all animals and include a group of large molecules that vary in size, shape, and interaction with other body substances. They have a structural role, and the structures of individual connective-tissue polysaccharides are related to specific animal functions; hyaluronic acid, for example, the major component of joint fluid in animals, functions as a lubricating agent and shock absorber.

The connective-tissue heteropolysaccharides contain acidic groups (uronic acids or sulfate groups) and can bind both water and inorganic metal ions. They can also play a role in other physiological functions; e.g., in the accumulation of calcium before bone formation. Ion-binding ability also appears to be related to the anticoagulant activity of the heteropolysaccharide heparin.

The size of the carbohydrate portion of glycoproteins such as gamma globulin or hen-egg albumin is usually between five and 10 monosaccharide units; several such units occur in some glycoprotein molecules. The function of the carbohydrate component has not yet been established except for glycoproteins associated with cell surfaces; in this case, they appear to act as antigenic determinants—i.e., they are capable of inducing the formation of specific antibodies.

Protein

Protein is a highly complex substance that is present in all living organisms. Proteins are of great nutritional value and are directly involved in the chemical processes essential for life.

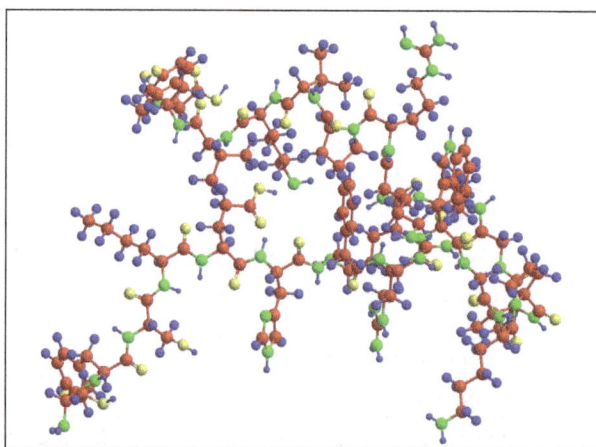

Peptide: The molecular structure of a peptide (a small protein) consists of a sequence of amino acids.

A protein molecule is very large compared with molecules of sugar or salt and consists of many amino acids joined together to form long chains, much as beads are arranged on a string. There are about 20 different amino acids that occur naturally in proteins. Proteins of similar function have similar amino acid composition and sequence. Although it is not yet possible to explain all of the functions of a protein from its amino acid sequence, established correlations between structure and function can be attributed to the properties of the amino acids that compose proteins.

Plants can synthesize all of the amino acids; animals cannot, even though all of them are essential for life. Plants can grow in a medium containing inorganic nutrients that provide nitrogen, potassium, and other substances essential for growth. They utilize the carbon dioxide in the air during the process of photosynthesis to form organic compounds such as carbohydrates. Animals, however, must obtain organic nutrients from outside sources. Because the protein content of most plants is low, very large amounts of plant material are required by animals, such as ruminants (e.g., cows), that eat only plant material to meet their amino acid requirements. Nonruminant animals, including humans, obtain proteins principally from animals and their products—e.g., meat, milk, and eggs. The seeds of legumes are increasingly being used to prepare inexpensive protein-rich food.

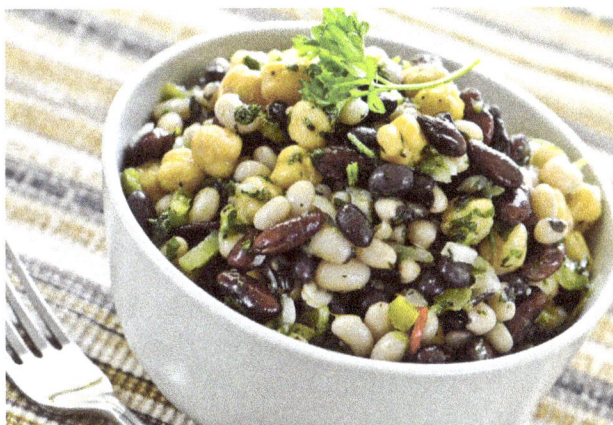

Legume amino acid: Legumes—such as beans, lentils, and peas—are high
in protein and contain many essential amino acids.

The protein content of animal organs is usually much higher than that of the blood plasma. Muscles, for example, contain about 30 percent protein, the liver 20 to 30 percent, and red blood cells 30 percent. Higher percentages of protein are found in hair, bones, and other organs and tissues with a low water content. The quantity of free amino acids and peptides in animals is much smaller than the amount of protein; protein molecules are produced in cells by the stepwise alignment of amino acids and are released into the body fluids only after synthesis is complete.

The high protein content of some organs does not mean that the importance of proteins is related to their amount in an organism or tissue; on the contrary, some of the most important proteins, such as enzymes and hormones, occur in extremely small amounts. The importance of proteins is related principally to their function. All enzymes identified thus far are proteins. Enzymes, which are the catalysts of all metabolic reactions, enable an organism to build up the chemical substances necessary for life—proteins, nucleic acids, carbohydrates, and lipids—to convert them into other substances, and to degrade them. Life without enzymes is not possible. There are several protein hormones with important regulatory functions. In all vertebrates, the respiratory protein hemoglobin acts as oxygen carrier in the blood, transporting oxygen from the lung to body organs and tissues. A large group of structural proteins maintains and protects the structure of the animal body.

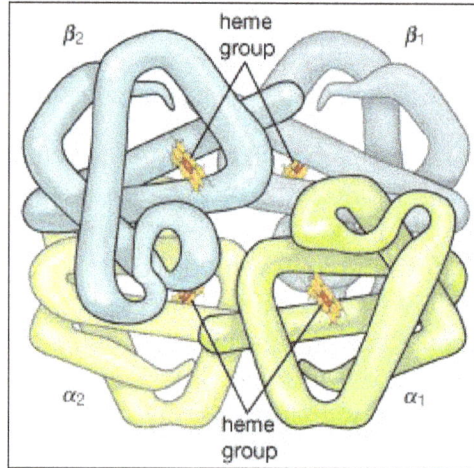

Hemoglobin is a protein made up of four polypeptide chains (α_1, α_2, β_1, and β_2). Each chain is attached to a heme group composed of porphyrin (an organic ringlike compound) attached to an iron atom. These iron-porphyrin complexes coordinate oxygen molecules reversibly, an ability directly related to the role of hemoglobin in oxygen transport in the blood.

Properties of Proteins

Amino Acid Composition of Proteins

The common property of all proteins is that they consist of long chains of α-amino (alpha amino) acids. The general structure of α-amino acids is shown in. The α-amino acids are so called because the α-carbon atom in the molecule carries an amino group ($-NH_2$); the α-carbon atom also carries a carboxyl group ($-COOH$).

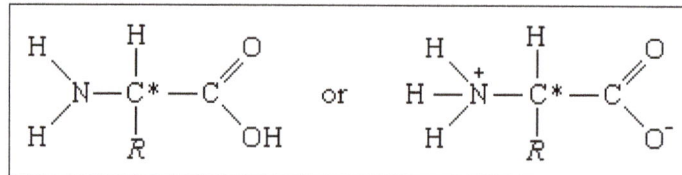

In acidic solutions, when the pH is less than 4, the $-COO$ groups combine with hydrogen ions (H^+) and are thus converted into the uncharged form ($-COOH$). In alkaline solutions, at pH above 9, the ammonium groups ($-NH_3^+$) lose a hydrogen ion and are converted into amino groups ($-NH_2$). In the pH range between 4 and 8, amino acids carry both a positive and a negative charge and therefore do not migrate in an electrical field. Such structures have been designated as dipolar ions, or zwitterions (i.e., hybrid ions).

Although more than 100 amino acids occur in nature, particularly in plants, only 20 types are commonly found in most proteins. In protein molecules the α-amino acids are linked to each other by peptide bonds between the amino group of one amino acid and the carboxyl group of its neighbour.

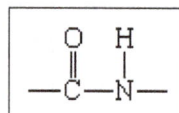

The condensation (joining) of three amino acids yields the tripeptide.

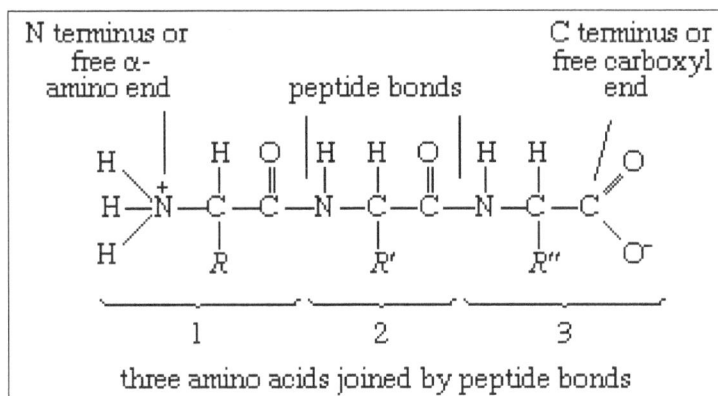

three amino acids joined by peptide bonds

It is customary to write the structure of peptides in such a way that the free α-amino group (also called the N terminus of the peptide) is at the left side and the free carboxyl group (the C terminus) at the right side. Proteins are macromolecular polypeptides—i.e., very large molecules (macromolecules) composed of many peptide-bonded amino acids. Most of the common ones contain more than 100 amino acids linked to each other in a long peptide chain. The average molecular weight (based on the weight of a hydrogen atom as 1) of each amino acid is approximately 100 to 125; thus, the molecular weights of proteins are usually in the range of 10,000 to 100,000 daltons (one dalton is the weight of one hydrogen atom). The species-specificity and organ-specificity of proteins result from differences in the number and sequences of amino acids. Twenty different amino acids in a chain 100 amino acids long can be arranged in far more than 10^{100} ways (10^{100} is the number one followed by 100 zeroes).

Structures of Common Amino Acids

The amino acids present in proteins differ from each other in the structure of their side (R) chains. The simplest amino acid is glycine, in which R is a hydrogen atom. In a number of amino acids, R represents straight or branched carbon chains. One of these amino acids is alanine, in which R is the methyl group ($-CH_3$). Valine, leucine, and isoleucine, with longer R groups, complete the alkyl side-chain series. The alkyl side chains (R groups) of these amino acids are nonpolar; this means that they have no affinity for water but some affinity for each other. Although plants can form all of the alkyl amino acids, animals can synthesize only alanine and glycine; thus valine, leucine, and isoleucine must be supplied in the diet.

Two amino acids, each containing three carbon atoms, are derived from alanine; they are serine and cysteine. Serine contains an alcohol group ($-CH_2OH$) instead of the methyl group of alanine, and cysteine contains a mercapto group ($-CH_2SH$). Animals can synthesize serine but not cysteine or cystine. Cysteine occurs in proteins predominantly in its oxidized form (oxidation in this sense meaning the removal of hydrogen atoms), called cystine. Cystine consists of two cysteine molecules linked by the disulfide bond ($-S-S-$) that results when a hydrogen atom is removed from the mercapto group of each of the cysteines. Disulfide bonds are important in protein structure because they allow the linkage of two different parts of a protein molecule to—and thus the formation of loops in—the otherwise straight chains. Some proteins contain small amounts of cysteine with free sulfhydryl ($-SH$) groups.

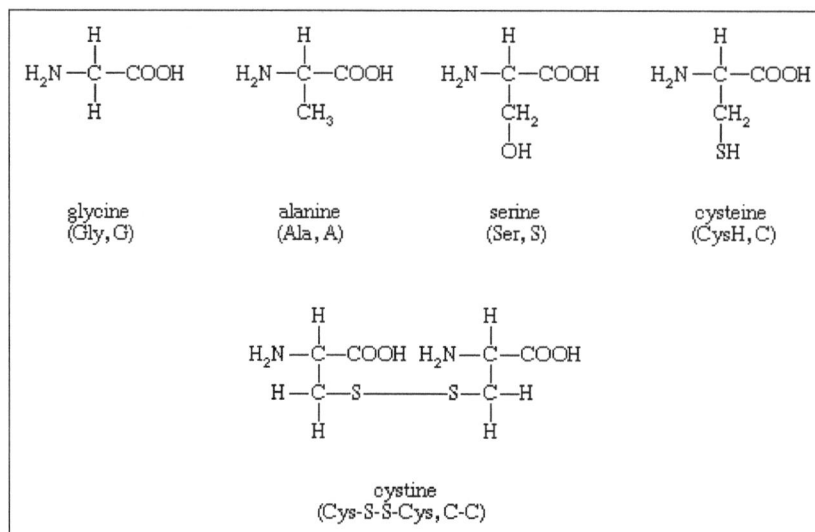

Four amino acids, each consisting of four carbon atoms, occur in proteins; they are aspartic acid, asparagine, threonine, and methionine. Aspartic acid and asparagine, which occur in large amounts, can be synthesized by animals. Threonine and methionine cannot be synthesized and thus are essential amino acids; i.e., they must be supplied in the diet. Most proteins contain only small amounts of methionine.

Proteins also contain an amino acid with five carbon atoms (glutamic acid) and a secondary amine (in proline), which is a structure with the amino group ($-NH_2$) bonded to the alkyl side chain, forming a ring. Glutamic acid and aspartic acid are dicarboxylic acids; that is, they have two carboxyl groups ($-COOH$).

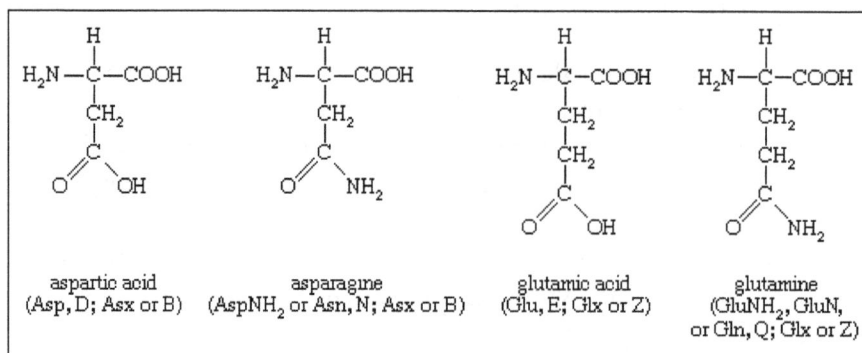

Glutamine is similar to asparagine in that both are the amides of their corresponding dicarboxylic acid forms; i.e., they have an amide group ($-CONH_2$) in place of the carboxyl ($-COOH$) of the side chain. Glutamic acid and glutamine are abundant in most proteins; e.g., in plant proteins they sometimes comprise more than one-third of the amino acids present. Both glutamic acid and glutamine can be synthesized by animals.

The amino acids proline and hydroxyproline occur in large amounts in collagen, the protein of the connective tissue of animals. Proline and hydroxyproline lack free amino ($-NH_2$) groups because the amino group is enclosed in a ring structure with the side chain; they thus cannot exist in a zwitterion form. Although the nitrogen-containing group (>NH) of these amino acids can form a peptide bond with the carboxyl group of another amino acid, the bond so formed gives rise to a kink in the peptide chain; i.e., the ring structure alters the regular bond angle of normal peptide bonds.

Proteins usually are almost neutral molecules; that is, they have neither acidic nor basic properties. This means that the acidic carboxyl ($-COO^-$) groups of aspartic and glutamic acid are about equal in number to the amino acids with basic side chains. Three such basic amino acids, each containing six carbon atoms, occur in proteins. The one with the simplest structure, lysine, is synthesized by plants but not by animals. Even some plants have a low lysine content. Arginine is found in all proteins; it occurs in particularly high amounts in the strongly basic protamines (simple proteins composed of relatively few amino acids) of fish sperm. The third basic amino acid is histidine. Both arginine and histidine can be synthesized by animals. Histidine is a weaker base than either lysine or arginine. The imidazole ring, a five-membered ring structure containing two nitrogen atoms in the side chain of histidine, acts as a buffer (i.e., a stabilizer of hydrogen ion concentration) by binding hydrogen ions (H^+) to the nitrogen atoms of the imidazole ring.

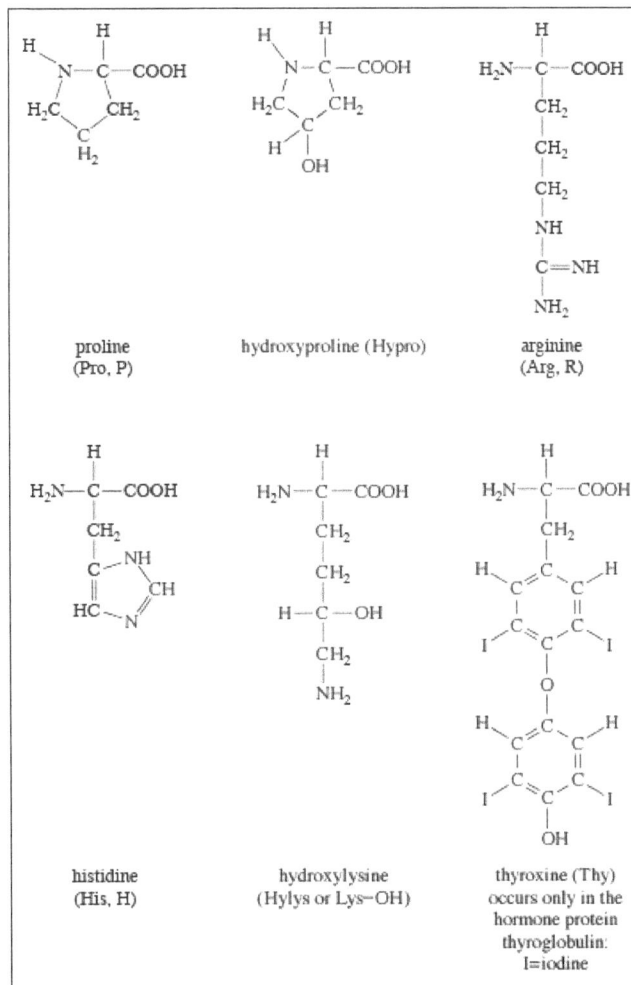

The remaining amino acids—phenylalanine, tyrosine, and tryptophan—have in common an aromatic structure; i.e., a benzene ring is present. These three amino acids are essential, and, while animals cannot synthesize the benzene ring itself, they can convert phenylalanine to tyrosine.

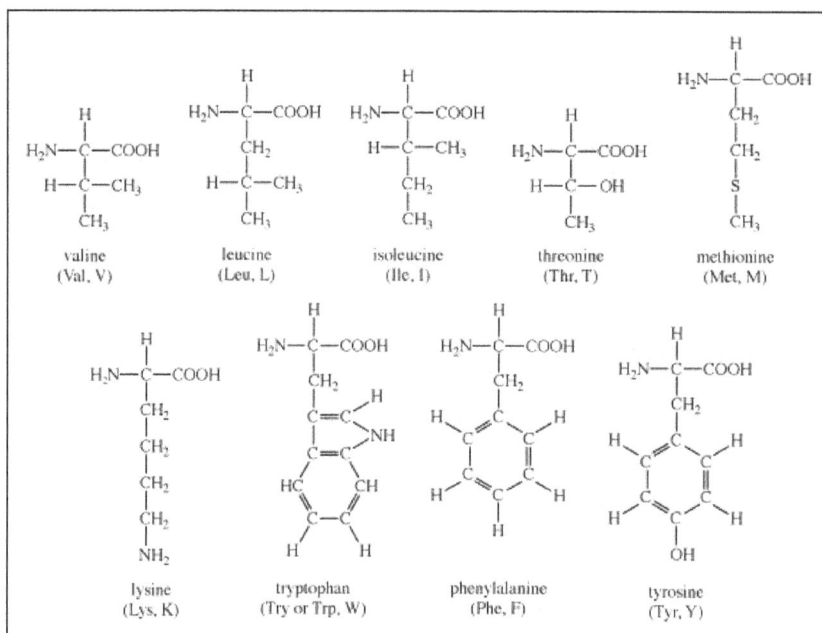

Because these amino acids contain benzene rings, they can absorb ultraviolet light at wavelengths between 270 and 290 nanometres (nm; 1 nanometre = 10^{-9} metre = 10 angstrom units). Phenylalanine absorbs very little ultraviolet light; tyrosine and tryptophan, however, absorb it strongly and are responsible for the absorption band most proteins exhibit at 280–290 nanometres. This absorption is often used to determine the quantity of protein present in protein samples.

Most proteins contain only the amino acids described above; however, other amino acids occur in proteins in small amounts. For example, the collagen found in connective tissue contains, in addition to hydroxyproline, small amounts of hydroxylysine. Other proteins contain some monomethyl-, dimethyl-, or trimethyllysine—i.e., lysine derivatives containing one, two, or three methyl groups ($-CH_3$). The amount of these unusual amino acids in proteins, however, rarely exceeds 1 or 2 percent of the total amino acids.

Physicochemical Properties of the Amino Acids

The physicochemical properties of a protein are determined by the analogous properties of the amino acids in it.

The α-carbon atom of all amino acids, with the exception of glycine, is asymmetric; this means that four different chemical entities (atoms or groups of atoms) are attached to it. As a result, each of the amino acids, except glycine, can exist in two different spatial, or geometric, arrangements (i.e., isomers), which are mirror images akin to right and left hands.

These isomers exhibit the property of optical rotation. Optical rotation is the rotation of the plane of polarized light, which is composed of light waves that vibrate in one plane, or direction, only. Solutions of substances that rotate the plane of polarization are said to be optically active, and the degree of rotation is called the optical rotation of the solution. The direction in which the light is rotated is generally designed as plus, or d, for dextrorotatory (to the right), or as minus, or l, for levorotatory (to the left). Some amino acids are dextrorotatory, others are levorotatory. With the exception of a few small proteins (peptides) that occur in bacteria, the amino acids that occur in proteins are L-amino acids.

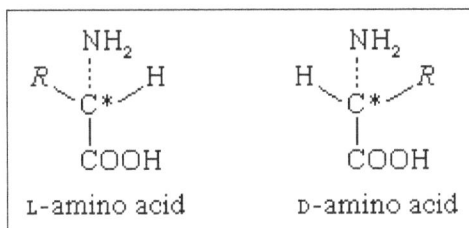

In bacteria, D-alanine and some other D-amino acids have been found as components of gramicidin and bacitracin. These peptides are toxic to other bacteria and are used in medicine as antibiotics. The D-alanine has also been found in some peptides of bacterial membranes.

In contrast to most organic acids and amines, the amino acids are insoluble in organic solvents. In aqueous solutions they are dipolar ions (zwitterions, or hybrid ions) that react with strong acids or bases in a way that leads to the neutralization of the negatively or positively charged ends, respectively. Because of their reactions with strong acids and strong bases, the amino acids act as buffers—stabilizers of hydrogen ion (H^+) or hydroxide ion (OH^-) concentrations. In fact, glycine is frequently used as a buffer in the pH range from 1 to 3 (acid solutions) and from 9 to 12 (basic solutions). In acid solutions, glycine has a positive charge and therefore migrates to the cathode (negative electrode of a direct-current electrical circuit with terminals in the solution). Its charge, however, is negative in alkaline solutions, in which it migrates to the anode (positive electrode). At pH 6.1 glycine does not migrate, because each molecule has one positive and one negative charge. The pH at which an amino acid does not migrate in an electrical field is called the isoelectric point. Most of the monoamino acids (i.e., those with only one amino group) have isoelectric points similar to that of glycine. The isoelectric points of aspartic and glutamic acids, however, are close to pH 3, and those of histidine, lysine, and arginine are at pH 7.6, 9.7, and 10.8, respectively.

Amino Acid Sequence in Protein Molecules

Since each protein molecule consists of a long chain of amino acid residues, linked to each other by peptide bonds, the hydrolytic cleavage of all peptide bonds is a prerequisite for the quantitative determination of the amino acid residues. Hydrolysis is most frequently accomplished by boiling the protein with concentrated hydrochloric acid. The quantitative determination of the amino acids is based on the discovery that amino acids can be separated from each other by chromatography on filter paper and made visible by spraying the paper with ninhydrin. The amino acids of the protein hydrolysate are separated from each other by passing the hydrolysate through a column of adsorbents, which adsorb the amino acids with different affinities and, on washing the column with buffer solutions, release them in a definite order. The amount of each of the amino acids can be determined by the intensity of the colour reaction with ninhydrin.

To obtain information about the sequence of the amino acid residues in the protein, the protein is degraded stepwise, one amino acid being split off in each step. This is accomplished by coupling the free α-amino group ($-NH_2$) of the N-terminal amino acid with phenyl isothiocyanate; subsequent mild hydrolysis does not affect the peptide bonds. The procedure, called the Edman degradation, can be applied repeatedly; it thus reveals the sequence of the amino acids in the peptide chain.

Unavoidable small losses that occur during each step make it impossible to determine the sequence of more than about 30 to 50 amino acids by this procedure. For this reason the protein is usually first hydrolyzed by exposure to the enzyme trypsin, which cleaves only peptide bonds formed by the carboxyl groups of lysine and arginine. The Edman degradation is then applied to each of the few resulting peptides produced by the action of trypsin. Further information can be gained by hydrolyzing another portion of the protein with another enzyme, for instance with chymotrypsin, which splits predominantly peptide bonds formed by the amino acids tyrosine, phenylalanine, and tryptophan. The combination of results obtained with two or more different proteolytic (protein degrading) enzymes was first applied by English biochemist Frederick Sanger, and it enabled him to elucidate the amino acid sequence of insulin. The amino acid sequences of many other proteins subsequently were determined in the same manner.

Levels of Structural Organization in Proteins

Primary Structure

Analytical and synthetic procedures reveal only the primary structure of the proteins—that is, the amino acid sequence of the peptide chains. They do not reveal information about the conformation (arrangement in space) of the peptide chain—that is, whether the peptide chain is present as a long straight thread or is irregularly coiled and folded into a globule. The configuration, or conformation, of a protein is determined by mutual attraction or repulsion of polar or nonpolar groups in the side chains (R groups) of the amino acids. The former have positive or negative charges in their side chains; the latter repel water but attract each other. Some parts of a peptide chain containing 100 to 200 amino acids may form a loop, or helix; others may be straight or form irregular coils.

The terms secondary, tertiary, and quaternary structure are frequently applied to the configuration of the peptide chain of a protein. A nomenclature committee of the International Union of Biochemistry (IUB) has defined these terms as follows: The primary structure of a protein is determined by its amino acid sequence without any regard for the arrangement of the peptide chain in space. The secondary structure is determined by the spatial arrangement of the main peptide chain without any regard for the conformation of side chains or other segments of the main chain. The tertiary structure is determined by both the side chains and other adjacent segments of the main chain, without regard for neighbouring peptide chains. Finally, the term quaternary structure is used for the arrangement of identical or different subunits of a large protein in which each subunit is a separate peptide chain.

Secondary Structure

The nitrogen and carbon atoms of a peptide chain cannot lie on a straight line, because of the magnitude of the bond angles between adjacent atoms of the chain; the bond angle is about 110°. Each of the nitrogen and carbon atoms can rotate to a certain extent, however, so that the chain has a limited flexibility. Because all of the amino acids, except glycine, are asymmetric L-amino acids, the peptide chain tends to assume an asymmetric helical shape; some of the fibrous proteins consist of elongated helices around a straight screw axis. Such structural features result from properties common to all peptide chains. The product of their effects is the secondary structure of the protein.

Tertiary Structure

The tertiary structure is the product of the interaction between the side chains (R) of the amino acids composing the protein. Some of them contain positively or negatively charged groups, others are polar, and still others are nonpolar. The number of carbon atoms in the side chain varies from zero in glycine to nine in tryptophan. Positively and negatively charged side chains have the tendency to attract each other; side chains with identical charges repel each other. The bonds formed by the forces between the negatively charged side chains of aspartic or glutamic acid on the one hand, and the positively charged side chains of lysine or arginine on the other hand, are called salt bridges. Mutual attraction of adjacent peptide chains also results from the formation of numerous hydrogen bonds.

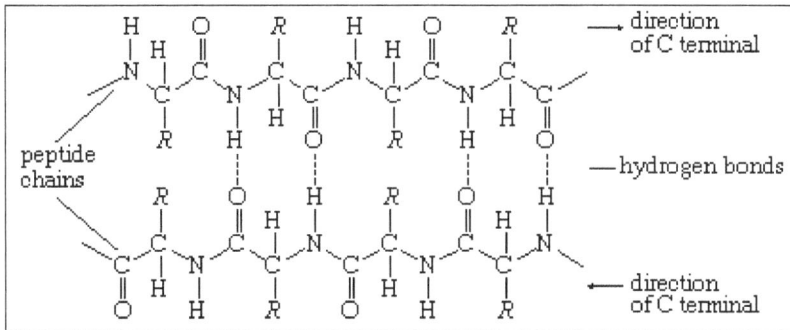

Hydrogen bonds form as a result of the attraction between the nitrogen-bound hydrogen atom (the imide hydrogen) and the unshared pair of electrons of the oxygen atom in the double bonded carbon—oxygen group (the carbonyl group). The result is a slight displacement of the imide hydrogen toward the oxygen atom of the carbonyl group. Although the hydrogen bond is much weaker than a covalent bond (i.e., the type of bond between two carbon atoms, which equally share the pair of bonding electrons between them), the large number of imide and carbonyl groups in peptide chains results in the formation of numerous hydrogen bonds. Another type of attraction is that between nonpolar side chains of valine, leucine, isoleucine, and phenylalanine; the attraction results in the displacement of water molecules and is called hydrophobic interaction.

In proteins rich in cystine, the conformation of the peptide chain is determined to a considerable extent by the disulfide bonds (−S−S−) of cystine. The halves of cystine may be located in different parts of the peptide chain and thus may form a loop closed by the disulfide bond.

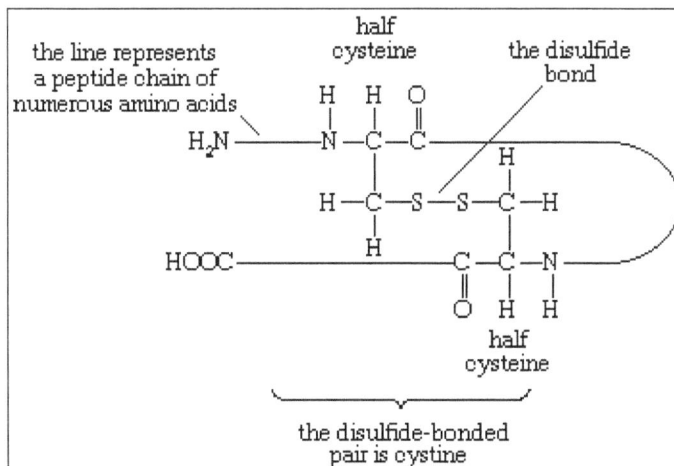

If the disulfide bond is reduced (i.e., hydrogen is added) to two sulfhydryl (−SH) groups, the tertiary structure of the protein undergoes a drastic change—closed loops are broken and adjacent disulfide-bonded peptide chains separate.

Quaternary Structure

The nature of the quaternary structure is demonstrated by the structure of hemoglobin. Each molecule of human hemoglobin consists of four peptide chains, two α-chains and two β-chains; i.e., it is a tetramer. The four subunits are linked to each other by hydrogen bonds and hydrophobic interaction. Because the four subunits are so closely linked, the hemoglobin tetramer is called a molecule, even though no covalent bonds occur between the peptide chains of the four subunits. In other proteins, the subunits are bound to each other by covalent bonds (disulfide bridges).

The amino acid sequence of porcine proinsulin is shown below. The arrows indicate the direction from the N terminus of the β-chain (B) to the C terminus of the α-chain (A).

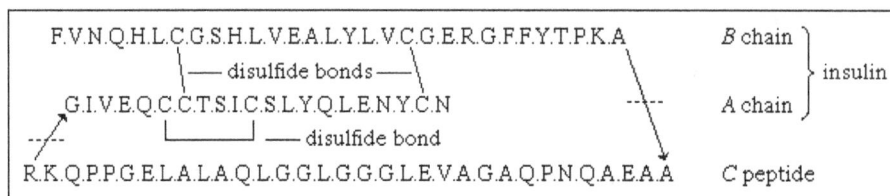

Isolation and Determination of Proteins

Animal material usually contains large amounts of protein and lipids and small amounts of carbohydrate; in plants, the bulk of the dry matter is usually carbohydrate. If it is necessary to determine the amount of protein in a mixture of animal foodstuffs, a sample is converted to ammonium salts by boiling with sulfuric acid and a suitable inorganic catalyst, such as copper sulfate (Kjeldahl method). The method is based on the assumption that proteins contain 16 percent nitrogen, and that nonprotein nitrogen is present in very small amounts. The assumption is justified for most tissues from higher animals but not for insects and crustaceans, in which a considerable portion of the body nitrogen is present in the form of chitin, a carbohydrate. Large amounts of nonprotein nitrogen are also found in the sap of many plants. In such cases, the precise quantitative analyses are made after the proteins have been separated from other biological compounds.

Proteins are sensitive to heat, acids, bases, organic solvents, and radiation exposure; for this reason, the chemical methods employed to purify organic compounds cannot be applied to proteins. Salts and molecules of small size are removed from protein solutions by dialysis—i.e., by placing the solution into a sac of semipermeable material, such as cellulose or acetylcellulose, which will allow small molecules to pass through but not large protein molecules, and immersing the sac in water or a salt solution. Small molecules can also be removed either by passing the protein solution through a column of resin that adsorbs only the protein or by gel filtration. In gel filtration, the large protein molecules pass through the column, and the small molecules are adsorbed to the gel.

Groups of proteins are separated from each other by salting out—i.e., the stepwise addition of sodium sulfate or ammonium sulfate to a protein solution. Some proteins, called globulins, become insoluble and precipitate when the solution is half-saturated with ammonium sulfate or when its sodium sulfate content exceeds about 12 percent. Other proteins, the albumins, can be precipitated from the supernatant solution (i.e., the solution remaining after a precipitation has taken place) by saturation with ammonium sulfate. Water-soluble proteins can be obtained in a dry state by freeze-drying (lyophilization), in which the protein solution is deep-frozen by lowering the temperature below –15 °C (5 °F) and removing the water; the protein is obtained as a dry powder.

Most proteins are insoluble in boiling water and are denatured by it—i.e., irreversibly converted into an insoluble material. Heat denaturation cannot be used with connective tissue because the principal structural protein, collagen, is converted by boiling water into water-soluble gelatin.

Fractionation (separation into components) of a mixture of proteins of different molecular weight can be accomplished by gel filtration. The size of the proteins retained by the gel depends upon the properties of the gel. The proteins retained in the gel are removed from the column by solutions of a suitable concentration of salts and hydrogen ions.

Many proteins were originally obtained in crystalline form, but crystallinity is not proof of purity; many crystalline protein preparations contain other substances. Various tests are used to determine whether a protein preparation contains only one protein. The purity of a protein solution can be determined by such techniques as chromatography and gel filtration. In addition, a solution of pure protein will yield one peak when spun in a centrifuge at very high speeds (ultracentrifugation) and will migrate as a single band in electrophoresis (migration of the protein in an electrical field). After these methods and others (such as amino acid analysis) indicate that the protein solution is pure, it can be considered so. Because chromatography, ultracentrifugation, and electrophoresis cannot be applied to insoluble proteins, little is known about them; they may be mixtures of many similar proteins.

Very small (microheterogeneous) differences in some of the apparently pure proteins are known to occur. They are differences in the amino acid composition of otherwise identical proteins and are transmitted from generation to generation; i.e., they are genetically determined. For example, some humans have two hemoglobins, hemoglobin A and hemoglobin S, which differ in one amino acid at a specific site in the molecule. In hemoglobin A the site is occupied by glutamic acid and in hemoglobin S by valine. Refinement of the techniques of protein analysis has resulted in the discovery of other instances of microheterogeneity.

The quantity of a pure protein can be determined by weighing or by measuring the ultraviolet absorbancy at 280 nanometres. The absorbency at 280 nanometres depends on the content of tyrosine and tryptophan in the protein. Sometimes the slightly less sensitive biuret reaction, a purple colour given by alkaline protein solutions upon the addition of copper sulfate, is used; its intensity depends only on the number of peptide bonds per gram, which is similar in all proteins.

Physicochemical Properties of Proteins

Molecular Weight of Proteins

The molecular weight of proteins cannot be determined by the methods of classical chemistry (e.g., freezing-point depression), because they require solutions of a higher concentration of protein than can be prepared.

If a protein contains only one molecule of one of the amino acids or one atom of iron, copper, or another element, the minimum molecular weight of the protein or a subunit can be calculated; for example, the protein myoglobin contains 0.34 gram of iron in 100 grams of protein. The atomic weight of iron is 56; thus the minimum molecular weight of myoglobin is $(56 \times 100)/0.34 =$ about 16,500. Direct measurements of the molecular weight of myoglobin yield the same value. The molecular weight of hemoglobin, however, which also contains 0.34 percent iron, has been found to be 66,000 or $4 \times 16,500$; thus hemoglobin contains four atoms of iron.

The method most frequently used to determine the molecular weight of proteins is ultracentrifugation—i.e., spinning in a centrifuge at velocities up to about 60,000 revolutions per minute. Centrifugal forces of more than 200,000 times the gravitational force on the surface of Earth are achieved at such velocities. The first ultracentrifuges, built in 1920, were used to determine the molecular weight of proteins. The molecular weights of a large number of proteins have been determined. Most consist of several subunits, the molecular weight of which is usually less than 100,000 and frequently ranges from 20,000 to 30,000. Proteins of very high molecular weights are found among hemocyanins, the copper-containing respiratory proteins of invertebrates; some range as high as several million. Although there is no definite lower limit for the molecular weight of proteins, short amino acid sequences are usually called peptides.

Shape of Protein Molecules

In the technique of X-ray diffraction, the X-rays are allowed to strike a protein crystal. The X-rays, diffracted (bent) by the crystal, impinge on a photographic plate, forming a pattern of spots. This method reveals that peptide chains can assume very complicated, apparently irregular shapes. Two extremes in shape include the closely folded structure of the globular proteins and the elongated, unidimensional structure of the threadlike fibrous proteins; both were recognized many years before the technique of X-ray diffraction was developed. Solutions of fibrous proteins are extremely viscous (i.e., sticky); those of the globular proteins have low viscosity (i.e., they flow easily). A 5 percent solution of a globular protein—ovalbumin, for example—easily flows through a narrow glass tube; a 5 percent solution of gelatin, a fibrous protein, however, does not flow through the tube, because it is liquid only at high temperatures and solidifies at room temperature. Even solutions containing only 1 or 2 percent of gelatin are highly viscous and flow through a narrow tube either very slowly or only under pressure.

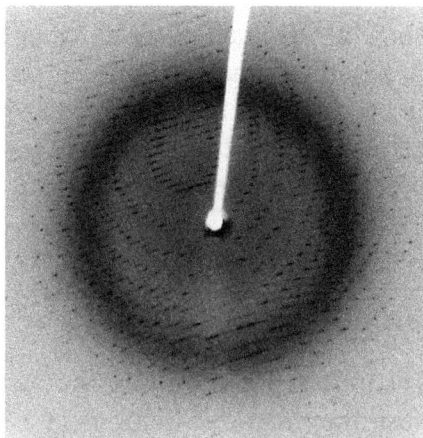

X-ray diffraction pattern of a crystallized enzyme.

The elongated peptide chains of the fibrous proteins can be imagined to become entangled not only mechanically but also by mutual attraction of their side chains, and in this way they incorporate large amounts of water. Most of the hydrophilic (water-attracting) groups of the globular proteins, however, lie on the surface of the molecules, and, as a result, globular proteins incorporate only a few water molecules. If a solution of a fibrous protein flows through a narrow tube, the elongated molecules become oriented parallel to the direction of the flow, and the solution thus becomes birefringent like a crystal; i.e., it splits a light ray into two components that travel at different velocities and are polarized at right angles to each other. Globular proteins do not show this phenomenon, which is called flow birefringence. Solutions of myosin, the contractile protein of muscles, show very high flow birefringence; other proteins with very high flow birefringence include solutions of fibrinogen, the clotting material of blood plasma, and solutions of tobacco mosaic virus. The gamma-globulins of the blood plasma show low flow birefringence, and none can be observed in solutions of serum albumin and ovalbumin.

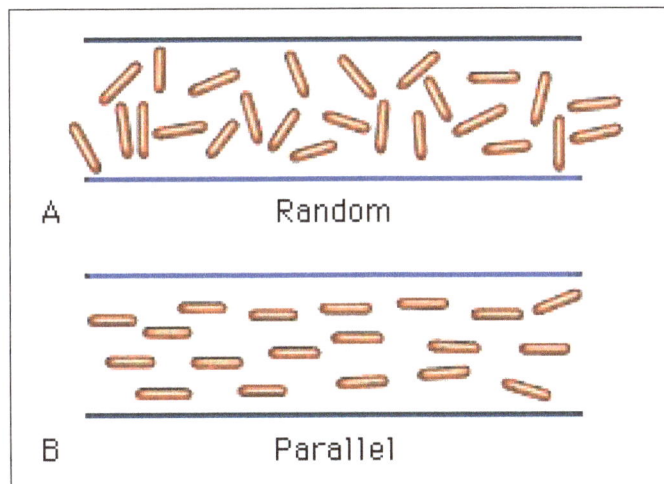

Flow birefringence: Orientation of elongated, rodlike macromolecules
(A) in resting solution, or (B) during flow through a horizontal tube.

Hydration of Proteins

When dry proteins are exposed to air of high water content, they rapidly bind water up to a maximum quantity, which differs for different proteins; usually it is 10 to 20 percent of the weight of the protein. The hydrophilic groups of a protein are chiefly the positively charged groups in the side chains of lysine and arginine and the negatively charged groups of aspartic and glutamic acid. Hydration (i.e., the binding of water) may also occur at the hydroxyl ($-OH$) groups of serine and threonine or at the amide ($-CONH_2$) groups of asparagine and glutamine.

The binding of water molecules to either charged or polar (partly charged) groups is explained by the dipolar structure of the water molecule; that is, the two positively charged hydrogen atoms form an angle of about 105°, with the negatively charged oxygen atom at the apex. The centre of the positive charges is located between the two hydrogen atoms; the centre of the negative charge of the oxygen atom is at the apex of the angle. The negative pole of the dipolar water molecule binds to positively charged groups; the positive pole binds negatively charged ones. The negative pole of the water molecule also binds to the hydroxyl and amino groups of the protein.

The water of hydration is essential to the structure of protein crystals; when they are completely dehydrated, the crystalline structure disintegrates. In some proteins this process is accompanied by denaturation and loss of the biological function.

In aqueous solutions, proteins bind some of the water molecules very firmly; others are either very loosely bound or form islands of water molecules between loops of folded peptide chains. Because the water molecules in such an island are thought to be oriented as in ice, which is crystalline water, the islands of water in proteins are called icebergs. Water molecules may also form bridges between the carbonyl and imino groups of adjacent peptide chains, resulting in structures similar to those of the pleated sheet but with a water molecule in the position of the hydrogen bonds of that configuration. The extent of hydration of protein molecules in aqueous solutions is important, because some of the methods used to determine the molecular weight of proteins yield the molecular weight of the hydrated protein. The amount of water bound to one gram of a globular protein in solution varies from 0.2 to 0.5 gram. Much larger amounts of water are mechanically immobilized between the elongated peptide chains of fibrous proteins; for example, one gram of gelatin can immobilize at room temperature 25 to 30 grams of water.

Hydration of proteins is necessary for their solubility in water. If the water of hydration of a protein dissolved in water is reduced by the addition of a salt such as ammonium sulfate, the protein is no longer soluble and is salted out, or precipitated. The salting-out process is reversible because the protein is not denatured (i.e., irreversibly converted to an insoluble material) by the addition of such salts as sodium chloride, sodium sulfate, or ammonium sulfate. Some globulins, called euglobulins, are insoluble in water in the absence of salts; their insolubility is attributed to the mutual interaction of polar groups on the surface of adjacent molecules, a process that results in the formation of large aggregates of molecules. Addition of small amounts of salt causes the euglobulins to become soluble. This process, called salting in, results from a combination between anions (negatively charged ions) and cations (positively charged ions) of the salt and positively and negatively charged side chains of the euglobulins. The combination prevents the aggregation of euglobulin molecules by preventing the formation of salt bridges between them. The addition of more sodium or ammonium sulfate causes the euglobulins to salt out again and to precipitate.

Electrochemistry of Proteins

Because the α-amino group and α-carboxyl group of amino acids are converted into peptide bonds in the protein molecule, there is only one α-amino group (at the N terminus) and one α-carboxyl group (at the C terminus) in a given protein molecule. The electrochemical character of a protein is affected very little by these two groups. Of importance, however, are the numerous positively charged ammonium groups ($-NH_3^+$) of lysine and arginine and the negatively charged carboxyl groups ($-COO^-$) of aspartic acid and glutamic acid. In most proteins, the number of positively and negatively charged groups varies from 10 to 20 per 100 amino acids.

Electrometric Titration

When measured volumes of hydrochloric acid are added to a solution of protein in salt-free water, the pH decreases in proportion to the amount of hydrogen ions added until it is about 4. Further addition of acid causes much less decrease in pH because the protein acts as a buffer at pH values of 3 to 4. The reaction that takes place in this pH range is the protonation of the carboxyl group—i.e., the conversion of −COO⁻ into −COOH. Electrometric titration of an isoelectric protein with potassium hydroxide causes a very slow increase in pH and a weak buffering action of the protein at pH 7; a very strong buffering action occurs in the pH range from 9 to 10. The buffering action at pH 7, which is caused by loss of protons (positively charged hydrogen) from the imidazolium groups (i.e., the five-member ring structure in the side chain) of histidine, is weak because the histidine content of proteins is usually low. The much stronger buffering action at pH values from 9 to 10 is caused by the loss of protons from the hydroxyl group of tyrosine and from the ammonium groups of lysine. Finally, protons are lost from the guanidinium groups (i.e., the nitrogen-containing terminal portion of the arginine side chains) of arginine at pH 12. Electrometric titrations of proteins yield similar curves. Electrometric titration makes possible the determination of the approximate number of carboxyl groups, ammonium groups, histidines, and tyrosines per molecule of protein.

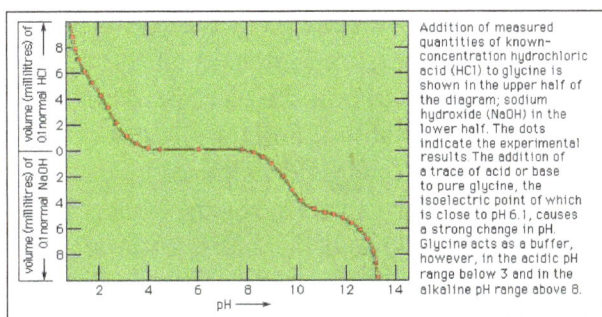

Electrometric titration of glycine.

Electrophoresis

The positively and negatively charged side chains of proteins cause them to behave like amino acids in an electrical field; that is, they migrate during electrophoresis at low pH values to the cathode (negative terminal) and at high pH values to the anode (positive terminal). The isoelectric point, the pH value at which the protein molecule does not migrate, is in the range of pH 5 to 7 for many proteins. Proteins such as lysozyme, cytochrome c, histone, and others rich in lysine and arginine, however, have isoelectric points in the pH range between 8 and 10. The isoelectric point of pepsin, which contains very few basic amino acids, is close to 1.

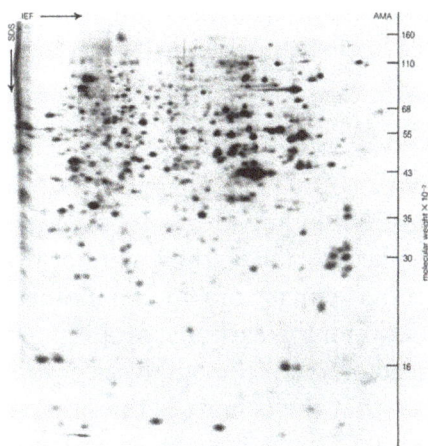

Two-dimensional gel electrophoresis: In two-dimensional gel electrophoresis, proteins are separated based on charge and size. Approaches commonly employed include isoelectric focusing (IEF) sodium dodecyl sulfate (SDS) polyacrylamide gel electrophoresis (PAGE) and immobilized pH gradient (IPG-Dalt) SDS-PAGE.

Free-boundary electrophoresis, the original method of determining electrophoretic migration, has been replaced in many instances by zone electrophoresis, in which the protein is placed in either a gel of starch, agar, or polyacrylamide or in a porous medium such as paper or cellulose acetate. The migration of hemoglobin and other coloured proteins can be followed visually. Colourless proteins are made visible after the completion of electrophoresis by staining them with a suitable dye.

Conformation of Globular Proteins

Results of X-ray Diffraction Studies

Most knowledge concerning secondary and tertiary structure of globular proteins has been obtained by the examination of their crystals using X-ray diffraction. In this technique, X-rays are allowed to strike the crystal; the X-rays are diffracted by the crystal and impinge on a photographic plate, forming a pattern of spots. The measured intensity of the diffraction pattern, as recorded on a photographic film, depends particularly on the electron density of the atoms in the protein crystal. This density is lowest in hydrogen atoms, and they do not give a visible diffraction pattern. Although carbon, oxygen, and nitrogen atoms yield visible diffraction patterns, they are present in such great number—about 700 or 800 per 100 amino acids—that the resolution of the structure of a protein containing more than 100 amino acids is almost impossible. Resolution is considerably improved by substituting into the side chains of certain amino acids very heavy atoms, particularly those of heavy metals. Mercury ions, for example, bind to the sulfhydryl ($-SH$) groups of cysteine. Platinum chloride has been used in other proteins. In the iron-containing proteins, the iron atom already in the molecule is adequate.

Although the X-ray diffraction technique cannot resolve the complete three-dimensional conformation (that is, the secondary and tertiary structure of the peptide chain), complete resolution has been obtained by combination of the results of X-ray diffraction with those of amino acid sequence analysis. In this way the complete conformation of such proteins as myoglobin, chymotrypsinogen, lysozyme, and ribonuclease has been resolved.

The X-ray diffraction method has revealed regular structural arrangements in proteins; one is an extended form of antiparallel peptide chains that are linked to each other by hydrogen bonds between the carbonyl and imino groups. This conformation, called the pleated sheet, or β-structure, is found in some fibrous proteins. Short strands of the β-structure have also been detected in some globular proteins.

A second important structural arrangement is the α-helix; it is formed by a sequence of amino acids wound around a straight axis in either a right-handed or a left-handed spiral. Each turn of the helix corresponds to a distance of 5.4 angstroms (= 0.54 nanometre) in the direction of the screw axis and contains 3.7 amino acids. Hence, the length of the α-helix per amino acid residue is 5.4 divided by 3.7, or 1.5 angstroms (1 angstrom = 0.1 nanometre). The stability of the α-helix is maintained by hydrogen bonds between the carbonyl and imino groups of neighbouring turns of the helix. It was once thought, based on data from analyses of the myoglobin molecule, more than half of which consists of α-helices, that the α-helix is the predominant structural element of the globular proteins; it is now known that myoglobin is exceptional in this respect. The other globular proteins for which the structures have been resolved by X-ray diffraction contain only small regions of α-helix. In most of them the peptide chains are folded in an apparently random fashion, for which the term random coil has been used. The term is misleading, however, because the folding is not random; rather, it is dictated by the primary structure and modified by the secondary and tertiary structures.

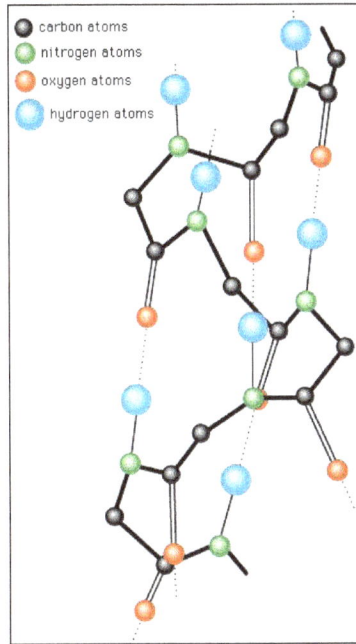

The α-helix in the structural arrangement of a protein.

The first proteins for which the internal structures were completely resolved are the iron-containing proteins myoglobin and hemoglobin. The investigation of the hydrated crystals of these proteins by Austrian-born British biochemist Max Perutz and British biochemist John C. Kendrew, who won the 1962 Nobel Prize for Chemistry for their work, revealed that the folding of the peptide chains is so tight that most of the water is displaced from the centre of the globular molecules. The amino acids that carry the ammonium ($-NH_3^+$) and carboxyl ($-COO^-$) groups were found to be shifted to the surface of the globular molecules, and the nonpolar amino acids were found to be concentrated in the interior.

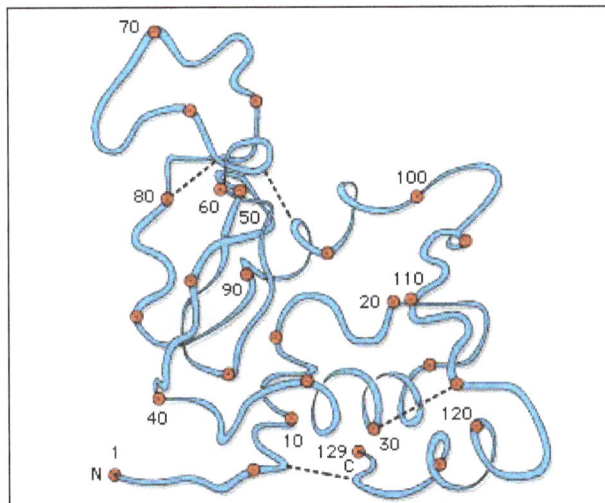

Lysozyme; protein conformation.

The simplified structure of lysozyme from hen's egg white has a single peptide chain of 129 amino acids. The amino acid residues are numbered from the terminal α group (N) to the terminal carboxyl group (C). Circles indicate every fifth residue, and every tenth residue is numbered. Broken lines indicate the four disulfide bridges. Alpha-helices are visible in the ranges 25 to 35, 90 to 100, and 120 to 125.

Other Approaches to the Determination of Protein Structure

None of the several other physical methods that have been used to obtain information on the secondary and tertiary structure of proteins provides as much direct information as the X-ray diffraction technique. Most of the techniques, however, are much simpler than X-ray diffraction, which requires, for the resolution of the structure of one protein, many years of work and equipment such as electronic computers. Some of the simpler techniques are based on the optical properties of proteins—refractivity, absorption of light of different wavelengths, rotation of the plane polarized light at different wavelengths, and luminescence.

Spectrophotometric Behaviour

Spectrophotometry of protein solutions (the measurement of the degree of absorbance of light by a protein within a specified wavelength) is useful within the range of visible light only with proteins that contain coloured prosthetic groups (the nonprotein components). Examples of such proteins include the red heme proteins of the blood, the purple pigments of the retina of the eye, green and yellow proteins that contain bile pigments, blue copper-containing proteins, and dark brown proteins called melanins. Peptide bonds, because of their carbonyl groups, absorb light energy at very short wavelengths (185–200 nanometres). The aromatic rings of phenylalanine, tyrosine, and tryptophan, however, absorb ultraviolet light between wavelengths of 280 and 290 nanometres. The absorbance of ultraviolet light by tryptophan is greatest, that of tyrosine is less, and that of phenylalanine is least. If the tyrosine or tryptophan content of the protein is known, therefore, the concentration of the protein solution can be determined by measuring its absorbance between 280 and 290 nanometres.

Optical Activity

It will be recalled that the amino acids, with the exception of glycine, exhibit optical activity. It is not surprising, therefore, that proteins also are optically active. They are usually levorotatory (i.e., they rotate the plane of polarization to the left) when polarized light of wavelengths in the visible range is used. Although the specific rotation (a function of the concentration of a protein solution and the distance the light travels in it) of most L-amino acids varies from −30° to +30°, the amino acid cystine has a specific rotation of approximately −300°. Although the optical rotation of a protein depends on all of the amino acids of which it is composed, the most important ones are cystine and the aromatic amino acids phenylalanine, tyrosine, and tryptophan. The contribution of the other amino acids to the optical activity of a protein is negligibly small.

Chemical Reactivity of Proteins

Information on the internal structure of proteins can be obtained with chemical methods that reveal whether certain groups are present on the surface of the protein molecule and thus able to react or whether they are buried inside the closely folded peptide chains and thus are unable to react. The chemical reagents used in such investigations must be mild ones that do not affect the structure of the protein.

The reactivity of tyrosine is of special interest. It has been found, for example, that only three of the six tyrosines found in the naturally occurring enzyme ribonuclease can be iodinated (i.e., reacted to accept an iodine atom). Enzyme-catalyzed breakdown of iodinated ribonuclease is used to identify the peptides in which the iodinated tyrosines are present. The three tyrosines that can be iodinated lie on the surface of ribonuclease; the others, assumed to be inaccessible, are said to be buried in the molecule. Tyrosine can also be identified by using other techniques—e.g., treatment with diazonium compounds or tetranitromethane. Because the compounds formed are coloured, they can easily be detected when the protein is broken down with enzymes.

Cysteine can be detected by coupling with compounds such as iodoacetic acid or iodoacetamide; the reaction results in the formation of carboxymethylcysteine or carbamidomethylcysteine, which can be detected by amino acid determination of the peptides containing them. The imidazole groups of certain histidines can also be located by coupling with the same reagents under different conditions. Unfortunately, few other amino acids can be labelled without changes in the secondary and tertiary structure of the protein.

Association of Protein Subunits

Many proteins with molecular weights of more than 50,000 occur in aqueous solutions as complexes: dimers, tetramers, and higher polymers—i.e., as chains of two, four, or more repeating basic structural units. The subunits, which are called monomers or protomers, usually are present as an even number. Less than 10 percent of the polymers have been found to have an odd number of monomers. The arrangement of the subunits is thought to be regular and may be cyclic, cubic, or tetrahedral. Some of the small proteins also contain subunits. Insulin, for example, with a molecular weight of about 6,000, consists of two peptide chains linked to each other by disulfide bridges (−S−S−). Similar interchain disulfide bonds have been found in the immunoglobulins. In other proteins, hydrogen bonds and hydrophobic bonds (resulting from the interaction between the amino acid side chains of valine, leucine, isoleucine, and phenylalanine) cause the formation of aggregates of the subunits. The subunits of some proteins are identical; those of others differ. Hemoglobin is a tetramer consisting of two α-chains and two β-chains.

Protein Denaturation

When a solution of a protein is boiled, the protein frequently becomes insoluble—i.e., it is denatured—and remains insoluble even when the solution is cooled. The denaturation of the proteins of egg white by heat—as when boiling an egg—is an example of irreversible denaturation. The denatured protein has the same primary structure as the original, or native, protein. The weak forces between charged groups and the weaker forces of mutual attraction of nonpolar groups are disrupted at elevated temperatures, however; as a result, the tertiary structure of the protein is lost. In some instances the original structure of the protein can be regenerated; the process is called renaturation.

Denaturation can be brought about in various ways. Proteins are denatured by treatment with alkaline or acid, oxidizing or reducing agents, and certain organic solvents. Interesting among denaturing agents are those that affect the secondary and tertiary structure without affecting the primary structure. The agents most frequently used for this purpose are urea and guanidinium chloride. These molecules, because of their high affinity for peptide bonds, break the hydrogen bonds and the salt bridges between positive and negative side chains, thereby abolishing the tertiary structure of the peptide chain. When denaturing agents are removed from a protein solution, the native protein re-forms in many cases. Denaturation can also be accomplished by reduction of the disulfide bonds of cystine—i.e., conversion of the disulfide bond ($-S-S-$) to two sulfhydryl groups ($-SH$). This, of course, results in the formation of two cysteines. Reoxidation of the cysteines by exposure to air sometimes regenerates the native protein. In other cases, however, the wrong cysteines become bound to each other, resulting in a different protein. Finally, denaturation can also be accomplished by exposing proteins to organic solvents such as ethanol or acetone. It is believed that the organic solvents interfere with the mutual attraction of nonpolar groups.

Some of the smaller proteins, however, are extremely stable, even against heat; for example, solutions of ribonuclease can be exposed for short periods of time to temperatures of 90 °C (194 °F) without undergoing significant denaturation. Denaturation does not involve identical changes in protein molecules. A common property of denatured proteins, however, is the loss of biological activity—e.g., the ability to act as enzymes or hormones.

Although denaturation had long been considered an all-or-none reaction, it is now thought that many intermediary states exist between native and denatured protein. In some instances, however, the breaking of a key bond could be followed by the complete breakdown of the conformation of the native protein.

Although many native proteins are resistant to the action of the enzyme trypsin, which breaks down proteins during digestion, they are hydrolyzed by the same enzyme after denaturation. The peptide bonds that can be split by trypsin are inaccessible in the native proteins but become accessible during denaturation. Similarly, denatured proteins give more intense colour reactions for tyrosine, histidine, and arginine than do the same proteins in the native state. The increased accessibility of reactive groups of denatured proteins is attributed to an unfolding of the peptide chains.

If denaturation can be brought about easily and if renaturation is difficult, how is the native conformation of globular proteins maintained in living organisms, in which they are produced stepwise, by incorporation of one amino acid at a time? Experiments on the biosynthesis of proteins from amino acids containing radioactive carbon or heavy hydrogen reveal that the protein molecule grows stepwise from the N terminus to the C terminus; in each step a single amino acid residue is incorporated. As soon as the growing peptide chain contains six or seven amino acid residues, the side chains interact with each other and thus cause deviations from the straight or β-chain configuration. Depending on the nature of the side chains, this may result in the formation of a α-helix or of loops closed by hydrogen bonds or disulfide bridges. The final conformation is probably frozen when the peptide chain attains a length of 50 or more amino acid residues.

Conformation of Proteins in Interfaces

Like many other substances with both hydrophilic and hydrophobic groups, soluble proteins tend to migrate into the interface between air and water or oil and water; the term oil here means a hydrophobic liquid such as benzene or xylene. Within the interface, proteins spread, forming thin films. Measurements of the surface tension, or interfacial tension, of such films indicate that tension is reduced by the protein film. Proteins, when forming an interfacial film, are present as a monomolecular layer—i.e., a layer one molecule in height. Although it was once thought that globular protein molecules unfold completely in the interface, it has now been established that many proteins can be recovered from films in the native state. The application of lateral pressure on a protein film causes it to increase in thickness and finally to form a layer with a height corresponding to the diameter of the native protein molecule. Protein molecules in an interface, because of Brownian motions (molecular vibrations), occupy much more space than do those in the film after the application of pressure. The Brownian motion of compressed molecules is limited to the two dimensions of the interface, since the protein molecules cannot move upward or downward.

The motion of protein molecules at the air–water interface has been used to determine the molecular weight of proteins. The technique involves measuring the force exerted by the protein layer on a barrier.

When a protein solution is vigorously shaken in air, it forms a foam, because the soluble proteins migrate into the air–water interface and persist there, preventing or slowing the reconversion of the foam into a homogeneous solution. Some of the unstable, easily modified proteins are denatured when spread in the air–water interface. The formation of a permanent foam when egg white is vigorously stirred is an example of irreversible denaturation by spreading in a surface.

Classification of Proteins

Classification by Solubility

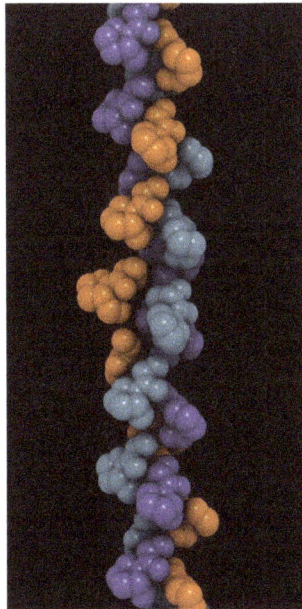

Collagen molecule

After two German chemists, Emil Fischer and Franz Hofmeister, independently stated in 1902 that proteins are essentially polypeptides consisting of many amino acids, an attempt was made to classify proteins according to their chemical and physical properties, because the biological function of proteins had not yet been established. Proteins were classified primarily according to their solubility in a number of solvents. This classification is no longer satisfactory, however, because proteins of quite different structure and function sometimes have similar solubilities; conversely, proteins of the same function and similar structure sometimes have different solubilities. The terms associated with the old classification, however, are still widely used.

Albumins are proteins that are soluble in water and in water half-saturated with ammonium sulfate. On the other hand, globulins are salted out (i.e., precipitated) by half-saturation with ammonium sulfate. Globulins that are soluble in salt-free water are called pseudoglobulins; those insoluble in salt-free water are euglobulins. Both prolamins and glutelins, which are plant proteins, are insoluble in water; the prolamins dissolve in 50 to 80 percent ethanol, the glutelins in acidified or alkaline solution. The term protamine is used for a number of proteins in fish sperm that consist of approximately 80 percent arginine and therefore are strongly alkaline. Histones, which are less alkaline, apparently occur only in cell nuclei, where they are bound to nucleic acids. The term scleroproteins has been used for the insoluble proteins of animal organs. They include keratin, the insoluble protein of certain epithelial tissues such as the skin or hair, and collagen, the protein of the connective tissue. A large group of proteins has been called conjugated proteins, because they are complex molecules of protein consisting of protein and nonprotein moieties. The nonprotein portion is called the prosthetic group. Conjugated proteins can be subdivided into mucoproteins, which, in addition to protein, contain carbohydrate; lipoproteins, which contain lipids; phosphoproteins, which are rich in phosphate; chromoproteins, which contain pigments such as iron-porphyrins, carotenoids, bile pigments, and melanin; and finally, nucleoproteins, which contain nucleic acid.

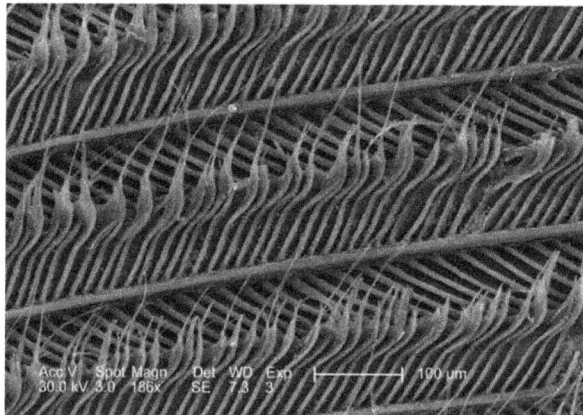

Keratin: Scanning electron micrograph showing strands of keratin in a feather, magnified 186×.

The weakness of the above classification lies in the fact that many, if not all, globulins contain small amounts of carbohydrate; thus there is no sharp borderline between globulins and mucoproteins. Moreover, the phosphoproteins do not have a prosthetic group that can be isolated; they are merely proteins in which some of the hydroxyl groups of serine are phosphorylated (i.e., contain phosphate). Finally, the globulins include proteins with quite different roles—enzymes, antibodies, fibrous proteins, and contractile proteins.

Classification by Biological Functions

In view of the unsatisfactory state of the old classification, it is preferable to classify the proteins according to their biological function. Such a classification is far from ideal, however, because one protein can have more than one function. The contractile protein myosin, for example, also acts as an ATPase (adenosine triphosphatase), an enzyme that hydrolyzes adenosine triphosphate (removes a phosphate group from ATP by introducing a water molecule). Another problem with functional classification is that the definite function of a protein frequently is not known. A protein cannot be called an enzyme as long as its substrate (the specific compound upon which it acts) is not known. It cannot even be tested for its enzymatic action when its substrate is not known.

Special Structure and Function of Proteins

Despite its weaknesses, a functional classification is used here in order to demonstrate, whenever possible, the correlation between the structure and function of a protein. The structural, fibrous proteins are presented first, because their structure is simpler than that of the globular proteins and more clearly related to their function, which is the maintenance of either a rigid or a flexible structure.

Scleroproteins

Collagen

Collagen is the structural protein of bones, tendons, ligaments, and skin. For many years collagen was considered to be insoluble in water. Part of the collagen of calf skin, however, can be extracted with citrate buffer at pH 3.7. A precursor of collagen called procollagen is converted in the body into collagen. Procollagen has a molecular weight of 120,000. Cleavage of one or a few peptide bonds of procollagen yields collagen, which has three subunits, each with a molecular weight of 95,000; therefore, the molecular weight of collagen is 285,000 (3 × 95,000). The three subunits are wound as spirals around an elongated straight axis. The length of each subunit is 2,900 angstroms, and its diameter is approximately 15 angstroms. The three chains are staggered, so that the trimer has no definite terminal limits.

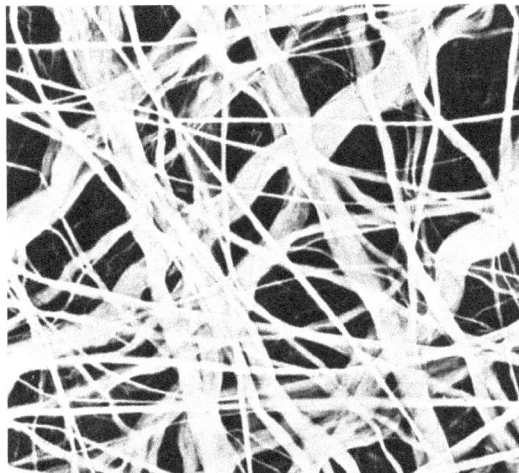

Randomly oriented collagenous fibres of varying size in a thin spread of loose areolar connective tissue (magnified about 370 ×).

Collagen differs from all other proteins in its high content of proline and hydroxyproline. Hydroxyproline does not occur in significant amounts in any other protein except elastin. Most of the proline in collagen is present in the sequence glycine–proline-X, in which X is frequently alanine or hydroxyproline. Collagen does not contain cystine or tryptophan and therefore cannot substitute for other proteins in the diet. The presence of proline causes kinks in the peptide chain and thus reduces the length of the amino acid unit from 3.7 angstroms in the extended chain of the β-structure to 2.86 angstroms in the collagen chain. In the intertwined triple helix, the glycines are inside, close to the axis; the prolines are outside.

Native collagen resists the action of trypsin but is hydrolyzed by the bacterial enzyme collagenase. When collagen is boiled with water, the triple helix is destroyed, and the subunits are partially hydrolyzed; the product is gelatin. The unfolded peptide chains of gelatin trap large amounts of water, resulting in a hydrated molecule.

When collagen is treated with tannic acid or with chromium salts, cross links form between the collagen fibres, and it becomes insoluble; the conversion of hide into leather is based on this tanning process. The tanned material is insoluble in hot water and cannot be converted to gelatin. On exposure to water at 62° to 63 °C (144° to 145 °F), however, the cross links formed by the tanning agents collapse, and the leather contracts irreversibly to about one-third its original volume.

Collagen seems to undergo an aging process in living organisms that may be caused by the formation of cross links between collagen fibres. They are formed by the conversion of some lysine side chains to aldehydes (compounds with the general structure RCHO), and the combination of the aldehydes with the ε-amino groups of intact lysine side chains. The protein elastin, which occurs in the elastic fibres of connective tissue, contains similar cross links and may result from the combination of collagen fibres with other proteins. When cross-linked collagen or elastin is degraded, products of the cross-linked lysine fragments, called desmosins and isodesmosins, are formed.

Keratin

Keratin, the structural protein of epithelial cells in the outermost layers of the skin, has been isolated from hair, nails, hoofs, and feathers. Keratin is completely insoluble in cold or hot water; it is not attacked by proteolytic enzymes (i.e., enzymes that break apart, or lyse, protein molecules), and therefore cannot replace proteins in the diet. The great stability of keratin results from the numerous disulfide bonds of cystine. The amino acid composition of keratin differs from that of collagen. Cystine may account for 24 percent of the total amino acids. The peptide chains of keratin are arranged in approximately equal amounts of antiparallel and parallel pleated sheets, in which the peptide chains are linked to each other by hydrogen bonds between the carbonyl and imino groups.

Reduction of the disulfide bonds to sulfhydryl groups results in dissociation of the peptide chains, the molecular weight of which is 25,000 to 28,000 each. The formation of permanent waves in the beauty treatment of hair is based on partial reduction of the disulfide bonds of hair keratin by thioglycol, or some other mild reducing agent, and subsequent oxidation of the sulfhydryl groups (−SH) in the reoriented hair to disulfide bonds (−S−S−) by exposure to the oxygen of the air.

The length of keratin fibres depends on their water content. They can bind approximately 16 percent of water; this hydration is accompanied by an increase in the length of the fibres of 10 to 12 percent.

The most thoroughly investigated keratin is hair keratin, particularly that of wool. It consists of a mixture of peptides with high and low cystine content. When wool is heated in water to about 90

°C (190 °F), it shrinks irreversibly. This is attributed to the breakage of hydrogen bonds and other noncovalent bonds; disulfide bonds do not seem to be affected.

The most thoroughly investigated scleroprotein has been fibroin, the insoluble material of silk. The raw silk comprising the cocoon of the silkworm consists of two proteins. One, sericin, is soluble in hot water; the other, fibroin, is not. The amino acid composition of the latter differs from that of all other proteins. It contains large amounts of glycine, alanine, tyrosine, and serine; small amounts of the other amino acids; and no sulfur-containing ones. The peptide chains are arranged in antiparallel β-structures. Fibroin is partly soluble in concentrated solutions of lithium thiocyanate or in mixtures of cupric salts and ethylene diamine. Such solutions contain a protein of molecular weight 170,000, which is a dimer of two subunits.

Little is known about either the scleroproteins of the marine sponges or the insoluble proteins of the cellular membranes of animal cells. Some of the membranes are soluble in detergents; others, however, are detergent-insoluble.

Muscle Proteins

The total amount of muscle proteins in mammals, including humans, exceeds that of any other protein. About 40 percent of the body weight of a healthy human adult weighing about 70 kilograms (150 pounds) is muscle, which is composed of about 20 percent muscle protein. Thus, the human body contains about 5 to 6 kilograms (11 to 13 pounds) of muscle protein. An albumin-like fraction of these proteins, originally called myogen, contains various enzymes—phosphorylase, aldolase, glyceraldehyde phosphate dehydrogenase, and others; it does not seem to be involved in contraction. The globulin fraction contains myosin, the contractile protein, which also occurs in blood platelets, small bodies found in blood. Similar contractile substances occur in other contractile structures; for example, in the cilia or flagella (whiplike organs of locomotion) of bacteria and protozoans. In contrast to the scleroproteins, the contractile proteins are soluble in salt solutions and susceptible to enzymatic digestion.

The energy required for muscle contraction is provided by the oxidation of carbohydrates or lipids. The term mechanochemical reaction has been used for this conversion of chemical into mechanical energy. The molecular process underlying the reaction is known to involve the fibrous muscle proteins, the peptide chains of which undergo a change in conformation during contraction.

Myosin, which can be removed from fresh muscle by adding it to a chilled solution of dilute potassium chloride and sodium bicarbonate, is insoluble in water. Myosin, solutions of which are highly viscous, consists of an elongated—probably double-stranded—peptide chain, which is coiled at both ends in such a way that a terminal globule is formed. The length of the molecule is approximately 160 nanometres and its average diameter 2.6 nanometres. The equivalent weight of each of the two terminal globules is approximately 30,000; the molecular weight of myosin is close to 500,000. Trypsin splits myosin into large fragments called meromyosin. Myosin contains many amino acids with positively and negatively charged side chains; they form 18 and 16 percent, respectively, of the total number of amino acids. Myosin catalyzes the hydrolytic cleavage of ATP (adenosine triphosphate). A smaller protein with properties similar to those of myosin is tropomyosin. It has a molecular weight of 70,000 and dimensions of 45 by 2 nanometres. More than 90 percent of its peptide chains are present in the α-helix form.

Myosin combines easily with another muscle protein called actin, the molecular weight of which is about 50,000; it forms 12 to 15 percent of the muscle proteins. Actin can exist in two forms—one, G-actin, is globular; the other, F-actin, is fibrous. Actomyosin is a complex molecule formed by one molecule of myosin and one or two molecules of actin. In muscle, actin and myosin filaments are oriented parallel to each other and to the long axis of the muscle. The actin filaments are linked to each other lengthwise by fine threads called S filaments. During contraction the S filaments shorten, so that the actin filaments slide toward each other, past the myosin filaments, thus causing a shortening of the muscle.

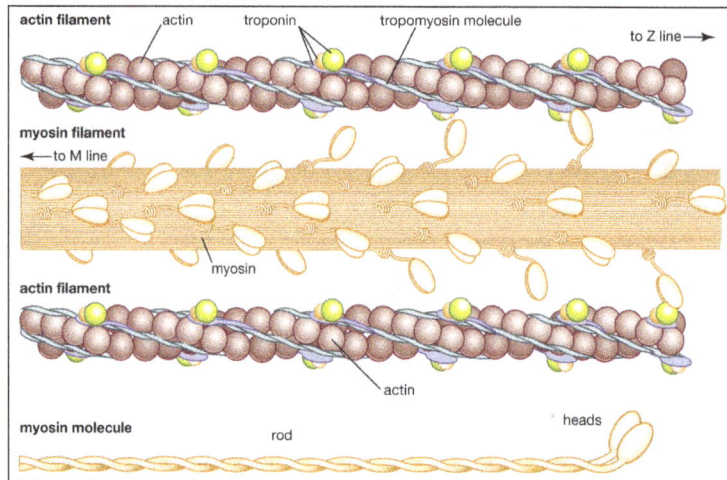

Muscle: The structure of actin and myosin filaments.

Fibrinogen and Fibrin

Fibrinogen, the protein of the blood plasma, is converted into the insoluble protein fibrin during the clotting process. The fibrinogen-free fluid obtained after removal of the clot, called blood serum, is blood plasma minus fibrinogen. The fibrinogen content of the blood plasma is 0.2 to 0.4 percent.

Fibrinogen can be precipitated from the blood plasma by half-saturation with sodium chloride. Fibrinogen solutions are highly viscous and show strong flow birefringence. In electron micrographs the molecules appear as rods with a length of 47.5 nanometres and a diameter of 1.5 nanometres; in addition, two terminal and a central nodule are visible. The molecular weight is 340,000. An unusually high percentage, about 36 percent, of the amino acid side chains are positively or negatively charged.

The clotting process is initiated by the enzyme thrombin, which catalyzes the breakage of a few peptide bonds of fibrinogen; as a result, two small fibrinopeptides with molecular weights of 1,900 and 2,400 are released. The remainder of the fibrinogen molecule, a monomer, is soluble and stable at pH values less than 6 (i.e., in acid solutions). In neutral solution (pH 7) the monomer is converted into a larger molecule, insoluble fibrin; this results from the formation of new peptide bonds. The newly formed peptide bonds form intermolecular and intramolecular cross links, thus giving rise to a large clot, in which all molecules are linked to each other. Clotting, which takes place only in the presence of calcium ions, can be prevented by compounds such as oxalate or citrate, which have a high affinity for calcium ions.

Albumins, Globulins and other Soluble Proteins

The blood plasma, the lymph, and other animal fluids usually contain one to seven grams of protein per 100 millilitres of fluid, which includes small amounts of hundreds of enzymes and a large number of protein hormones.

Proteins of the Blood Serum

Human blood serum contains about 7 percent protein, two-thirds of which is in the albumin fraction; the other third is in the globulin fraction. Electrophoresis of serum reveals a large albumin peak and three smaller globulin peaks, the alpha-, beta-, and gamma-globulins. The amounts of alpha-, beta-, and gamma-globulin in normal human serum are approximately 1.5, 1.9, and 1.1 percent, respectively. Each globulin fraction is a mixture of many different proteins, as has been demonstrated by immunoelectrophoresis. In this method, serum from an animal (e.g., a rabbit) injected with human serum is allowed to diffuse into the four protein bands—albumin, alpha-, beta-, and gamma-globulin—obtained from the electrophoresis of human serum. Because the animal has previously been injected with human serum, its blood contains antibodies (substances formed in response to a foreign substance introduced into the body) against each of the human serum proteins; each antibody combines with the serum protein (antigen) that caused its formation in the animal. The result is the formation of about 20 regions of insoluble antigen-antibody precipitate, which appear as white arcs in the transparent gel of the electrophoresis medium. Each region corresponds to a different human serum protein.

Serum albumin is much less heterogeneous (i.e., contains fewer distinct proteins) than are the globulins; in fact, it is one of the few serum proteins that can be obtained in a crystalline form. Serum albumin combines easily with many acidic dyes (e.g., Congo red and methyl orange); with bilirubin, the yellow bile pigment; and with fatty acids. It seems to act, in living organisms, as a carrier for certain biological substances. Present in blood serum in relatively high concentration, serum albumin also acts as a protective colloid, a protein that stabilizes other proteins. Albumin (molecular weight of 68,000) has a single free sulfhydryl ($-SH$) group, which on oxidation forms a disulfide bond with the sulfhydryl group of another serum albumin molecule, thus forming a dimer. The isoelectric point of serum albumin is pH 4.7.

The alpha-globulin fraction of blood serum is a mixture of several conjugated proteins. The best known are an α-lipoprotein (combination of lipid and protein) and two mucoproteins (combinations of carbohydrate and protein). One mucoprotein is called orosomucoid, or α_1-acid glycoprotein; the other is called haptoglobin because it combines specifically with globin, the protein component of hemoglobin. Haptoglobin contains about 20 percent carbohydrate. The beta-globulin fraction of serum contains, in addition to lipoproteins and mucoproteins, two metal-binding proteins, transferrin and ceruloplasmin, which bind iron and copper, respectively. They are the principal iron and copper carriers of the blood.

The gamma-globulins are the most heterogeneous globulins. Although most have a molecular weight of approximately 150,000, that of some, called macroglobulins, is as high as 800,000. Because typical antibodies are of the same size and exhibit the same electrophoretic behaviour as γ-globulins, they are called immunoglobulins. The designation IgM or gamma M (γM) is used for the macroglobulins; the designation IgG or gamma G (γG) is used for γ–globulins of molecular weight 150,000.

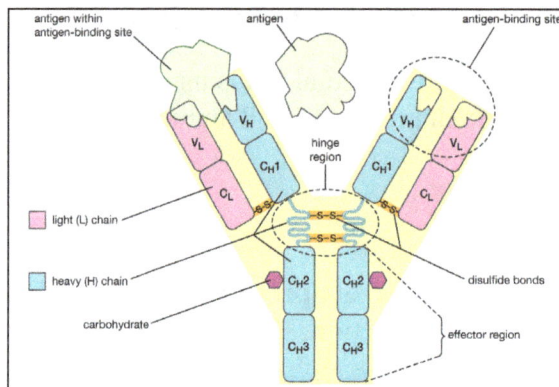

The four-chain structure of an antibody, or immunoglobulin, molecule: The basic unit is composed of two identical light (L) chains and two identical heavy (H) chains, which are held together by disulfide bonds to form a flexible Y shape. Each chain is composed of a variable (V) region and a constant (C) region.

Milk Proteins

Milk contains the following: an albumin, α-lactalbumin; a globulin, beta-lactoglobulin; and a phosphoprotein, casein. If acid is added to milk, casein precipitates. The remaining watery liquid (the supernatant solution), or whey, contains α-lactalbumin and β-lactoglobulin. Both have been obtained in crystalline form; in bovine milk, their molecular weights are approximately 14,000 and 18,400, respectively. Lactoglobulin also occurs as a dimer of molecular weight 37,000. Genetic variations can produce small variations in the amino acid composition of lactoglobulin. The amino acid composition and the tertiary structure of lactalbumin resemble that of lysozyme, an egg protein.

Casein is precipitated not only by the addition of acid but also by the action of the enzyme rennin, which is found in gastric juice. Rennin from calf stomachs is used to precipitate casein, from which cheese is made. Milk fat precipitates with casein; milk sugar, however, remains in the supernatant (whey). Casein is a mixture of several similar phosphoproteins, called α-, β-, γ-, and κ-casein, all of which contain some serine side chains combined with phosphoric acid. Approximately 75 percent of casein is α-casein. Cystine has been found only in κ-casein. In milk, casein seems to form polymeric globules (micelles) with radially arranged monomers, each with a molecular weight of 24,000; the acidic side chains occur predominantly on the surface of the micelle, rather than inside.

Egg Proteins

About 50 percent of the proteins of egg white are composed of ovalbumin, which is easily obtained in crystals. Its molecular weight is 46,000 and its amino acid composition differs from that of serum albumin. Other proteins of egg white are conalbumin, lysozyme, ovoglobulin, ovomucoid, and avidin. Lysozyme is an enzyme that hydrolyzes the carbohydrates found in the capsules certain bacteria secrete around themselves; it causes lysis (disintegration) of the bacteria. The molecular weight of lysozyme is 14,100. Its three-dimensional structure is similar to that of α-lactalbumin, which stimulates the formation of lactose by the enzyme lactose synthetase. Lysozyme has also been found in the urine of patients suffering from leukemia, meningitis, and renal disease.

Avidin is a glycoprotein that combines specifically with biotin, a vitamin. In animals fed large amounts of raw egg white, the action of avidin results in "egg-white injury." The molecular weight of avidin, which forms a tetramer, is 16,200. Its amino acid sequence is known.

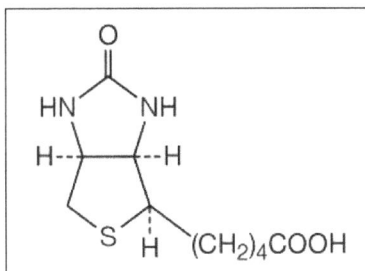

Egg-yolk proteins contain a mixture of lipoproteins and livetins. The latter are similar to serum albumin, α-globulin, and β-globulin. The yolk also contains a phosphoprotein, phosvitin. Phosvitin, which has also been found in fish sperm, has a molecular weight of 40,000 and an unusual amino acid composition; one third of its amino acids are phosphoserine.

Protamines and Histones

Protamines are found in the sperm cells of fish. The most thoroughly investigated protamines are salmine from salmon sperm and clupeine from herring sperm. The protamines are bound to deoxyribonucleic acid (DNA), forming nucleoprotamines. The amino acid composition of the protamines is simple; they contain, in addition to large amounts of arginine, small amounts of five or six other amino acids. The composition of the salmine molecule, for example, is: Arg_{51}, Ala_4, Val_4, Ile_1, Pro_7, and Ser_6, in which the subscript numbers indicate the number of each amino acid in the molecule. Because of the high arginine content, the isoelectric points of the protamines are at pH values of 11 to 12; i.e., the protamines are alkaline. The molecular weights of salmine and clupeine are close to 6,000. All of the protamines investigated thus far are mixtures of several similar proteins.

The histones are less basic than the protamines. They contain high amounts of either lysine or arginine and small amounts of aspartic acid and glutamic acid. Histones occur in combination with DNA as nucleohistones in the nuclei of the body cells of animals and plants, but not in animal sperm. The molecular weights of histones vary from 10,000 to 22,000. In contrast to the protamines, the histones contain most of the 20 amino acids, with the exception of tryptophan and the sulfur-containing ones. Like the protamines, histone preparations are heterogeneous mixtures. The amino acid sequence of some of the histones has been determined.

Plant Proteins

Plant proteins, mostly globulins, have been obtained chiefly from the protein-rich seeds of cereals and legumes. Small amounts of albumins are found in seeds. The best known globulins, insoluble in water, can be extracted from seeds by treatment with 2 to 10 percent solutions of sodium chloride. Many plant globulins have been obtained in crystalline form; they include edestin from hemp, molecular weight 310,000; amandin from almonds, 330,000; concanavalin A (42,000) and B (96,000); and canavalin (113,000) from jack beans. They are polymers of smaller subunits; edestin, for example, is a hexamer of a subunit with a molecular weight of 50,000, and concanavalin B a trimer of a subunit with a molecular weight of 30,000. After extraction of lipids from cereal seeds by ether and alcohol, further extraction with water containing 50 to 80 percent of alcohol yields proteins that are insoluble in water but soluble in water–ethanol mixtures and have been called prolamins. Their solubility in aqueous ethanol may result from their high proline and glutamine content. Gliadin, the prolamin from wheat, contains 14 grams of proline and 46 grams of glutamic acid in 100 grams of protein; most of the glutamic acid is in the form of glutamine. The total amounts of the basic amino acids (arginine, lysine, and histidine) in gliadin are only 5 percent of the weight of gliadin. Because the glysine content is either low or nonexistent, human populations dependent on grain as a sole protein source suffer from lysine deficiency.

Conjugated Proteins

Combination of Proteins with Prosthetic Groups

The link between a protein molecule and its prosthetic group is a covalent bond (an electron-sharing bond) in the glycoproteins, the biliproteins, and some of the heme proteins. In lipoproteins, nucleoproteins, and some heme proteins, the two components are linked by noncovalent bonds; the bonding results from the same forces that are responsible for the tertiary structure of proteins: hydrogen bonds, salt bridges between positively and negatively charged groups, disulfide bonds, and mutual interaction of hydrophobic groups. In the metalloproteins (proteins with a metal element as a prosthetic group), the metal ion usually forms a centre to which various groups are bound.

Mucoproteins and Glycoproteins

The prosthetic groups in mucoproteins and glycoproteins are oligosaccharides (carbohydrates consisting of a small number of simple sugar molecules) usually containing from four to 12 sugar molecules; the most common sugars are galactose, mannose, glucosamine, and galactosamine. Xylose, fucose, glucuronic acid, sialic acid, and other simple sugars sometimes also occur. Some mucoproteins contain 20 percent or more of carbohydrate, usually in several oligosaccharides attached to different parts of the peptide chain. The designation mucoprotein is used for proteins with more than 3 to 4 percent carbohydrate; if the carbohydrate content is less than 3 percent, the protein is sometimes called a glycoprotein or simply a protein.

Mucoproteins, highly viscous proteins originally called mucins, are found in saliva, in gastric juice, and in other animal secretions. Mucoproteins occur in large amounts in cartilage, synovial fluid (the lubricating fluid of joints and tendons), and egg white. The mucoprotein of cartilage is formed by the combination of collagen with chondroitinsulfuric acid, which is a polymer of either glucuronic or iduronic acid and acetylhexosamine or acetylgalactosamine. It is not yet clear whether or not chondroitinsulfate is bound to collagen by covalent bonds.

Lipoproteins and Proteolipids

The bond between the protein and the lipid portion of lipoproteins and proteolipids is a noncovalent one. It is thought that some of the lipid is enclosed in a meshlike arrangement of peptide chains and becomes accessible for reaction only after the unfolding of the chains by denaturing agents. Although lipoproteins in the α- and β-globulin fraction of blood serum are soluble in water (but insoluble in organic solvents), some of the brain lipoproteins, because they have a high lipid content, are soluble in organic solvents; they are called proteolipids. The β-lipoprotein of human blood serum is a macroglobulin with a molecular weight of about 1,300,000, 70 percent of which is lipid; of the lipid, about 30 percent is phospholipid and 40 percent cholesterol and compounds derived from it.

Because of their lipid content, the lipoproteins have the lowest density (mass per unit volume) of all proteins and are usually classified as low- and high-density lipoproteins (LDL and HDL).

Coloured lipoproteins are formed by the combination of protein with carotenoids. Crustacyanin, the pigment of lobsters, crayfish, and other crustaceans, contains astaxanthin, which is a compound derived from carotene. Among the most interesting of the coloured lipoproteins are the pigments of the retina of the eye. They contain retinal, which is a compound derived from carotene and which is formed by the oxidation of vitamin A. In rhodopsin, the red pigment of the retina, the aldehyde group $(-CHO)$ of retinal forms a covalent bond with an amino $(-NH_2)$ group of opsin, the protein carrier. Colour vision is mediated by the presence of several visual pigments in the retina that differ from rhodopsin either in the structure of retinal or in that of the protein carrier.

Metalloproteins

Proteins in which heavy metal ions are bound directly to some of the side chains of histidine, cysteine, or some other amino acid are called metalloproteins. Two metalloproteins, transferrin and ceruloplasmin, occur in the globulin fractions of blood serum; they act as carriers of iron and copper, respectively. Transferrin has a molecular weight of about 80,000 and consists of two identical subunits, each of which contains one ferric ion (Fe^{3+}) that seems to be bound to tyrosine. Several genetic variants of transferrin are known to occur in humans. Another iron protein, ferritin, which contains 20 to 22 percent iron, is the form in which iron is stored in animals; it has been obtained in crystalline form from liver and spleen. A molecule consisting of 20 subunits, its molecular weight is approximately 480,000. The iron can be removed by reduction from the ferric (Fe^{3+}) to the ferrous (Fe^{2+}) state. The iron-free protein, apoferritin, is synthesized in the body before the iron is incorporated.

Green plants and some photosynthetic and nitrogen-fixing bacteria (i.e., bacteria that convert atmospheric nitrogen, N_2, into amino acids and proteins) contain various ferredoxins. They are small proteins containing 50 to 100 amino acids and a chain of iron and disulfide units (FeS_2), in which some of the sulfur atoms are contributed by cysteine; others are sulfide ions (S^{2-}). The number of FeS_2 units per ferredoxin molecule varies from five in the ferredoxin of spinach to 10 in the ferredoxin of certain bacteria. Ferredoxins act as electron carriers in photosynthesis and in nitrogen fixation.

Ceruloplasmin is a copper-containing globulin that has a molecular weight of 151,000; the molecule consists of eight subunits, each containing one copper ion. Ceruloplasmin is the principal carrier of copper in organisms, although copper can also be transported by the iron-containing globulin transferrin. Another copper-containing protein, copper-zinc superoxide dismutase (formerly known as erythrocuprein), has been isolated from red blood cells; it has also been found in the liver and in the brain. The molecule, which consists of two subunits of similar size, contains copper ions and zinc ions. Because of their copper content, ceruloplasmin and copper-zinc superoxide dismutase possess catalytic activity in oxidation-reduction reactions.

Many animal enzymes contain zinc ions, which are usually bound to the sulfur of cysteine. Horse kidneys contain the protein metallothionein, which contain zinc and cadmium; both are bound to sulfur. A vanadium-protein complex (hemovanadin) has been found in surprisingly high amounts in yellowish-green cells (vanadocytes) of tunicates, which are marine invertebrates.

Heme Proteins and other Chromoproteins

Although the heme proteins contain iron, they are usually not classified as metalloproteins, because their prosthetic group is an iron-porphyrin complex in which the iron is bound very firmly. The intense red or brown colour of the heme proteins is not caused by iron but by porphyrin, a complex cyclic structure. All porphyrin compounds absorb light intensely at or close to 410 nanometres. Porphyrin consists of four pyrrole rings (five-membered closed structures containing one nitrogen and four carbon atoms) linked to each other by methine groups ($-CH=$). The iron atom is kept in the centre of the porphyrin ring by interaction with the four nitrogen atoms. The iron atom can combine with two other substituents; in oxyhemoglobin, one substituent is a histidine of the protein carrier, the other is an oxygen molecule. In some heme proteins, the protein is also bound covalently to the side chains of porphyrin. Heme proteins are described below.

The chromoprotein melanin, a pigment found in dark skin, dark hair, and melanotic tumours, occurs in every major group of living organisms and appears to be remarkably diverse in structure. In humans, melanin produced by melanocytes may be dark brown (eumelanin) or pale red or yellowish (phaeomelanin). The different types are synthesized via different pathways, though they share the same initial step—the oxidation of tyrosine.

Green chromoproteins called biliproteins are found in many insects, such as grasshoppers, and also in the eggshells of many birds. The biliproteins are derived from the bile pigment biliverdin, which in turn is formed from porphyrin; biliverdin contains four pyrrole rings and three of the four methine groups of porphyrin. Large amounts of biliproteins have been found in red algae and blue-green algae; the red protein is called phycoerythrin, the blue one phycocyanobilin.

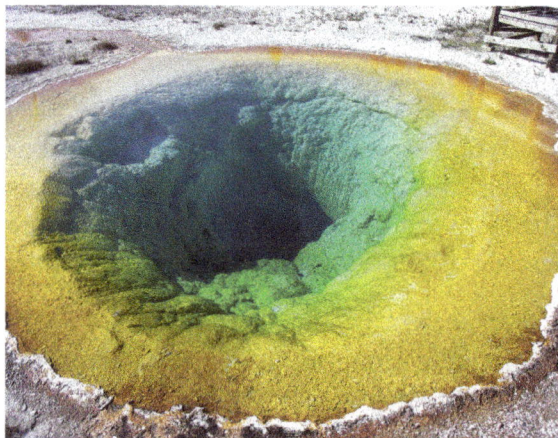

Blue-green algae in Morning Glory Pool, Yellowstone National Park, Wyoming.

Nucleoprotein

When a protein solution is mixed with a solution of a nucleic acid, the phosphoric acid component of the nucleic acid combines with the positively charged ammonium groups ($-NH_3^+$) of the protein to form a protein–nucleic acid complex. The nucleus of a cell contains predominantly deoxyribonucleic acid (DNA) and the cytoplasm predominantly ribonucleic acid (RNA); both parts of the cell also contain protein. Protein–nucleic acid complexes, therefore, form in living cells.

The only nucleoproteins for which some evidence for specificity exists are nucleoprotamines, nucleohistones, and some RNA and DNA viruses. The nucleoprotamines are the form in which protamines occur in the sperm cells of fish; the histones of the thymus and of pea seedlings and other plant material apparently occur predominantly as nucleohistones. Both nucleoprotamines and nucleohistones contain only DNA.

Some of the simplest viruses consist of a specific RNA, which is coated by protein. One of the best known RNA viruses, tobacco mosaic virus (TMV), has the shape of a rod. RNA comprises only 5.1 percent of the mass of the virus. The complete sequence of the virus protein, which consists of about 2,130 identical peptide chains, each containing 158 amino acids, has been determined. The protein is arranged in a spiral around the RNA core.

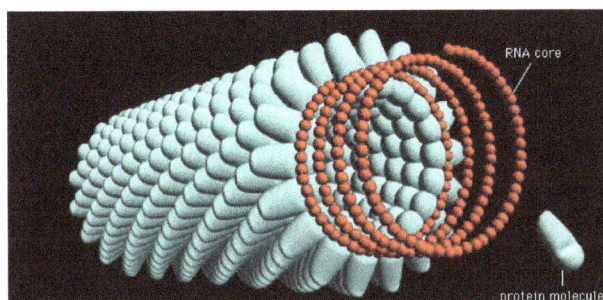

Schematic structure of the tobacco mosaic virus: The cutaway section shows the helical ribonucleic acid associated with protein molecules in a ratio of three nucleotides per protein molecule.

Respiratory Proteins

Hemoglobin

Hemoglobin is the oxygen carrier in all vertebrates and some invertebrates. In oxyhemoglobin (HbO_2), which is bright red, the ferrous ion (Fe^{2+}) is bound to the four nitrogen atoms of porphyrin; the other two substituents are an oxygen molecule and the histidine of globin, the protein component of hemoglobin. Deoxyhemoglobin (deoxy-Hb), as its name implies, is oxyhemoglobin minus oxygen (i.e., reduced hemoglobin); it is purple in colour. Oxidation of the ferrous ion of hemoglobin yields a ferric compound, methemoglobin, sometimes called hemiglobin or ferrihemoglobin. The oxygen of oxyhemoglobin can be displaced by carbon monoxide, for which hemoglobin has a much greater affinity, preventing oxygen from reaching the body tissues.

The hemoglobins of all mammals, birds, and many other vertebrates are tetramers of two α- and two β-chains. The molecular weight of the tetramer is 64,500; the molecular weight of the α- and β-chains is approximately 16,100 each, and the four subunits are linked to each other by noncovalent interactions. If hemin (the ferric porphyrin component) is removed from globin (the protein component), two molecules of globin, each consisting of one α- and one β-chain, are obtained; the molecular weight of globin is 32,200. In contrast to hemoglobin, globin is an unstable protein that is easily denatured. If native globin is incubated with a solution of hemin at pH values of 8 to 9, native hemoglobin is reconstituted. Myoglobin, the red pigment of mammalian muscles, is a monomer with a molecular weight of 16,000.

The mammalian hemoglobins differ from each other in their amino acid composition and therefore in their secondary and tertiary structure. Rat and horse hemoglobins crystallize very easily, but those of humans, cattle, and sheep, because they are more soluble, are difficult to crystallize. The shape of hemoglobin crystals varies in different species; moreover, decomposition and denaturation occur at different rates in different species. It was also found that the blood of human newborns contains two different hemoglobins: about 20 percent of their hemoglobin is an adult hemoglobin (hemoglobin A) and 80 percent is a fetal hemoglobin (hemoglobin F). Hemoglobin F persists in the infant for the first seven months of life. The same hemoglobin F has also been found in the blood of patients suffering from thalassemia, an anemia with a high incidence in regions surrounding the Mediterranean Sea. Hemoglobin F contains, as does hemoglobin A, two α-chains; the two β-chains, however, have been replaced by two quite different γ-chains. When the technique of electrophoresis was first applied to the hemoglobin of blacks suffering from sickle cell anemia in 1949, a new hemoglobin (hemoglobin S) was discovered. More than 200 different human hemoglobins have been discovered since. They differ from normal hemoglobin A in the amino acid composition of either the α- or the β-chain.

The hemoglobins of some of the lowest fishes are monomers containing one iron atom per molecule. Hemoglobin-like respiratory proteins have been found in some invertebrates. The red hemoglobin of insects, mollusks, and protozoans is called erythrocruorin. It differs from vertebrate hemoglobin by its high molecular weight.

Although green plants contain no hemoglobin, a red protein, called leghemoglobin, has been discovered in the root nodules of leguminous plants. It seems to be produced by the nitrogen-fixing bacteria of the root nodules and may be involved in the reduction of atmospheric nitrogen to ammonia and amino acids.

Other Respiratory Proteins

A green respiratory protein, chlorocruorin, has been found in the blood of marine worms in the genera Serpula and Spirographis. It has the same high molecular weight as erythrocruorin but differs from hemoglobin in its prosthetic group. A red metalloprotein, hemerythrin, acts as a respiratory protein in marine worms of the phylum Sipuncula. The molecule consists of eight subunits with a molecular weight of 13,500 each. Hemerythrin contains no porphyrins and therefore is not a heme protein.

A metalloprotein containing copper is the respiratory protein of crustaceans (shrimps, crabs, etc.) and of some gastropods (snails). The protein, called hemocyanin, is pale yellow when not combined with oxygen, and blue when combined with oxygen. The molecular weights of hemocyanins vary from 300,000 to 9,000,000. Each animal investigated thus far apparently has a species-specific hemocyanin.

Protein Hormones

Some hormones that are products of endocrine glands are proteins or peptides, others are steroids. None of the hormones has any enzymatic activity. Each has a target organ in which it elicits some biological action—e.g., secretion of gastric or pancreatic juice, production of milk, production of steroid hormones. The mechanism by which the hormones exert their effects is not fully understood. Cyclic adenosine monophosphate is involved in the transmittance of the hormonal stimulus to the cells whose activity is specifically increased by the hormone.

Hormones of the Thyroid Gland

Thyroglobulin, the active groups of which are two molecules of the iodine-containing compound thyroxine, has a molecular weight of 670,000. Thyroglobulin also contains thyroxine with two and three iodine atoms instead of four and tyrosine with one and two iodine atoms. Injection of the hormone causes an increase in metabolism; lack of it results in a slowdown.

Another hormone, calcitonin, which lowers the calcium level of the blood, occurs in the thyroid gland. The amino acid sequences of calcitonin from pig, beef, and salmon differ from human calcitonin in some amino acids. All of them, however, have the half-cystines (C) and the prolinamide (P) in the same position.

C.S.N.L.S.T.C.V.L.S.A.Y.W.K.D.L.N.N.Y.H.R.F.S.G.M.G.F.G.P.E.T.P.(CONH$_2$)

Parathyroid hormone (parathormone), produced in small glands that are embedded in or lie behind the thyroid gland, is essential for maintaining the calcium level of the blood. A decrease in its production results in hypocalcemia (a reduction of calcium levels in the bloodstream below the normal range). Bovine parathormone has a molecular weight of 8,500; it contains no cystine or cysteine and is rich in aspartic acid, glutamic acid, or their amides.

Hormones of the Pancreas

Although the amino acid structure of insulin has been known since 1949, repeated attempts to synthesize it gave very poor yields because of the failure of the two peptide chains to combine forming the correct disulfide bridge. The ease of the biosynthesis of insulin is explained by the discovery in the pancreas of proinsulin, from which insulin is formed. The single peptide chain of proinsulin loses a peptide consisting of 33 amino acids and called the connecting peptide, or C peptide, during its conversion to insulin. The disulfide bridges of proinsulin connect the A and B chains.

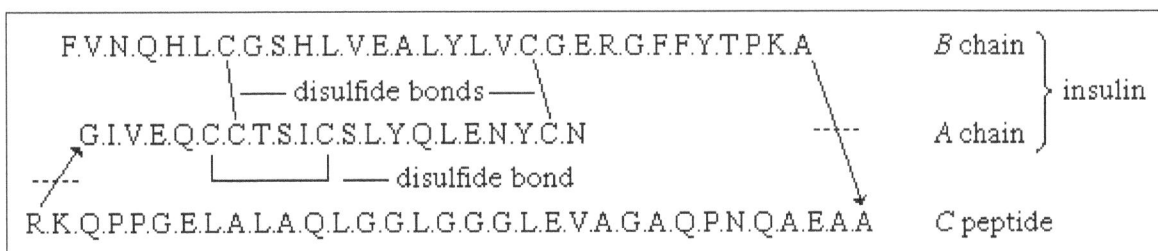

In aqueous solutions, insulin exists predominantly as a complex of six subunits, each of which contains an A and a B chain. The insulins of several species have been isolated and analyzed; their amino acid sequences have been found to differ somewhat, but all apparently contain the same disulfide bridges between the two chains.

Although the injection of insulin lowers the blood sugar, administration of glucagon, another pancreas hormone, raises the blood sugar level. Glucagon consists of a straight peptide chain of 29 amino acids. It has been synthesized; the synthetic product has the full biological activity of natural glucagon. The structure of glucagon is free of cystine and isoleucine.

The pituitary gland has an anterior lobe, a posterior lobe, and an intermediate portion; they differ in cellular structure and in the structure and action of the hormones they form. The posterior lobe produces two similar hormones, oxytocin and vasopressin. The former causes contraction of the pregnant uterus; the latter raises the blood pressure. Both are octapeptides formed by a ring of five amino acids (the two cystine halves count as one amino acid) and a side chain of three amino acids. The two cystine halves are linked to each other by a disulfide bond, and the C terminal amino acid is glycinamide. The structure has been established and confirmed. Human vasopressin differs from oxytocin in that isoleucine is replaced by phenylalanine and leucine by arginine.

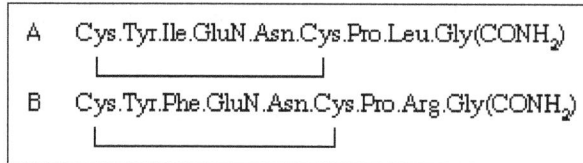

A   Cys.Tyr.Ile.GluN.Asn.Cys.Pro.Leu.Gly(CONH$_2$)

B   Cys.Tyr.Phe.GluN.Asn.Cys.Pro.Arg.Gly(CONH$_2$)

The intermediate part of the pituitary gland produces the melanocyte-stimulating hormone (MSH), which causes expansion of the pigmented melanophores (cells) in the skin of frogs and other batrachians. Two hormones, called α-MSH and β-MSH, have been prepared from hog pituitary glands. The first, α-MSH, consists of 13 amino acids; its N terminal serine is acetylated (i.e., the acetyl group, CH$_3$CO, of acetic acid is attached), and its C terminal valine residue is present as valinamide. The second, β-MSH, contains in its 18 amino acids many of those occurring in α-MSH.

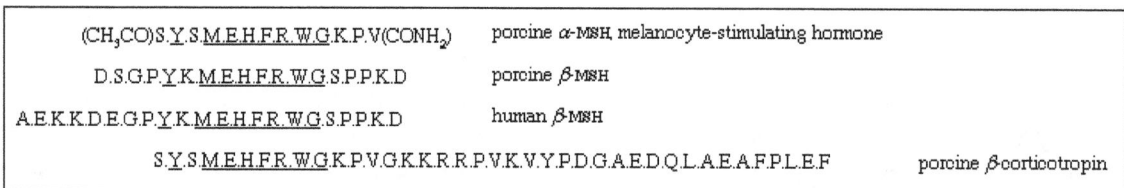

(CH$_3$CO)S.Y.S.M.E.H.F.R.W.G.K.P.V(CONH$_2$)	porcine α-MSH, melanocyte-stimulating hormone
D.S.G.P.Y.K.M.E.H.F.R.W.G.S.P.P.K.D	porcine β-MSH
A.E.K.K.D.E.G.P.Y.K.M.E.H.F.R.W.G.S.P.P.K.D	human β-MSH
S.Y.S.M.E.H.F.R.W.G.K.P.V.G.K.K.R.R.P.V.K.V.Y.P.D.G.A.E.D.Q.L.A.E.A.F.P.L.E.F	porcine β-corticotropin

The anterior pituitary lobe produces several protein hormones—a thyroid-stimulating hormone (thyrotropin), molecular weight 28,000; a lactogenic hormone, molecular weight 22,500; a growth hormone, molecular weight 21,500; a luteinizing hormone, molecular weight 30,000; and a follicle-stimulating hormone, molecular weight 29,000. The thyroid-stimulating hormone consists of α and β subunits with a composition similar to the subunits of luteinizing hormone. When separated, neither of the two subunits has hormonal activity; when combined, however, they regain about 50 percent of the original activity. The lactogenic hormone (prolactin) from sheep pituitary glands contains 190 amino acids. Their sequence has been elucidated; a similar peptide chain of 188 amino acids that has been synthesized not only has 10 percent of the biological activity of the natural hormone but also some activity of the growth hormone. The amino acid sequence of the growth hormone (somatotropic hormone) is also known; it seems to stimulate the synthesis of RNA and in this way to accelerate growth. The luteinizing hormone, a mucoprotein containing about 12 percent carbohydrate, consists of two subunits, each with a molecular weight of approximately 15,000; when separated, the subunits recombine spontaneously. The urine of pregnant women contains chorionic gonadotropin, the presence of which makes possible early diagnosis of pregnancy. The amino acid sequence is known. The sequence of 160 of its 190 amino acids is identical with those of the growth hormone; 100 of these also occur in the same sequence as in lactogenic hormone. The different pituitary hormones and the chorionic gonadotropin thus may have been derived from a common substance that, during evolution, underwent differentiation.

Peptides with Hormonelike Activity

Small peptides have been discovered that, like hormones, act on certain target organs. One peptide, angiotensin (angiotonin or hypertensin), is formed in the blood from angiotensinogen by the action of renin, an enzyme of the kidney. It is an octapeptide and increases blood pressure. Similar peptides include bradykinin, which stimulates smooth muscles; gastrin, which stimulates secretion of hydrochloric acid and pepsin in the stomach; secretin, which stimulates the flow of pancreatic juice; and kallikrein, the activity of which is similar to bradykinin.

Immunoglobulins and Antibodies

Antibodies, proteins that combat foreign substances in the body, are associated with the globulin fraction of the immune serum. when the serum globulins are separated into α-, β-, and γ- fractions, antibodies are associated with the γ-globulins. Antibodies can be purified by precipitation with the antigen (i.e., the foreign substance) that caused their formation, followed by separation of the antigen-antibody complex. Antibodies prepared in this way consist of a mixture of many similar antibody molecules, which differ in molecular weight, amino acid composition, and other properties. The same differences are found in the γ-globulins of normal blood serums. The γ-globulin of normal blood serum is thought to consist of a mixture of hundreds of different γ-globulins, each of which occurs in amounts too small for isolation. Because the physical and chemical properties of normal γ-globulins are the same as those of antibodies, the γ-globulins are frequently called immunoglobulins. They may be considered to be antibodies against unknown antigens. If solutions of γ-globulin are resolved by gel filtration through dextran, the first fraction has a molecular weight of 900,000. This fraction is called IgM or γM; Ig is an abbreviation for immunoglobulin and M for macroglobulin. The next two fractions are IgA (γA) and IgG (γG), with molecular weights of about 320,000 and 150,000 respectively. Two other immunoglobulins, known as IgD and IgE, have also been detected in much smaller amounts in some immune sera.

The bulk of the immunoglobulins is found in the IgG fraction, which also contains most of the antibodies. The IgM molecules are apparently pentamers—aggregates of five of the IgG molecules. Electron microscopy shows their five subunits to be linked to each other by disulfide bonds in the form of a pentagon. The IgA molecules are found principally in milk and in secretions of the intestinal mucosa. Some of them contain, in addition to a dimer of IgG, a "secretory piece" that enables the passage of IgA molecules between tissue and fluid; the structure of the secretory piece is not yet known. The IgM and IgA immunoglobulins and antibodies contain 10 to 15 percent carbohydrate; the carbohydrate content of the IgG molecules is 2 to 3 percent.

IgG molecules treated with the enzyme papain split into three fragments of almost identical molecular weight of 50,000. Two of these, called Fab fragments, are identical; the third is abbreviated Fc. Reduction to sulfhydryl groups of some of the disulfide bonds of IgG results in the formation of two heavy, or H, chains (molecular weight 55,000) and two light, or L, chains (molecular weight 22,000). They are linked by disulfide bonds in the order L−H−H−L. Each H chain contains four intrachain disulfide bonds, and each L chain contains two.

Antibody preparations of the IgG type, even after removal of IgM and IgA antibodies, are heterogeneous. The H and L chains consist of a large number of different L chains and a variety of H chains.

Pure IgG, IgM, and IgA immunoglobulins, however, occur in the blood serum of patients suffering from myelomas, which are malignant tumours of the bone marrow. The tumours produce either an IgG, an IgM, or an IgA protein, but rarely more than one class. A protein called the Bence-Jones protein, which is found in the urine of patients suffering from myeloma tumours, is identical with the L chains of the myeloma protein. Each patient has a different Bence-Jones protein; no two of the more than 100 Bence-Jones proteins that have been analyzed thus far are identical. It is thought that one lymphoid cell among hundreds of thousands becomes malignant and multiplies rapidly, forming the mass of a myeloma tumour that produces one γ-globulin.

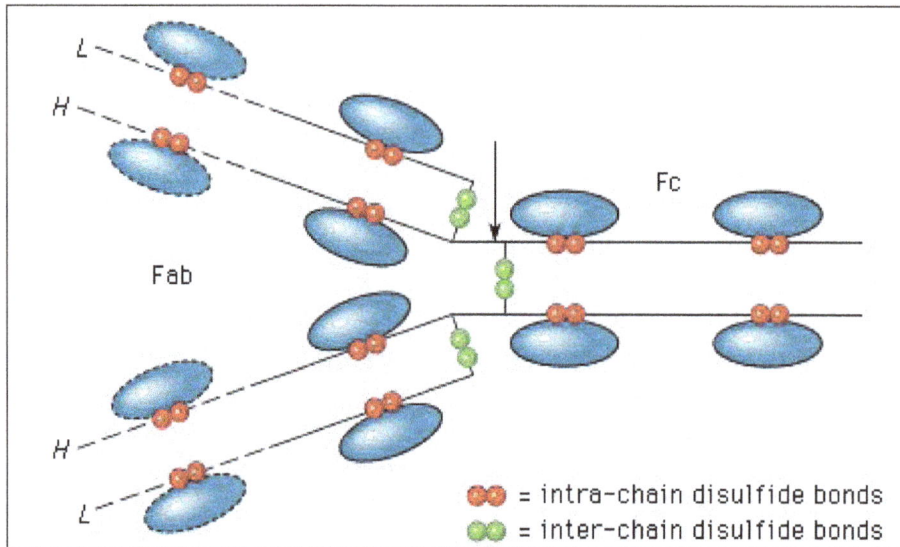

Diagram of an IgG immunoglobulin.

Analyses of the Bence-Jones proteins have revealed that the L chains of humans and other mammals are of two quite different types, kappa (κ) and lambda (λ). Both consist of approximately 220 amino acids. The N–terminal halves of κ- and λ-chains are variable, differing in each Bence-Jones protein. The C–terminal halves of these same L chains have a constant amino acid sequence of either the κ- or the λ-type. The fact that one half of a peptide chain is variable and the other half invariant is contradictory to the view that the amino acid sequence of each peptide chain is determined by one gene. Evidently, two genes, one of them variable, the other invariant, fuse to form the gene for the single peptide chain of the L chains. Whereas the normal human L chains are always mixtures of the κ- and λ-types, the H chains of IgG, IgM, and IgA are different. They have been designated as gamma (γ), mu (μ), and alpha (α) chains, respectively. The N-terminal quarter of the H chains has a variable amino acid sequence; the C-terminal three-quarters of the H chains have a constant amino acid sequence.

Some of the amino acid sequences in the L and H chains are transmitted from generation to generation. As a result, the constant portion of the human L chains of the κ-type has in position 191 either valine or leucine. They correspond to two alleles (character-determining portions) of a gene; the two types are called allotypes. The valine-containing genetic type has been designated as In-V(a⁺), the leucine-containing type as InV(b⁺). Many more allotypes, called Gm allotypes, have been found in the gamma chains of the human IgG immunoglobulins; more than 20 Gm allotypes are known. Certain combinations of Gm types occur. For example, the combination of Gm types 5, 6, and 11 has been found in Caucasians and African Americans but not in Chinese; the combination of 1, 2, and 17 has not been found in African Americans; and the combination of 1, 4, and 17 has not been found in Caucasians. Allotypes have also been discovered to occur in a number of other animals, including rabbits and mice.

It is understandable from the occurrence of a large number of allotypes that antibodies, even if produced in response to a single antigen, are mixtures of different allotypes. The existence of several classes of antibodies, of different allotypes, and of adaptation of the variable portions of antibodies to different regions of an antigen molecule results in a multiplicity of antibody molecules even if only a single antigen is administered. For this reason it has not yet been possible to unravel the amino acid sequence in the variable portion of antibody molecules. Much of the amino acid sequence in the constant regions of the L and H chains of humans and rabbit immunoglobulins, however, has been resolved.

Lipid

Lipids are important molecules that serve different roles in the human body. A common misconception is that fat is simply fattening. However, fat is probably the reason we are all here. Throughout history, there have been many instances when food was scarce. Our ability to store excess caloric energy as fat for future usage allowed us to continue as a species during these times of famine. So, normal fat reserves are a signal that metabolic processes are efficient and a person is healthy.

Lipids are a family of organic compounds that are mostly insoluble in water. Composed of fats and oils, lipids are molecules that yield high energy and have a chemical composition mainly of carbon, hydrogen, and oxygen. Lipids perform three primary biological functions within the body: they serve as structural components of cell membranes, function as energy storehouses, and function as important signaling molecules.

The three main types of lipids are triglycerides, phospholipids, and sterols. Triglycerides make up more than 95 percent of lipids in the diet and are commonly found in fried foods, vegetable oil, butter, whole milk, cheese, cream cheese, and some meats. Naturally occurring triglycerides are found in many foods, including avocados, olives, corn, and nuts. We commonly call the triglycerides in our food "fats" and "oils." Fats are lipids that are solid at room temperature, whereas oils are liquid. As with most fats, triglycerides do not dissolve in water. The terms fats, oils, and triglycerides are discretionary and can be used interchangeably.

Phospholipids make up only about 2 percent of dietary lipids. They are water-soluble and are found in both plants and animals. Phospholipids are crucial for building the protective barrier, or membrane, around your body's cells. In fact, phospholipids are synthesized in the body to form cell and organelle membranes. In blood and body fluids, phospholipids form structures in which fat is enclosed and transported throughout the bloodstream.

Sterols are the least common type of lipid. Cholesterol is perhaps the best well-known sterol. Though cholesterol has a notorious reputation, the body gets only a small amount of its cholesterol through food—the body produces most of it. Cholesterol is an important component of the cell membrane and is required for the synthesis of sex hormones, vitamin D, and bile salts.

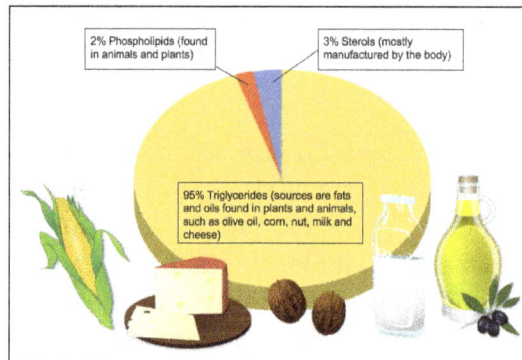

Types of Lipids

Lipoproteins

Lipoproteins are lipid-protein complexes that allow all lipids derived from food or synthesized in specific organs to be transported throughout the body by the circulatory system. The basic structure of these aggregates is that of an oil droplet made up of triglycerides and cholesteryl esters surrounded by a layer of proteins and amphipathic lipids—very similar to that of a micelle. If the concentration of one or another lipoprotein becomes too high, then a fraction of the complex becomes insoluble and is deposited on the walls of arteries and capillaries. This buildup of deposits is called atherosclerosis and ultimately results in blockage of critical arteries to cause a heart attack or stroke.

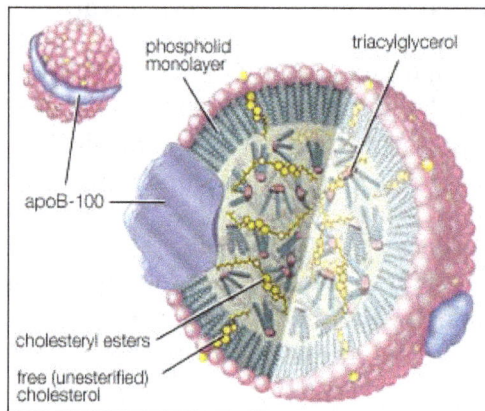

Cutaway view of a low-density lipoprotein (LDL) complex: The LDL complex is essentially a droplet of triacylglycerols and cholesteryl esters encased in a sphere made up of phospholipid, free cholesterol, and protein molecules known as apoprotein B-100 (ApoB-100). The LDL complex is the principal vehicle for delivering cholesterol to body tissues through the blood.

Classification and Formation

There are four major classes of circulating lipoproteins, each with its own characteristic protein and lipid composition. They are chylomicrons, very low-density lipoproteins (VLDL), low-density lipoproteins (LDL), and high-density lipoproteins (HDL). Within all these classes of complexes, the various molecular components are not chemically linked to each other but are simply associated in such a way as to minimize hydrophobic contacts with water. The most distinguishing feature of each class is the relative amounts of lipid and protein. Because the lipid and protein composition is reflected in the density of each lipoprotein (lipid molecules being less dense than proteins), density, an easily measured attribute, forms the operational basis of defining the lipoprotein classes. Measuring density also provides the basis of separating and purifying lipoproteins from plasma for study and diagnosis. The table gives a summary of the characteristics of the lipoprotein classes and shows the correlation between composition and density.

Human plasma lipoproteins					
	chylomicron	VLDL	IDL	LDL	HDL
Density (g/ml)	<0.95	0.950–1.006	1.006–1.019	1.019–1.063	1.063–1.210
Components (% dry weight)					
	2	7	15	20	40–55
Triglycerides	83	50	31	10	8
Free cholesterol	2	7	7	8	4
Cholesteryl esters	3	12	23	42	12–20
Phospholipids	7	20	22	22	22
Apoprotein composition	A-I, A-II, B-48, C-I, C-II, C-III	B-100, C-I, C-II, C-III, E	B-100, C-I, C-II, C-III, E	B-100	A-I, A-II, . C-I, C-II, C-III, D, E

The principal lipid components are triglycerides, cholesterol, cholesteryl esters, and phospholipids. The hydrophobic core of the particle is formed by the triglycerides and cholesteryl esters. The fatty acyl chains of these components are unsaturated, and so the core structure is liquid at body temperature. The table gives more details about the nine different protein components, called apoproteins, of the lipoprotein classes. With the exception of LDL, which contains only one type of apoprotein, all classes have multiple apoprotein components. All the apoproteins, like phospholipids, are amphipathic and interact favourably with both lipids and water. A more-detailed consideration of the character and functions of these lipoprotein particles follows.

Human plasma apolipoproteins		
Apolipoprotein	Molecular weight	Lipoprotein distribution
apoA-I	28,331	HDL
apoA-II	17,380	HDL
apoB-48	241,000	chylomicrons
apoB-100	500,000	VLDL, LDL
apoC-I	7,000	HDL, VLDL
apoC-II	8,837	chylomicrons, VLDL, HDL
apoC-III	8,750	chylomicrons, VLDL, HDL
apoD	33,000	HDL
apoE	34,145	chylomicrons, VLDL, HDL

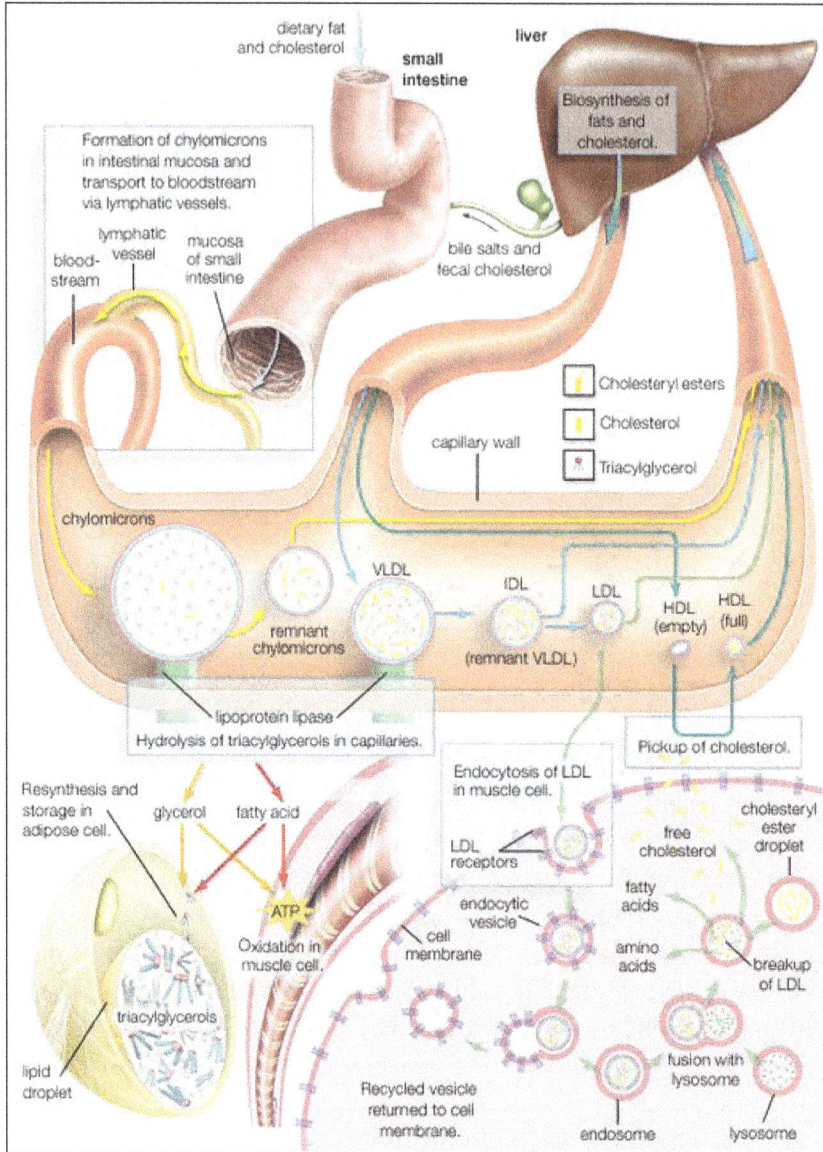

Synthesis of lipoprotein complexes in the small intestine, liver, and blood plasma and their delivery to peripheral tissues of the body.

Chylomicrons

Chylomicrons are the largest lipoproteins, with diameters of 75–600 nanometres (nm; $1\,nm = 10^{-9}$ metre). They have the lowest protein-to-lipid ratio (being about 90 percent lipid) and therefore the lowest density. Chylomicrons are synthesized by the absorptive cells of the intestinal lining and are secreted by these cells into the lymphatic system, which joins the blood circulation at the subclavian vein. The triglyceride, cholesteryl ester, and free cholesterol content of these particles is derived from the digestion of dietary fat. Their primary destinations in peripheral areas are heart muscle, skeletal muscle, adipose tissue, and lactating mammary tissue. The transfer of triglycerides and cholesteryl esters to the tissues depletes the lipid-protein aggregates of these substances and leaves remnant chylomicrons, which are eventually taken up by the liver. The lipid and protein remnants are used to form VLDL and LDL, described below.

Very Low-density Lipoproteins (VLDL)

VLDL is a lipoprotein class synthesized by the liver that is analogous to the chylomicrons secreted by the intestine. Its purpose is also to deliver triglycerides, cholesteryl esters, and cholesterol to peripheral tissues. VLDL is largely depleted of its triglyceride content in these tissues and gives rise to an intermediate-density lipoprotein (IDL) remnant, which is returned to the liver in the bloodstream. As might be expected, the same proteins are present in both VLDL and IDL.

Low-density Lipoproteins (LDL)

Low-density lipoproteins are derived from VLDL and IDL in the plasma and contain a large amount of cholesterol and cholesteryl esters. Their principal role is to deliver these two forms of cholesterol to peripheral tissues. Almost two-thirds of the cholesterol and its esters found in plasma (blood free of red and white cells) is associated with LDL.

High-density Lipoproteins (HDL)

Lipoproteins of this class are the smallest, with a diameter of 10.8 nm and the highest protein-to-lipid ratio. The resulting high density gives this class its name. HDL plays a primary role in the removal of excess cholesterol from cells and returning it to the liver, where it is metabolized to bile acids and salts that are eventually eliminated through the intestine. LDL and HDL together are the major factors in maintaining the cholesterol balance of the body. Because of the high correlation between blood cholesterol levels and atherosclerosis, high ratios of HDL to cholesterol (principally as found in LDL) correlate well with a lower incidence of this disease in humans.

Functions, Origins and Recycling of Apolipoproteins

The nine classes of apoproteins listed in the table are synthesized in the mucosal cells of the intestine and in the liver, with the liver accounting for about 80 percent of production.

Chylomicrons are synthesized in the intestinal mucosa. The cells of this tissue, although able to make most apoproteins, are the principal source of apoB (the B-48 form) and apoA-I. The apoC-II component of chylomicrons is an activator for a plasma enzyme that hydrolyzes the triglyceride of these complexes. This enzyme, called lipoprotein lipase, resides on the cell surface and makes the fatty acids of triglycerides available to the cell for energy metabolism. To some degree, the enzyme is also activated by apoC-II, present in minor amounts in chylomicrons.

VLDL, the lipoprotein carrier for triglycerides synthesized in the liver and destined for use in the heart and muscle, has a complement of five apoproteins. Among them are apoB-100, a protein performing a structural role in the complex, and apoC-I, -II, and -III. The first two of these activate the enzymes lecithin cholesterol acyltransferase (LCAT) and lipoprotein lipase. Curiously, apoC-III, a minor component of both chylomicrons and VLDL, inhibits lipoprotein lipase. Following discharge of the triglycerides, the remnants of VLDL return to the liver.

LDL contains a single apoprotein and is the principal carrier of cholesterol to the peripheral tissue as both the free sterol and esters. The discharge of the lipid contents of this complex requires the recognition of the LDL B-100 apoprotein by a receptor located on the surface of recipient cells. When the protein is bound to the receptor, the receptor-LDL complex is engulfed by the cell in a process known as endocytosis. The endocytosed LDL discharges its contents within the cell, and B-100 is degraded to free amino acids that are used to synthesize new proteins or are metabolized as an energy source.

The primary function of HDL with its complement of apoproteins is to take up cholesterol from the cells of the body and deliver it to the liver for its ultimate excretion as bile acids and salts. The major apoproteins are A-I, an LCAT activator, and A-II. All of the HDL apoproteins have their biosynthetic origin in the liver. When HDL is secreted by this organ, it is a small, flattened discoid devoid of cholesterol but containing phospholipids and the apoproteins. In the peripheral tissues, HDL picks up cholesterol from the surface membranes of cells and, through the agency LCAT, converts it into esters using acyl chains from phosphatidylcholine.

Biological Functions of Lipids

The majority of lipids in biological systems function either as a source of stored metabolic energy or as structural matrices and permeability barriers in biological membranes. Very small amounts of special lipids act as both intracellular messengers and extracellular messengers such as hormones and pheromones. Amphipathic lipids, the molecules that allow membranes to form compartments, must have been among the progenitors of living beings. This theory is supported by studies of several simple, single-cell organisms, in which up to one-third of the genome is thought to code for membrane proteins and the enzymes of membrane lipid biosynthesis.

Cellular Energy Source

Fatty acids that are stored in adipose tissue as triglycerides are a major energy source in higher animals, as is glucose, a simple six-carbon carbohydrate. In healthy, well-fed humans only about 2 percent of the energy is derived from the metabolism of protein. Large amounts of lipids are stored in adipose tissue. In the average American male about 25 percent of body weight is fat, whereas only 1 percent is accounted for by glycogen (a polymer of glucose). In addition, the energy available to the body from oxidative metabolism of 1 gram of triglyceride is more than twice that produced by the oxidation of an equal weight of carbohydrate such as glycogen.

Storage of Triglyceride in Adipose Cells

In higher animals and humans, adipose tissue consisting of adipocytes (fat cells) is widely distributed over the body—mainly under the skin, around deep blood vessels, and in the abdominal cavity and to a lesser degree in association with muscles. Bony fishes have adipose tissue mainly distributed among muscle fibres, but sharks and other cartilaginous fishes store lipids in the liver. The fat stored in adipose tissue arises from the dietary intake of fat or carbohydrate in excess of the energy requirements of the body. A dietary excess of 1 gram of triglyceride is stored as 1 gram of fat, but only about 0.3 gram of dietary excess carbohydrate can be stored as triglyceride. The reverse process, the conversion of excess fat to carbohydrate, is metabolically impossible. In humans, excessive dietary intake can make adipose tissue the largest mass in the body.

Excess triglyceride is delivered to the adipose tissue by lipoproteins in the blood. There the triglycerides are hydrolyzed to free fatty acids and glycerol through the action of the enzyme lipoprotein lipase, which is bound to the external surface of adipose cells. Apoprotein C-II activates this enzyme, as do the quantities of insulin that circulate in the blood following ingestion of food. The liberated free fatty acids are then taken up by the adipose cells and resynthesized into triglycerides, which accumulate in a fat droplet in each cell.

Mobilization of Fatty Acids

In times of stress when the body requires energy, fatty acids are released from adipose cells and mobilized for use. The process begins when levels of glucagon and adrenaline in the blood increase and these hormones bind to specific receptors on the surface of adipose cells. This binding action starts a cascade of reactions in the cell that results in the activation of yet another lipase that hydrolyzes triglyceride in the fat droplet to produce free fatty acids. These fatty acids are released into the circulatory system and delivered to skeletal and heart muscle as well as to the liver. In the blood the fatty acids are bound to a protein called serum albumin; in muscle tissue they are taken up by the cells and oxidized to carbon dioxide (CO_2) and water to produce energy, as described below. It is not clear whether a special transport mechanism is required for enabling free fatty acids to enter cells from the circulation.

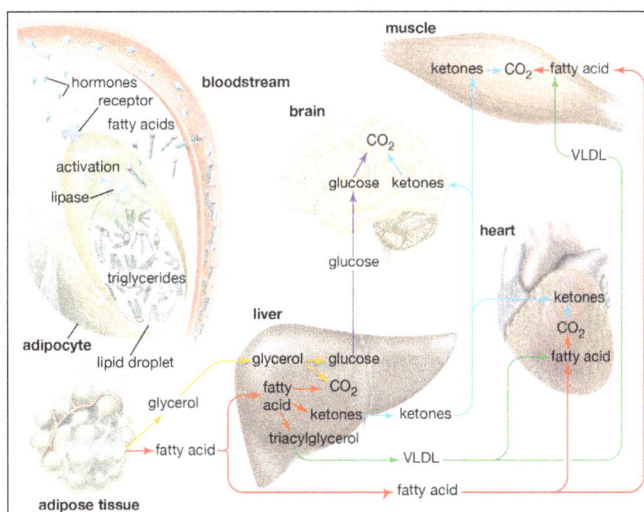

When hormones signal the need for energy, fatty acids and glycerol are released from triglycerides stored in fat cells (adipocytes) and are delivered to organs and tissues in the body.

The liver takes up a large fraction of the fatty acids. There they are in part resynthesized into triglycerides and are transported in VLDL lipoproteins to muscle and other tissues. A fraction is also converted to small ketone molecules that are exported via the circulation to peripheral tissues, where they are metabolized to yield energy.

Oxidation of Fatty Acids

Inside the muscle cell, free fatty acids are converted to a thioester of a molecule called coenzyme A, or CoA. (A thioester is a compound in which the linking oxygen in an ester is replaced by a sulfur atom.) Oxidation of the fatty acid–CoA thioesters actually takes place in discrete vesicular bodies called mitochondria. Most cells contain many mitochondria, each roughly the size of a bacterium, ranging from 0.5 to 10 m (micrometre; 1 m = one-millionth of a metre) in diameter; their size and shape differ depending on the cell type in which they occur. The mitochondrion is surrounded by a double membrane system enclosing a fluid interior space called the matrix. In the matrix are found the enzymes that convert the fatty acid–CoA thioesters into CO_2 and water (the chemical waste products of oxidation) and also adenosine triphosphate (ATP), the energy currency of living systems. The process consists of four sequential steps.

The first step is the transport of the fatty acid across the innermost of the two concentric mitochondrial membranes. The outer membrane is very porous so that the CoA thioesters freely permeate through it. The impermeable inner membrane is a different matter; here the fatty acid chains are transported across in the following way. On the cytoplasmic side of the membrane, an enzyme catalyzes the transfer of the fatty acid from CoA to a molecule of carnitine, a hydroxy amino acid. The carnitine ester is transported across the membrane by a transferase protein located in the membrane, and on the matrix side a second enzyme catalyzes the transfer of the fatty acid from carnitine back to CoA. The carnitine that is re-formed by loss of the attached fatty acid is transferred back to the cytoplasmic side of the mitochondrial membrane to be reused. The transfer of a fatty acid from the cytoplasm to the mitochondrial matrix thus occurs without the transfer of CoA itself from one compartment to the other. No energy is generated or consumed in this transport process, although energy is required for the initial formation of the fatty acid–CoA thioester in the cytoplasm.

The second step is the oxidation of the fatty acid to a set of two-carbon acetate fragments with thioester linkages to CoA. This series of reactions, known as β-oxidation, takes place in the matrix of the mitochondrion. Since most biological fatty acids have an even number of carbons, the number of acetyl-CoA fragments derived from a specific fatty acid is equal to one-half the number of carbons in the acyl chain. For example, palmitic acid (C_{16}) yields eight acetyl-CoA thioesters. In the case of rare unbranched fatty acids with an odd number of carbons, one three-carbon CoA ester is formed as well as the two-carbon acetyl-CoA thioesters. Thus, a C_{17} acid yields seven acetyl and one three-carbon CoA thioester. The energy in the successive oxidation steps is conserved by chemical reduction (the opposite of oxidation) of molecules that can subsequently be used to form ATP. ATP is the common fuel used in all the machinery of the cell (e.g., muscle, nerves, membrane transport systems, and biosynthetic systems for the formation of complex molecules such as DNA and proteins).

The two-carbon residues of acetyl-CoA are oxidized to CO_2 and water, with conservation of chemical energy in the form of $FADH_2$ and NADH and a small amount of ATP. This process is carried out in a series of nine enzymatically catalyzed reactions in the mitochondrial matrix space. The reactions form a closed cycle, often called the citric acid, tricarboxylic acid, or Krebs cycle (after its discoverer, Nobelist Sir Hans Krebs).

The final stage is the conversion of the chemical energy in NADH and $FADH_2$ formed in the second and third steps into ATP by a process known as oxidative phosphorylation. All the participating enzymes are located inside the mitochondrial inner membrane—except one, which is trapped in the space between the inner and outer membranes. In order for the process to produce ATP, the inner membrane must be impermeable to hydrogen ions (H^+). In the course of oxidative phosphorylation, molecules of NADH and $FADH_2$ are subjected to a series of linked oxidation-reduction reactions. NADH and $FADH_2$ are rich in electrons and give up these electrons to the first member of the reaction chain. The electrons then pass down the series of oxidation-reduction reactions and in the last reaction reduce molecular oxygen (O_2) to water (H_2O). This part of oxidative phosphorylation is called electron transport.

The chemical energy available in these electron-transfer reactions is conserved by pumping H^+ across the mitochondrial inner membrane from matrix to cytoplasm. Essentially an electrical battery is created, with the cytoplasm acting as the positive pole and the mitochondrial matrix as the negative pole. The net effect of electron transport is thus to convert the chemical energy of oxidation into the electrical energy of the transmembrane "battery." The energy stored in this battery is in turn used to generate ATP from adenosine diphosphate (ADP) and inorganic phosphate by the action of a complex enzyme called ATP synthase, also located on the inner mitochondrial membrane. Peter Mitchell received the Nobel Prize for Chemistry in 1978 for his discovery of the conversion of electron transport energy into a transmembrane battery and the use of this battery to generate ATP. It is interesting that a similar process forms the basis of photosynthesis—the mechanism by which green plants convert light energy from the Sun into carbohydrates and fats, the basic foods of both plants and animals. Many of the molecular details of the oxidative phosphorylation system are now known, but there is still much to learn about it and the equally complex process of photosynthesis.

The β-oxidation also occurs to a minor extent within small subcellular organelles called peroxisomes in animals and glyoxysomes in plants. In these cases fatty acids are oxidized to CO_2 and water, but the energy is released as heat. The biochemical details and physiological functions of these organelles are not well understood.

Regulation of Fatty Acid Oxidation

The rate of utilization of acetyl-CoA, the product of β-oxidation, and the availability of free fatty acids are the determining factors that control fatty acid oxidation. The concentrations of free fatty acids in the blood are hormone-regulated, with glucagon stimulating and insulin inhibiting fatty acid release from adipose tissue. The utilization in muscle of acetyl-CoA depends upon the activity of the citric acid cycle and oxidative phosphorylation—whose rates in turn reflect the demand for ATP.

In the liver the metabolism of free fatty acids reflects the metabolic state of the animal. In well-fed animals the liver converts excess carbohydrates to fatty acids, whereas in fasting animals fatty acid oxidation is the predominant activity, along with the formation of ketones. Although the details are not completely understood, it is clear that in the liver the metabolism of fatty acids is tightly linked to fatty acid synthesis so that a wasteful closed cycle of fatty acid synthesis from and metabolism back to acetyl-CoA is prevented.

Lipids in Biological Membranes

Biological membranes separate the cell from its environment and compartmentalize the cell interior. The various membranes playing these vital roles are composed of roughly equal weight percent protein and lipid, with carbohydrates constituting less than 10 percent in a few membranes. Although many hundreds of molecular species are present in any one membrane, the general organization of the generic components is known. All the lipids are amphipathic, with their hydrophilic (polar) and hydrophobic (nonpolar) portions located at separate parts of each molecule. As a result, the lipid components of membranes are arranged in what may be called a continuous bimolecular leaflet, or bilayer. The polar portions of the constituent molecules lie in the two bilayer faces, while the nonpolar portions constitute the interior of the bilayer. The lipid bilayer structure forms an impermeable barrier for essential water-soluble substances in the cell and provides the basis for the compartmentalizing function of biological membranes.

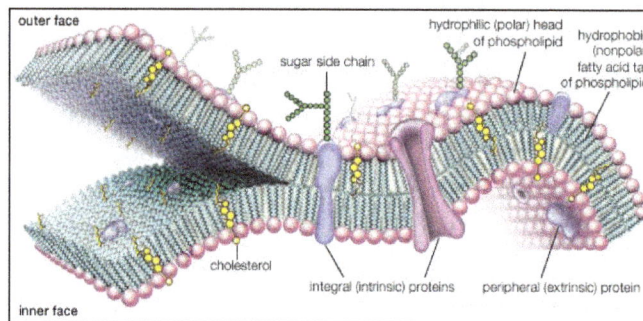

Molecular view of the cell membrane

Intrinsic proteins penetrate and bind tightly to the lipid bilayer, which is made up largely of phospholipids and cholesterol and which typically is between 4 and 10 nanometers (nm; 1 nm = 10^{-9} metre) in thickness. Extrinsic proteins are loosely bound to the hydrophilic (polar) surfaces, which face the watery medium both inside and outside the cell. Some intrinsic proteins present sugar side chains on the cell's outer surface.

Some protein components are inserted into the bilayer, and most span this structure. These so-called integral, or intrinsic, membrane proteins have amino acids with nonpolar side chains at the interface between the protein and the nonpolar central region of the lipid bilayer. A second class of proteins is associated with the polar surfaces of the bilayer and with the intrinsic membrane proteins. The protein components are specific for each type of membrane and determine their predominant physiological functions. The lipid component, apart from its critical barrier function, is for the most part physiologically silent, although derivatives of certain membrane lipids can serve as intracellular messengers.

The most remarkable feature of the general biomembrane structure is that the lipid and the protein components are not covalently bonded to one another or to molecules of the other group. This sheetlike structure, formed only by molecular associations, is less than 10 nm in thickness but many orders of magnitude larger in its other two dimensions. Membranes are surprisingly strong mechanically, yet they exhibit fluidlike properties. Although the surfaces of membranes contain polar units, they act as an electric insulator and can withstand several hundred thousand volts without breakdown. Experimental and theoretical studies have established that the structure and these unusual properties are conferred on biological membranes by the lipid bilayer.

Composition of the Lipid Bilayer

Most biological membranes contain a variety of lipids, including the various glycerophospholipids such as phosphatidyl-choline, -ethanolamine, -serine, -inositol, and -glycerol as well as sphingomyelin and, in some membranes, glycosphingolipids. (These compounds are described in the section Fatty acid derivatives.) Cholesterol, ergosterol, and sitosterol (described in the section Cholesterol and its derivatives) are sterols found in many membranes. The relative amounts of these lipids differ even in the same type of cell in different organisms, as shown in the table on the lipid composition of red blood cell membranes from different mammalian species. Even in a single cell, the lipid compositions of the membrane surrounding the cell (the plasma membrane) and the membranes of the various organelles within the cell (such as the microsomes, mitochondria, and nucleus) are different, as shown in the table on various membranes in a rat liver cell.

Organelle membrane lipid composition by weight percent of rat liver cells					
	membrane				
Lipid	Plasma membrane	Microsome	Inner mitochondria	Outer mitochondria	Nuclear
Cholesterol	28.0	6.0	<1.0	6.0	5.1
Phosphatidylcholine	31.0	55.20	37.9	42.70	58.30
Sphingomyelin	16.6	3.7	00.8	4.1	3.0
Phosphatidylethanolamine	14.3	24.00	38.3	28.60	21.50
Phosphatidylserine	02.7	—	<1.0	<1.00	3.4
Phosphatidylinositol	04.7	7.7	02.0	7.9	8.2
Phosphatidic acid and cardiolipin	01.4	1.5	20.4	8.9	<1.00
Lysophosphatidylcholine	01.3	1.9	00.6	1.7	1.4

Plasma membrane lipid composition by weight percent of mammalian red blood cells						
	Species					
Lipid	Pig	Human	Cat	Rabbit	Horse	Rat
Cholesterol	26.8	26.0	26.8	28.9	24.5	24.7
Phosphatidylcholine	13.9	17.5	18.7	22.3	22.0	31.8
Sphingomyelin	15.8	16.0	16.0	12.5	07.0	08.6
Phosphatidylethanolamine	17.7	16.6	13.6	21.0	12.6	14.4
Phosphatidylserine	10.6	07.9	08.1	08.0	09.4	07.2
Phosphatidylinositol	01.1	01.2	04.5	01.0	<0.2	02.3
Phosphatidic acid	<0.2	00.6	00.5	01.0	<0.2	<0.2
Lysophosphatidylcholine	00.5	00.9	<0.2	<0.2	00.9	02.6
Glycosphingolipids	13.4	11.0	11.9	05.3	23.5	08.3

On the other hand, the lipid compositions of all the cells of a specific type in a specific organism at a given time in its life are identical and thus characteristic. During the life of an organism, there may be changes in the lipid composition of some membranes; the physiological significance of these age-related changes is unknown, however.

Physical Characteristics of Membranes

One of the most surprising characteristics of biological membranes is the fact that both the lipid and the protein molecules, like molecules in any viscous liquid, are constantly in motion. Indeed, the membrane can be considered a two-dimensional liquid in which the protein components ride like boats. However, the lipid molecules in the bilayer must always be oriented with their polar ends at the surface and their nonpolar parts in the central region of the bilayer. The bilayer structure thus has the molecular orientation of a crystal and the fluidity of a liquid. In this liquid-crystalline state, thermal energy causes both lipid and protein molecules to diffuse laterally and also to rotate about an axis perpendicular to the membrane plane. In addition, the lipids occasionally flip from one face of the membrane bilayer to the other and attach and detach from the surface of the bilayer at very slow but measurable rates. Although these latter motions are forbidden to intrinsic proteins, both lipids and proteins can exhibit limited bobbing motions. Within this seemingly random, dynamic mixture of components, however, there is considerable order in the plane of the membrane. This order takes the form of a "fluid mosaic" of molecular association complexes of both lipids and proteins in the membrane plane. The plane of the biological membrane is thus compartmentalized by domain structures much as the three-dimensional space of the cell is compartmentalized by the membranes themselves. The domain mosaics run in size from tens of nanometres (billionths of a metre) to micrometres (millionths of a metre) and are stable over time intervals of nanoseconds to minutes. In addition to this in-plane domain structure, the two lipid monolayers making up the membrane bilayer frequently have different compositions. This asymmetry, combined with the fact that intrinsic membrane proteins do not rotate about an axis in the membrane plane, makes the two halves of the bilayer into separate domains.

An interesting class of proteins is attached to biological membranes by a lipid that is chemically linked to the protein. Many of these proteins are involved in intra- and intercellular signaling. In some cases defects in their structure render the cells cancerous, presumably because growth-limiting signals are blocked by the structural error.

Intracellular and Extracellular Messengers

In multicellular organisms (eukaryotes), the internal mechanisms that control and coordinate basic biochemical reactions are connected to other cells by means of nerves and chemical "messengers." The overall process of receiving these messages and converting the information they contain into metabolic and physiological effects is known as signal transduction. Many of the chemical messengers are lipids and are thus of special interest here. There are several types of external messengers. The first of these are hormones such as insulin and glucagon and the lipids known collectively as steroid hormones. A second class of lipid molecules is eicosanoids, which are produced in tissues and elicit cellular responses close to their site of origin. They are produced in very low levels and are turned over very rapidly (in seconds). Hormones have sites of action that are remote from their cells of origin and remain in the circulation for long periods (minutes to hours).

Steroid Hormones

Lipid hormones invoke changes in gene expression; that is, their action is to turn on or off the instructions issued by deoxyribonucleic acid (DNA) to produce proteins that regulate the biosynthesis of other important proteins. Steroids are carried in the circulation bound singly to specific carrier proteins that target them to the cells in particular organs. After permeating the external membranes of these cells, the steroid interacts with a specific carrier protein in the cytoplasm. This soluble complex migrates into the cell nucleus, where it interacts with the DNA to activate or repress transcription, the first step in protein biosynthesis.

All five major classes of steroid hormones produced from cholesterol contain the characteristic five rings of carbon atoms of the parent molecule. Progestins are a group of steroids that regulate events during pregnancy and are the precursors of the other steroid hormones. The glucocorticoids, cortisol, and corticosterones promote the biosynthesis of glucose and act to suppress inflammation. The mineralocorticoids regulate ion balances between the interior and the exterior of the cell. Androgens regulate male sexual characteristics, and estrogens perform an analogous function in females. The target organs for these hormones are listed in the table.

Organs affected by steroid hormones	
Hormone class	Target organs
Glucocorticoids	Liver, retina, kidney, oviduct, pituitary
Estrogens	Oviduct, liver
Progesterone	Oviduct, uterus
Androgens	Prostate, kidney, oviduct

Eicosanoids

Three types of locally acting signaling molecules are derived biosynthetically from C_{20} polyunsaturated fatty acids, principally arachidonic acid. Twenty-carbon fatty acids are all known collectively as eicosanoic acids. The three chemically similar classes are prostaglandins, thromboxanes, and leukotrienes. The eicosanoids interact with specific cell surface receptors to produce a variety of different effects on different tissues, but generally they cause inflammatory responses and changes in blood pressure, and they also affect the clotting of blood. Little is known about how these effects are produced within the cells of target tissues. However, it is known that aspirin and other anti-inflammatory drugs inhibit either an enzyme in the biosynthesis pathway or the eicosanoid receptor on the cell surface.

Intracellular Second Messengers

With the exception of the steroid hormones, most hormones such as insulin and glucagon interact with a receptor on the cell surface. The activated receptor then generates so-called second messengers within the cell that transmit the information to the biochemical systems whose activities must be altered to produce a particular physiological effect. The magnitude of the end effect is generally proportional to the concentration of the second messengers.

An important intracellular second-messenger signaling system, the phosphatidylinositol system, employs two second-messenger lipids, both of which are derived from phosphatidylinositol. One is diacylglycerol (diglyceride), the other is triphosphoinositol. In this system a membrane receptor acts upon an enzyme, phospholipase C, located on the inner surface of the cell membrane. Activation of this enzyme by one of the agents listed in the table causes the hydrolysis of a minor membrane phospholipid, phosphatidylinositol bisphosphate. Without leaving the membrane bilayer, the diacylglycerol next activates a membrane-bound enzyme, protein kinase C, that in turn catalyzes the addition of phosphate groups to a soluble protein. This soluble protein is the first member of a reaction sequence leading to the appropriate physiological response in the cell. The other hydrolysis product of phospholipase C, triphosphoinositol, causes the release of calcium from intracellular stores. Calcium is required, in addition to triacylglycerol, for the activation of protein kinase C.

Tissue affected by phosphoinositide second-messenger system		
Extracellular signal	Target tissue	Cellular response
Acetylcholine	Pancreas pancreas (islet cells) smooth muscle	Amylase secretion insulin release contraction
Vasopressin	Liver kidney	Glycogenolysis
Thrombin	Blood platelets	Platelet aggregation
Antigens	Lymphoblasts mast cells	DNA synthesis histamine secretion
Growth factors	Fibroblasts	Dna synthesis
Spermatozoa	Eggs (sea urchin)	Fertilization
Light	Photoreceptors (horseshoe crab)	Phototransduction
Thyrotropin-releasing hormone	Pituitary anterior lobe	Prolactin secretion

Vitamin

Vitamins are organic (carbon-containing) nutrients obtained through the diet and essential in small amounts for normal metabolic reactions.

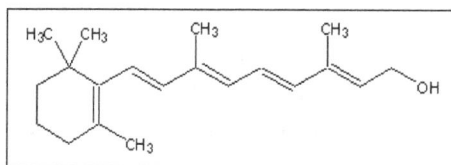

Retinol (Vitamin A)

Vitamins can act both as catalysts and participants in the chemical reaction. A catalyst is a substance that increases the rate of a reaction—by decreasing the activation energy required—without itself being permanently changed at the end of the chemical reaction. The body typically assembles vitamin-dependent catalysts from a variety of building blocks, including amino acids, sugars, phosphates, and vitamins. Each vitamin is typically used in multiple different catalysts and therefore has multiple functions.

Like enzymes, which are also catalysts, vitamins are essential in small quantities. However, enzymes are made by the body, whereas vitamins are normally obtained through the foods that we eat. Vitamins are normally converted in the body to coenzymes. Coenzymes are organic, non-protein molecules that are functional parts of an enzyme, which are generally proteins.

Vitamins show the importance of balance in human life. One can consume animals and drink water to address one's hunger and quench one's thirst. But without balance in one's diet, one will suffer from disease. For example, one needs to consume plants, such as fruits and vegetables, to obtain sufficient amounts of essential vitamin C, as sailors discovered when they failed to take fresh foods on their voyages.

Vitamins can be classified as either water soluble, which means they dissolve easily in water, or fat soluble, which means they are absorbed through the intestinal tract with the help of lipids.

Until the 1900s, vitamins could only be obtained by eating food. However, they are now commercially available. There are a few vitamins that we obtain by other means than directly from the diet: for example, microorganisms in the intestine—commonly known as gut flora—produce vitamin K and biotin, while one form of vitamin D is synthesized in the skin with the help of natural ultraviolet sunlight. Some vitamins can also be obtained from precursors that can be obtained in the diet. Examples include vitamin A, which can be produced from beta carotene and niacin from the amino acid tryptophan.

The term vitamin does not encompass other essential nutrients, such as dietary minerals, essential fatty acids, or essential amino acids, nor is it used for the large number of other nutrients that merely promote health, but are not strictly essential.

Biological Significance of Vitamins

Regulatory Role

The vitamins regulate reactions that occur in metabolism, in contrast to other dietary components known as macronutrients (e.g., fats, carbohydrates, proteins), which are the compounds utilized in the reactions regulated by the vitamins. Absence of a vitamin blocks one or more specific metabolic reactions in a cell and eventually may disrupt the metabolic balance within a cell and in the entire organism as well.

With the exception of vitamin C (ascorbic acid), all of the water-soluble vitamins have a catalytic function; i.e., they act as coenzymes of enzymes that function in energy transfer or in the metabolism of fats, carbohydrates, and proteins. The metabolic importance of the water-soluble vitamins is reflected by their presence in most plant and animal tissues involved in metabolism.

Some of the fat-soluble vitamins form part of the structure of biological membranes or assist in maintaining the integrity (and therefore, indirectly, the function) of membranes. Some fat-soluble vitamins also may function at the genetic level by controlling the synthesis of certain enzymes. Unlike the water-soluble ones, fat-soluble vitamins are necessary for specific functions in highly differentiated and specialized tissues; therefore, their distribution in nature tends to be more selective than that of the water-soluble vitamins.

Vitamins, which are found in all living organisms either because they are synthesized in the organism or are acquired from the environment, are not distributed equally throughout nature. Some are absent from certain tissues or species; for example, beta-carotene, which can be converted to vitamin A, is synthesized in plant tissues but not in animal tissues. On the other hand, vitamins A and D_3 (cholecalciferol) occur only in animal tissues. Both plants and animals are important natural vitamin sources for human beings. Since vitamins are not distributed equally in foodstuffs, the more restricted the diet of an individual, the more likely it is that he will lack adequate amounts of one or more vitamins. Food sources of vitamin D are limited, but it can be synthesized in the skin through ultraviolet radiation (from the Sun); therefore, with adequate exposure to sunlight, the dietary intake of vitamin D is of little significance.

All vitamins can be either synthesized or produced commercially from food sources and are available for human consumption in pharmaceutical preparations. Commercial processing of food (e.g., milling of grains) frequently destroys or removes considerable amounts of vitamins.

In most such instances, however, the vitamins are replaced by chemical methods. Some foods are fortified with vitamins not normally present in them (e.g., vitamin D is added to milk). Loss of vitamins may also occur when food is cooked; for instance, heat destroys vitamin A, and water-soluble vitamins may be extracted from food to water and lost. Certain vitamins (e.g., B vitamins, vitamin K) can be synthesized by microorganisms normally present in the intestines of some animals; however, the microorganisms usually do not supply the host animal with an adequate quantity of a vitamin.

Water-Soluble Vitamins

Basic Properties

Although the vitamins included in this classification are all water-soluble, the degree to which they dissolve in water is variable. This property influences the route of absorption, their excretion, and their degree of tissue storage and distinguishes them from fat-soluble vitamins, which are handled and stored differently by the body. The active forms and the accepted nomenclature of individual vitamins in each vitamin group are given in the table. The water-soluble vitamins are vitamin C (ascorbic acid) and the B vitamins, which include thiamin (vitamin B_1), riboflavin (vitamin B_2), vitamin B_6, niacin (nicotinic acid), vitamin B_{12}, folic acid, pantothenic acid, and biotin. These relatively simple molecules contain the elements carbon, hydrogen, and oxygen; some also contain nitrogen, sulfur, or cobalt.

The water-soluble vitamins, inactive in their so-called free states, must be activated to their coenzyme forms; addition of phosphate groups occurs in the activation of thiamin, riboflavin, and vitamin B_6; a shift in structure activates biotin, and formation of a complex between the free vitamin and parts of other molecules is involved in the activation of niacin, pantothenic acid, folic acid, and vitamin B_{12}. After an active coenzyme is formed, it must combine with the proper protein component (called an apoenzyme) before enzyme-catalyzed reactions can occur.

Functions

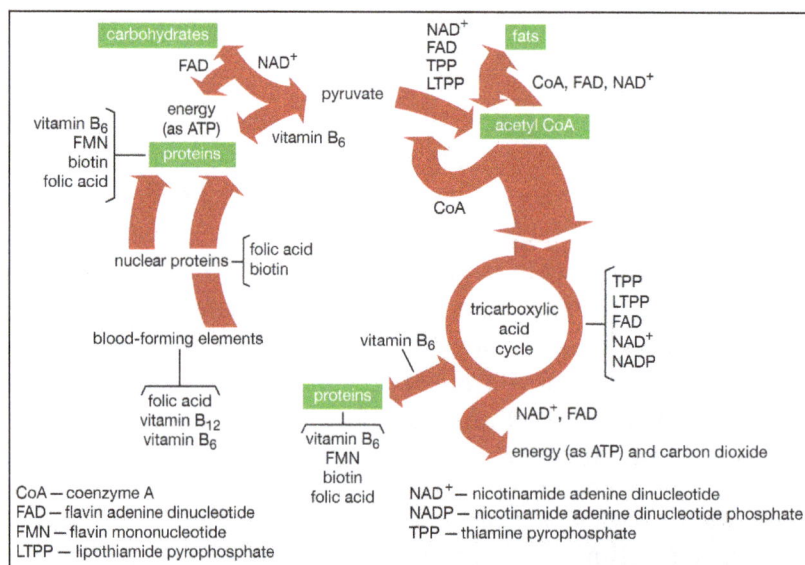

Functions of B-vitamin coenzymes in metabolism.

The B-vitamin coenzymes function in enzyme systems that transfer certain groups between molecules; as a result, specific proteins, fats, and carbohydrates are formed and may be utilized to produce body tissues or to store or release energy. The pantothenic acid coenzyme functions in the tricarboxylic acid cycle (also called the Krebs, or citric acid, cycle), which interconnects carbohydrate, fat, and protein metabolism; this coenzyme (coenzyme A) acts at the hub of these reactions and thus is an important molecule in controlling the interconversion of fats, proteins, and carbohydrates and their conversion into metabolic energy. Thiamin and vitamin B_6 coenzymes control the conversion of carbohydrates and proteins respectively into metabolic energy during the citric acid cycle. Niacin and riboflavin coenzymes facilitate the transfer of hydrogen ions or electrons (negatively charged particles), which occurs during the reactions of the tricarboxylic acid cycle. All of these coenzymes also function in transfer reactions that are involved in the synthesis of structural compounds; these reactions are not part of the tricarboxylic acid cycle.

Although vitamin C participates in some enzyme-catalyzed reactions, it has not yet been established that the vitamin is a coenzyme. Its function probably is related to its properties as a strong reducing agent (i.e., it readily gives electrons to other molecules).

Metabolism

The water-soluble vitamins are absorbed in the animal intestine, pass directly to the blood, and are carried to the tissues in which they will be utilized. Vitamin B_{12} requires a substance known as intrinsic factor in order to be absorbed.

Some of the B vitamins can occur in forms that cannot be used by an animal. Most of the niacin in some cereal grains (wheat, corn, rice, barley, bran), for example, is bound to another substance, forming a complex called niacytin that cannot be absorbed in the animal intestine. Biotin can be bound by the protein avidin, which is found in raw egg white; this complex also cannot be absorbed or broken down by digestive-tract enzymes, and thus the biotin cannot be utilized. In animal products (e.g., meat), biotin, vitamin B_6, and folic acid are bound to other molecules to form complexes or conjugated molecules; although none is active in the complex form, the three vitamins normally are released from the bound forms by the enzymes of the intestinal tract (for biotin and vitamin B_6) or in the tissues (for folic acid) and thus can be utilized. The B vitamins are distributed in most metabolizing tissues of plants and animals.

Water-soluble vitamins usually are excreted in the urine of humans. Thiamin, riboflavin, vitamin B_6, vitamin C, pantothenic acid, and biotin appear in urine as free vitamins (rather than as coenzymes); however, little free niacin is excreted in the urine. Products (also called metabolites) that are formed during the metabolism of thiamin, niacin, and vitamin B_6 also appear in the urine. Urinary metabolites of biotin, riboflavin, and pantothenic acid also are formed. Excretion of these vitamins (or their metabolites) is low when intake is sufficient for proper body function. If intake begins to exceed minimal requirements, excess vitamins are stored in the tissues. Tissue storage capacity is limited, however, and, as the tissues become saturated, the rate of excretion increases sharply. Unlike the other water-soluble vitamins, however, vitamin B_{12} is excreted solely in the feces. Some folic acid and biotin also are normally excreted in this way. Although fecal excretion of water-soluble vitamins (other than vitamin B_{12}, folic acid, and biotin) occurs, their source probably is the intestinal bacteria that synthesize the vitamins, rather than vitamins that have been eaten and utilized by the animal.

The water-soluble vitamins generally are not considered toxic if taken in excessive amounts. There is, however, one exception in humans: large amounts (50–100 mg; 1 mg = 0.001 gram) of niacin produce dilation of blood vessels; in larger amounts, the effects are more serious and may result in impaired liver function. Thiamin given to animals in amounts 100 times the requirement (i.e., about 100 mg) can cause death from respiratory failure. Therapeutic doses (100–500 mg) of thiamin have no known toxic effects in humans (except rare instances of anaphylactic shock in sensitive individuals). There is no known toxicity for any other B vitamins.

Fat-Soluble Vitamins

The four fat-soluble vitamin groups are A, D, E, and K; they are related structurally in that all have as a basic structural unit of the molecule a five-carbon isoprene segment, which is:

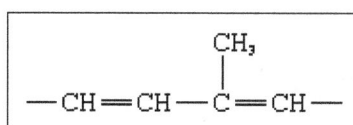

$$-CH=CH-\overset{\overset{\displaystyle CH_3}{|}}{C}=CH-$$

Each of the fat-soluble vitamin groups contains several related compounds that have biological activity. The active forms and the accepted nomenclature of individual vitamins in each vitamin group are given in the table. The potency of the active forms in each vitamin group varies, and not all of the active forms now known are available from dietary sources; i.e., some are produced synthetically.

Chemical Properties

The chemical properties of fat-soluble vitamins determine their biological activities, functions, metabolism, and excretion. However, while the substances in each group of fat-soluble vitamins are related in structure, indicating that they share similar chemical properties, they do have important differences. These differences impart to the vitamins unique qualities, chemical and biological, that affect attributes ranging from the manner in which the vitamins are stored to the species in which they are active.

Vitamin A Group

Ten carotenes, coloured molecules synthesized only in plants, show vitamin A activity; however, only the alpha- and beta-carotenes and cryptoxanthin are important to humans, and beta-carotene is the most active. Retinol (vitamin A alcohol) is considered the primary active form of the vitamin, although retinal, or vitamin A aldehyde, is the form involved in the visual process in the retina of the eye. A metabolite of retinol with high biological activity may be an even more direct active form than retinol. The ester form of retinol is the storage form of vitamin A; presumably, it must be converted to retinol before it is utilized. Retinoic acid is a short-lived product of retinol; only retinoic acid of the vitamin A group is not supplied by the diet.

Vitamin D Group

Although about 10 compounds have vitamin D activity, the two most important ones are ergocalciferol (vitamin D_2) and cholecalciferol (vitamin D_3). Vitamin D_3 represents the dietary source, while vitamin D_2 occurs in yeasts and fungi. Both can be formed from their respective provitamins by ultraviolet irradiation; in humans and other animals the provitamin (7-dehydrocholesterol), which is found in skin, can be converted by sunlight to vitamin D_3 and thus is an important source of the vitamin. Both vitamin D_2 and vitamin D_3 can be utilized by rats and humans; however, chicks cannot use vitamin D_2 effectively. The form of the vitamin probably active in humans is calcitriol.

Vitamin E Group

The tocopherols are a closely related group of biologically active compounds that vary only in number and position of methyl ($-CH_3$) groups in the molecule; however, these structural differences influence the biological activity of the various molecules. The active tocopherols are named in order of their potency; i.e., alpha-tocopherol is the most active. Some metabolites of alpha-tocopherol (such as alpha-tocopherolquinone and alphatocopheronolactone) have activity in some mammals (e.g., rats, rabbits); however, these metabolites do not support all the functions attributed to vitamin E.

Vitamin K Group

Vitamin K_1 (20), or phylloquinone, is synthesized by plants; the members of the vitamin K_2 (30), or menaquinone, series are of microbial origin. Vitamin K_2 (20) is the important form in mammalian tissue; all other forms are converted to K_2 (20) from vitamin K_3 (menadione). Since vitamin K_3 does not accumulate in tissue, it does not furnish any dietary vitamin K.

Functions

The vitamin A group is essential for the maintenance of the linings of the body surfaces (e.g., skin, respiratory tract, cornea), for sperm formation, and for the proper functioning of the immune system. In the retina of the eye, retinal is combined with a protein called opsin; the complex molecules formed as a result of this combination and known as rhodopsin (or visual purple) are involved in dark vision. The vitamin D group is required for growth (especially bone growth or calcification). The vitamin E group also is necessary for normal animal growth; without vitamin E, animals are not fertile and develop abnormalities of the central nervous system, muscles, and organs (especially the liver). The vitamin K group is required for normal metabolism, including the conversion of food into cellular energy in certain biological membranes; vitamin K also is necessary for the proper clotting of blood.

Mineral

Mineral nutrients (also called dietary elements and dietary minerals) are inorganic substances that are essential for life. While they're often referred to as minerals, mineral nutrients are correctly classified as elements. All living cells and organisms require these elements in addition to the four basic elements oxygen, hydrogen, nitrogen, and carbon. Minerals are classified into two groups: Major Minerals and Trace Minerals.

Major Minerals

Major minerals are classified as minerals that are required in the diet each day in amounts larger than 100 milligrams. These include sodium, potassium, chloride, calcium, phosphorus, magnesium, and sulfur. These major minerals can be found in various foods. For example, in Guam, the major mineral, calcium, is consumed in the diet not only through dairy, a common source of calcium, but also through through the mixed dishes, desserts and vegetables that they consume. Consuming a varied diet significantly improves an individual's ability to meet their nutrient needs.

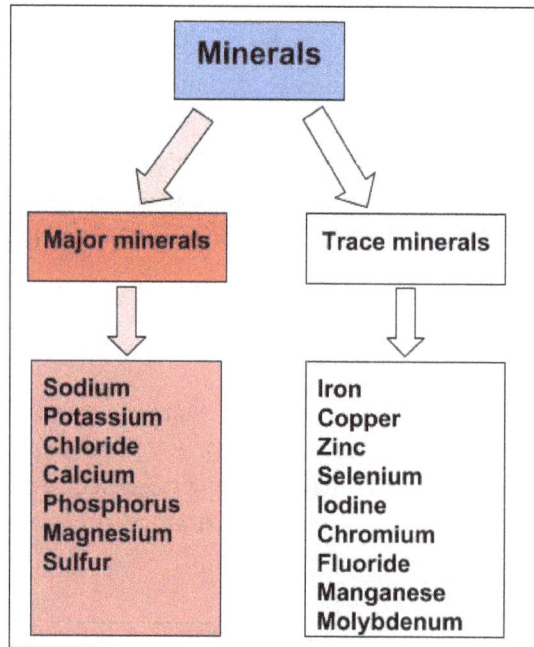

The Major Minerals

Bioavailability

Minerals are not as efficiently absorbed as most vitamins and so the bioavailability of minerals can be very low. Plant-based foods often contain factors, such as oxalate and phytate, that bind to minerals and inhibit their absorption. In general, minerals are better absorbed from animal-based foods. In most cases, if dietary intake of a particular mineral is increased, absorption will decrease. Some minerals influence the absorption of others. For instance, excess zinc in the diet can impair iron and copper absorption. Conversely, certain vitamins enhance mineral absorption. For example, vitamin C boosts iron absorption, and vitamin D boosts calcium and magnesium absorption. As is the case with vitamins, certain gastrointestinal disorders and diseases, such as Crohn's disease and kidney disease, as well as the aging process, impair mineral absorption, putting people with malabsorption conditions and the elderly at higher risk for mineral deficiencies.

Calcium

Calcium's Functional Roles

Calcium is the most abundant mineral in the body and greater than 99 percent of it is stored in bone tissue. Although only 1 percent of the calcium in the human body is found in the blood and soft tissues, it is here that it performs the most critical functions. Blood calcium levels are rigorously controlled so that if blood levels drop the body will rapidly respond by stimulating bone resorption, thereby releasing stored calcium into the blood. Thus, bone tissue sacrifices its stored calcium to maintain blood calcium levels. This is why bone health is dependent on the intake of dietary calcium and also why blood levels of calcium do not always correspond to dietary intake.

Calcium plays a role in a number of different functions in the body like bone and tooth formation. The most well-known calcium function is to build and strengthen bones and teeth. Recall that when bone tissue first forms during the modeling or remodeling process, it is unhardened, protein-rich osteoid tissue. In the osteoblast-directed process of bone mineralization, calcium phosphates (salts) are deposited on the protein matrix. The calcium salts typically make up about 65 percent of bone tissue. When your diet is calcium deficient, the mineral content of bone decreases causing it to become brittle and weak. Thus, increased calcium intake helps to increase the mineralized content of bone tissue. Greater mineralized bone tissue corresponds to a greater BMD, and to greater bone strength. The remaining calcium plays a role in nerve impulse transmission by facilitating electrical impulse transmission from one nerve cell to another. Calcium in muscle cells is essential for muscle contraction because the flow of calcium ions are needed for the muscle proteins (actin and myosin) to interact. Calcium is also essential in blood clotting by activating clotting factors to fix damaged tissue.

In addition to calcium's four primary functions calcium has several other minor functions that are also critical for maintaining normal physiology. For example, without calcium, the hormone insulin could not be released from cells in the pancreas and glycogen could not be broken down in muscle cells and used to provide energy for muscle contraction.

Maintaining Calcium Levels

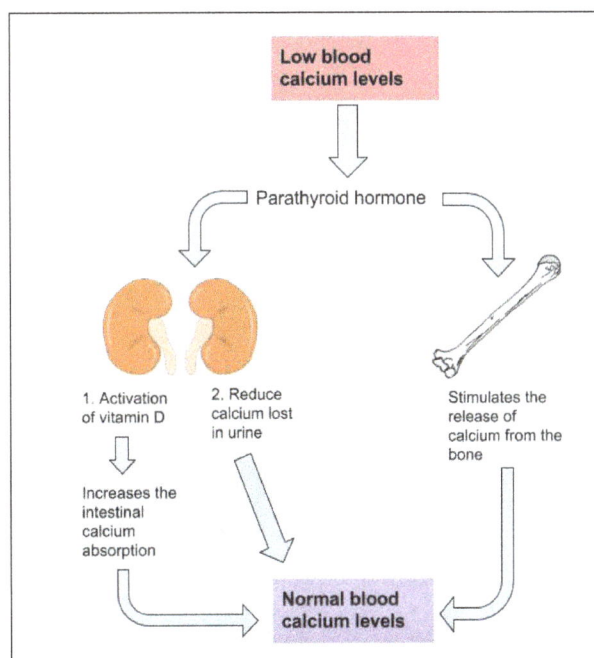

Maintaining Blood Calcium Levels

Because calcium performs such vital functions in the body, blood calcium level is closely regulated by the hormones parathyroid hormone (PTH), calcitriol, and calcitonin. When blood calcium levels are low, PTH is secreted to increase blood calcium levels via three different mechanisms. First, PTH stimulates the release of calcium stored in the bone. Second, PTH acts on kidney cells to increase calcium reabsorption and decrease its excretion in the urine. Third, PTH stimulates enzymes in the kidney that activate vitamin D to calcitriol. Calcitriol is the active hormone that acts on the intestinal cells and increases dietary calcium absorption. When blood calcium levels become too high, the hormone calcitonin is secreted by certain cells in the thyroid gland and PTH secretion stops. At higher nonphysiological concentrations, calcitonin lowers blood calcium levels by increasing calcium excretion in the urine, preventing further absorption of calcium in the gut and by directly inhibiting bone resorption.

Other Health Benefits of Calcium in the Body

Besides forming and maintaining strong bones and teeth, calcium has been shown to have other health benefits for the body, including:

- Cancer: The National Cancer Institute reports that there is enough scientific evidence to conclude that higher intakes of calcium decrease colon cancer risk and may suppress the growth of polyps that often precipitate cancer. Although higher calcium consumption protects against colon cancer, some studies have looked at the relationship between calcium and prostate cancer and found higher intakes may increase the risk for prostate cancer; however the data is inconsistent and more studies are needed to confirm any negative association.

- Blood pressure: Multiple studies provide clear evidence that higher calcium consumption reduces blood pressure. A review of twenty-three observational studies concluded that for every 100 milligrams of calcium consumed daily, systolic blood pressure is reduced 0.34 millimeters of mercury (mmHg) and diastolic blood pressure is decreased by 0.15 mmHg.

- Cardiovascular health: There is emerging evidence that higher calcium intakes prevent against other risk factors for cardiovascular disease, such as high cholesterol and obesity, but the scientific evidence is weak or inconclusive.

Calcium's Effect on Aging.

- Kidney stones: Another health benefit of a high-calcium diet is that it blocks kidney stone formation. Calcium inhibits the absorption of oxalate, a chemical in plants such as parsley and spinach, which is associated with an increased risk for developing kidney stones. Calcium's protective effects on kidney stone formation occur only when you obtain calcium from dietary sources. Calcium supplements may actually increase the risk for kidney stones in susceptible people.

Calcium inadequacy is most prevalent in adolescent girls and the elderly. Proper dietary intake of calcium is critical for proper bone health.

Despite the wealth of evidence supporting the many health benefits of calcium (particularly bone health), the average American diet falls short of achieving the recommended dietary intakes of calcium. In fact, in females older than nine years of age, the average daily intake of calcium is only about 70 percent of the recommended intake. Here we will take a closer look at particular groups of people who may require extra calcium intake.

- Adolescent teens: A calcium-deficient diet is common in teenage girls as their dairy consumption often considerably drops during adolescence.

- Amenorrheic women and the "female athlete triad": Amenorrhea refers to the absence of a menstrual cycle. Women who fail to menstruate suffer from reduced estrogen levels, which can disrupt and have a negative impact on the calcium balance in their bodies. The "female athlete triad" is a combination of three conditions characterized by amenorrhea, disrupted eating patterns, and osteoporosis. Exercise-induced amenorrhea and anorexia nervosa-related amenorrhea can decrease bone mass. In female athletes, as well as active women in the military, low BMD, menstrual irregularities, and individual dietary habits together with a history of previous stress issues are related to an increased susceptibility to future stress fractures.

- The elderly: As people age, calcium bioavailability is reduced, the kidneys lose their capacity to convert vitamin D to its most active form, the kidneys are no longer efficient in retaining calcium, the skin is less effective at synthesizing vitamin D, there are changes in overall dietary patterns, and older people tend to get less exposure to sunlight. Thus the risk for calcium inadequacy is great.

- Postmenopausal women: Estrogen enhances calcium absorption. The decline in this hormone during and after menopause puts postmenopausal women especially at risk for calcium deficiency. Decreases in estrogen production are responsible for an increase in bone resorption and a decrease in calcium absorption. During the first years of menopause, annual decreases in bone mass range from 3–5 percent. After age sixty-five, decreases are typically less than 1 percent.

- Lactose-intolerant people: Groups of people, such as those who are lactose intolerant, or who adhere to diets that avoid dairy products, may not have an adequate calcium intake.

- Vegans: Vegans typically absorb reduced amounts of calcium because their diets favor plant-based foods that contain oxalates and phytates.

In addition, because vegans avoid dairy products, their overall consumption of calcium-rich foods may be less.

If you are lactose intolerant, have a milk allergy, are a vegan, or you simply do not like dairy products, remember that there are many plant-based foods that have a good amount of calcium and there are also some low-lactose and lactose-free dairy products on the market.

Calcium Supplements: Which One to Buy?

Many people choose to fulfill their daily calcium requirements by taking calcium supplements. Calcium supplements are sold primarily as calcium carbonate, calcium citrate, calcium lactate, and calcium phosphate, with elemental calcium contents of about 200 milligrams per pill. It is important to note that calcium carbonate requires an acidic environment in the stomach to be used effectively. Although this is not a problem for most people, it may be for those on medication to reduce stomach-acid production or for the elderly who may have a reduced ability to secrete acid in the stomach. For these people, calcium citrate may be a better choice. Otherwise, calcium carbonate is the cheapest. The body is capable of absorbing approximately 30 percent of the calcium from these forms.

Beware of Lead

There is public health concern about the lead content of some brands of calcium supplements, as supplements derived from natural sources such as oyster shell, bone meal, and dolomite (a type of rock containing calcium magnesium carbonate) are known to contain high amounts of lead. In one study conducted on twenty-two brands of calcium supplements, it was proven that eight of the brands exceeded the acceptable limit for lead content. This was found to be the case in supplements derived from oyster shell and refined calcium carbonate. The same study also found that brands claiming to be lead-free did, in fact, show very low lead levels. Because lead levels in supplements are not disclosed on labels, it is important to know that products not derived from oyster shell or other natural substances are generally low in lead content. In addition, it was also found that one brand did not disintegrate as is necessary for absorption, and one brand contained only 77 percent of the stated calcium content.

Diet, Supplements and Chelated Supplements

In general, calcium supplements perform to a lesser degree than dietary sources of calcium in providing many of the health benefits linked to higher calcium intake. This is partly attributed to the fact that dietary sources of calcium supply additional nutrients with health-promoting activities. It is reported that chelated forms of calcium supplements are easier to absorb as the chelation process protects the calcium from oxalates and phytates that may bind with the calcium in the intestines. However, these are more expensive supplements and only increase calcium absorption up to 10 percent. In people with low dietary intakes of calcium, calcium supplements have a negligible benefit on bone health in the absence of a vitamin D supplement. However, when calcium supplements are taken along with vitamin D, there are many benefits to bone health: peak bone mass is increased in early adulthood, BMD is maintained throughout adulthood, the risk of developing osteoporosis is reduced, and the incidence of fractures is decreased in those who already had osteoporosis. Calcium and vitamin D pills do not have to be taken at the same time for effectiveness.

But remember that vitamin D has to be activated and in the bloodstream to promote calcium absorption. Thus, it is important to maintain an adequate intake of vitamin D.

Calcium Debate

A recent study published in the British Medical Journal reported that people who take calcium supplements at doses equal to or greater than 500 milligrams per day in the absence of a vitamin D supplement had a 30 percent greater risk for having a heart attack.

Does this mean that calcium supplements are bad for you? If you look more closely at the study, you will find that 5.8 percent of people (143 people) who took calcium supplements had a heart attack, but so did 5.5 percent of the people (111) people who took the placebo. While this is one study, several other large studies have not shown that calcium supplementation increases the risk for cardiovascular disease. While the debate over this continues in the realm of science, we should focus on the things we do know:

- There is overwhelming evidence that diets sufficient in calcium prevent osteoporosis and cardiovascular disease.

- People with risk factors for osteoporosis are advised to take calcium supplements if they are unable to get enough calcium in their diet. The National Osteoporosis Foundation advises that adults age fifty and above consume 1,200 milligrams of calcium per day. This includes calcium both from dietary sources and supplements.

- Consuming more calcium than is recommended is not better for your health and can prove to be detrimental. Consuming too much calcium at any one time, be it from diet or supplements, impairs not only the absorption of calcium itself, but also the absorption of other essential minerals, such as iron and zinc. Since the GI tract can only handle about 500 milligrams of calcium at one time, it is recommended to have split doses of calcium supplements rather than taking a few all at once to get the RDA of calcium.

Dietary Reference Intake for Calcium

The recommended dietary allowances (RDA) for calcium are listed in Table "Dietary Reference Intakes for Calcium". The RDA is elevated to 1,300 milligrams per day during adolescence because this is the life stage with accelerated bone growth. Studies have shown that a higher intake of calcium during puberty increases the total amount of bone tissue that accumulates in a person. For women above age fifty and men older than seventy-one, the RDAs are also a bit higher for several reasons including that as we age, calcium absorption in the gut decreases, vitamin D3 activation is reduced, and maintaining adequate blood levels of calcium is important to prevent an acceleration of bone tissue loss (especially during menopause). Currently, the dietary intake of calcium for females above age nine is, on average, below the RDA for calcium. The Institute of Medicine (IOM) recommends that people do not consume over 2,500 milligrams per day of calcium as it may cause adverse effects in some people.

Age Group	RDA (mg/day)	UL (mg/day)
Infants (0–6 months)	200	–
Infants (6–12 months)	260	–

Children (1–3 years)	700	2,500
Children (4–8 years)	1,000	2,500
Children (9–13 years)	1,300	2,500
Adolescents (14–18 years)	1,300	2,500
Adults (19–50 years)	1,000	2,500
Adult females (50–71 years)	1,200	2,500
Adults, male & female (> 71 years)	1,200	2,500

Dietary Sources of Calcium

In the typical American diet, calcium is obtained mostly from dairy products, primarily cheese. A slice of cheddar or Swiss cheese contains just over 200 milligrams of calcium. One cup of non-fat milk contains approximately 300 milligrams of calcium, which is about a third of the RDA for calcium for most adults. Foods fortified with calcium such as cereals, soy milk, and orange juice also provide one third or greater of the calcium RDA. Although the typical American diet relies mostly on dairy products for obtaining calcium, there are other good non-dairy sources of calcium.

Food	Serving	Calcium (mg)	Percent Daily Value
Yogurt, low fat	8 oz.	415	42
Mozzarella	1.5 oz.	333	33
Sardines, canned with bones	3 oz.	325	33
Cheddar Cheese	1.5 oz.	307	31
Milk, nonfat	8 oz.	299	30
Soymilk, calcium fortified	8 oz.	299	30
Orange juice, calcium fortified	6 oz.	261	26
Tofu, firm, made with calcium sulfate	½ c.	253	25
Salmon, canned with bones	3 oz.	181	18
Turnip, boiled	½ c.	99	10
Kale, cooked	1 c.	94	9
Vanilla Ice Cream	½ c.	84	8
White bread	1 slice	73	7
Kale, raw	1 c.	24	2
Broccoli, raw	½ c.	21	2

Calcium Bioavailability

In the small intestine, calcium absorption primarily takes place in the duodenum (first section of the small intestine) when intakes are low, but calcium is also absorbed passively in the jejunum and ileum (second and third sections of the small intestine), especially when intakes are higher. The body doesn't completely absorb all the calcium in food. Interestingly, the calcium in some vegetables such as kale, brussel sprouts, and bok choy is better absorbed by the body than are dairy products. About 30 percent of calcium is absorbed from milk and other dairy products.

The greatest positive influence on calcium absorption comes from having an adequate intake of vitamin D. People deficient in vitamin D absorb less than 15 percent of calcium from the foods they eat. The hormone estrogen is another factor that enhances calcium bioavailability. Thus, as a woman ages and goes through menopause, during which estrogen levels fall, the amount of calcium absorbed decreases and the risk for bone disease increases. Some fibers, such as inulin, found in jicama, onions, and garlic, also promote calcium intestinal uptake.

Chemicals that bind to calcium decrease its bioavailability. These negative effectors of calcium absorption include the oxalates in certain plants, the tannins in tea, phytates in nuts, seeds, and grains, and some fibers. Oxalates are found in high concentrations in spinach, parsley, cocoa, and beets. In general, the calcium bioavailability is inversely correlated to the oxalate content in foods. High-fiber, low-fat diets also decrease the amount of calcium absorbed, an effect likely related to how fiber and fat influence the amount of time food stays in the gut. Anything that causes diarrhea, including sickness, medications, and certain symptoms related to old age, decreases the transit time of calcium in the gut and therefore decreases calcium absorption. As we get older, stomach acidity sometimes decreases, diarrhea occurs more often, kidney function is impaired, and vitamin D absorption and activation is compromised, all of which contribute to a decrease in calcium bioavailability.

Phosphorus

Phosphorus's Functional Role

Phosphorus is present in our bodies as part of a chemical group called a phosphate group. These phosphate groups are essential as a structural component of cell membranes (as phospholipids), DNA and RNA, energy production (ATP), and regulation of acid-base homeostasis. Phosphorus however is mostly associated with calcium as a part of the mineral structure of bones and teeth. Blood phosphorus levels are not controlled as strictly as calcium so the PTH stimulates renal excretion of phosphate so that it does not accumulate to toxic levels.

Dietary Sources of Phosphorus

Table: Phosphorus Content of Various Foods.

Foods	Serving	Phosphorus (mg)	Percent Daily Value 1000
Salmon	3 oz.	315	32
Yogurt, non-fat	8 oz.	306	31
Turkey, light meat	3 oz.	217	22
Chicken, light meat	3 oz.	135	14
Beef	3 oz.	179	18
Lentils	½ c.	178	18
Almonds	1 oz.	136	14

Mozzarella	1 oz.	131	13
Peanuts*	1 oz.	108	11
Whole wheat bread	1 slice	68	7
Egg	1 large	86	9
Carbonated cola drink	12 oz.	41	4
Bread, enriched	1 slice	25	3

Sulfur

Sulfur is incorporated into protein structures in the body. Amino acids, methionine and cysteine contain sulfur which are essential for the antioxidant enzyme glutathione peroxidase. Some vitamins like thiamin and biotin also contain sulfur which are important in regulating acidity in the body. Sulfur is a major mineral with no recommended intake or deficiencies when protein needs are met. Sulfur is mostly consumed as a part of dietary proteins and sulfur containing vitamins.

Magnesium

Magnesium's Functional Role

Approximately 60 percent of magnesium in the human body is stored in the skeleton, making up about 1 percent of mineralized bone tissue. Magnesium is not an integral part of the hard mineral crystals, but it does reside on the surface of the crystal and helps maximize bone structure. Observational studies link magnesium deficiency with an increased risk for osteoporosis. A magnesium-deficient diet is associated with decreased levels of parathyroid hormone and the activation of vitamin D, which may lead to an impairment of bone remodeling. A study in nine hundred elderly women and men did show that higher dietary intakes of magnesium correlated to an increased BMD in the hip. Only a few clinical trials have evaluated the effects of magnesium supplements on bone health and their results suggest some modest benefits on BMD.

In addition to participating in bone maintenance, magnesium has several other functions in the body. In every reaction involving the cellular energy molecule, ATP, magnesium is required. More than three hundred enzymatic reactions require magnesium. Magnesium plays a role in the synthesis of DNA and RNA, carbohydrates, and lipids, and is essential for nerve conduction and muscle contraction. Another health benefit of magnesium is that it may decrease blood pressure.

Many Americans do not get the recommended intake of magnesium from their diets. Some observational studies suggest mild magnesium deficiency is linked to increased risk for cardiovascular disease. Signs and symptoms of severe magnesium deficiency may include tremor, muscle spasms, loss of appetite, and nausea.

Dietary Reference Intake and Food Sources for Magnesium

The RDAs for magnesium for adults between ages nineteen and thirty are 400 milligrams per day for males and 310 milligrams per day for females. For adults above age thirty, the RDA increases slightly to 420 milligrams per day for males and 320 milligrams for females.

Dietary Sources of Magnesium

Magnesium is part of the green pigment, chlorophyll, which is vital for photosynthesis in plants; therefore green leafy vegetables are a good dietary source for magnesium. Magnesium is also found in high concentrations in fish, dairy products, meats, whole grains, and nuts. Additionally chocolate, coffee, and hard water contain a good amount of magnesium. Most people in America do not fulfill the RDA for magnesium in their diets. Typically, Western diets lean toward a low fish intake and the unbalanced consumption of refined grains versus whole grains.

Table: Magnesium Content of Various Foods.

Food	Serving	Magnesium (mg)	Percent Daily Value
Almonds	1 oz.	80	20
Cashews	1 oz.	74	19
Soymilk	1 c.	61	15
Black beans	½ c.	60	15
Edamame	½ c.	50	13
Bread	2 slices	46	12
Avocado	1 c.	44	11
Brown rice	½ c.	42	11
Yogurt	8 oz.	42	11
Oatmeal, instant	1 packet	36	9
Salmon	3 oz.	26	7
Chicken breasts	3 oz.	22	6
Apple	1 medium	9	2

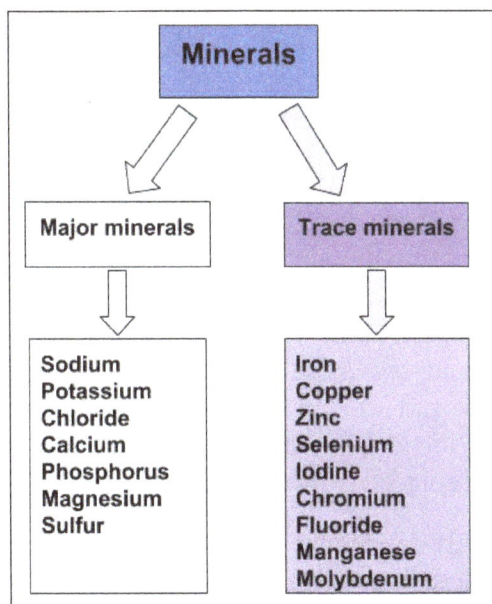

The Trace Minerals.

Trace minerals are classified as minerals required in the diet each day in smaller amounts, specifically 100 milligrams or less. These include copper, zinc, selenium, iodine, chromium, fluoride, manganese, molybdenum, and others. Although trace minerals are needed in smaller amounts it is important to remember that a deficiency in a trace mineral can be just as detrimental to your health as a major mineral deficiency.

Iron

Red blood cells contain the oxygen-carrier protein hemoglobin. It is composed of four globular peptides, each containing a heme complex. In the center of each heme, lies iron. Iron is needed for the production of other iron-containing proteins such as myoglobin. Myoglobin is a protein found in the muscle tissues that enhances the amount of available oxygen for muscle contraction. Iron is also a key component of hundreds of metabolic enzymes. Many of the proteins of the electron-transport chain contain iron–sulfur clusters involved in the transfer of high-energy electrons and ultimately ATP synthesis. Iron is also involved in numerous metabolic reactions that take place mainly in the liver and detoxify harmful substances. Moreover, iron is required for DNA synthesis. The great majority of iron used in the body is that recycled from the continuous breakdown of red blood cells.

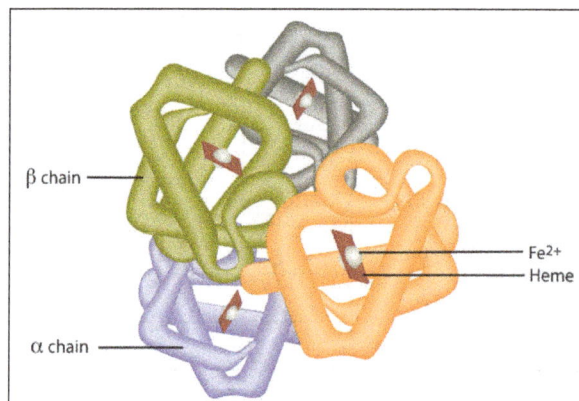

The Structure of Hemoglobin

Hemoglobin is composed of four peptides. Each contains a heme group with iron in the center. The iron in hemoglobin binds to oxygen in the capillaries of the lungs and transports it to cells where the oxygen is released. If iron level is low hemoglobin is not synthesized in sufficient amounts and the oxygen-carrying capacity of red blood cells is reduced, resulting in anemia. When iron levels are low in the diet the small intestine more efficiently absorbs iron in an attempt to compensate for the low dietary intake, but this process cannot make up for the excessive loss of iron that occurs with chronic blood loss or low intake. When blood cells are decommissioned for use, the body recycles the iron back to the bone marrow where red blood cells are made. The body stores some iron in the bone marrow, liver, spleen, and skeletal muscle. A relatively small amount of iron is excreted when cells lining the small intestine and skin cells die and in blood loss, such as during menstrual bleeding. The lost iron must be replaced from dietary sources.

The bioavailability of iron is highly dependent on dietary sources. In animal-based foods about 60 percent of iron is bound to hemoglobin, and heme iron is more bioavailable than nonheme iron. The other 40 percent of iron in animal-based foods is nonheme, which is the only iron source in plant-based foods. Some plants contain chemicals (such as phytate, oxalates, tannins, and polyphenols) that inhibit iron absorption. Although, eating fruits and vegetables rich in vitamin C at the same time as iron-containing foods markedly increases iron absorption.

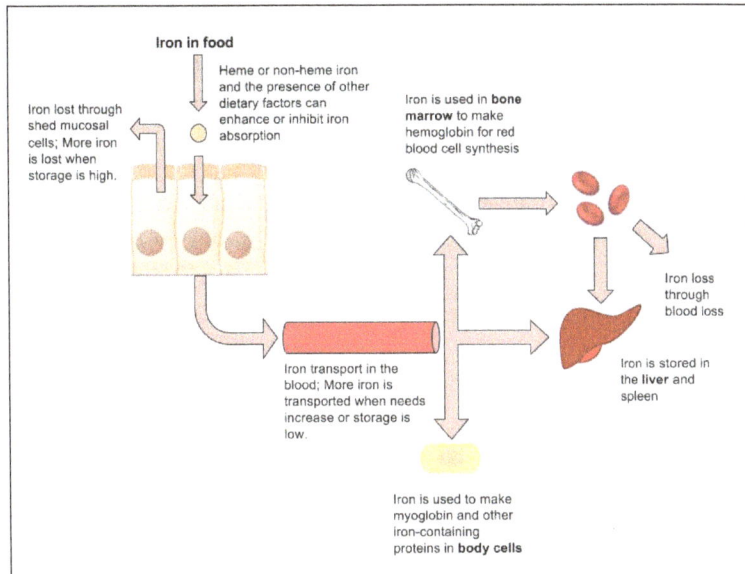

Iron Absorption, Functions and Loss

Dietary Sources of Iron

Table: Iron Content of Various Foods.

Food	Serving	Iron (mg)	Percent Daily Value
Breakfast cereals, fortified	1 serving	18	100
Oysters	3 oz.	8	44
Dark chocolate	3 oz.	7	39
Beef liver	3 oz.	5	28
Lentils	½ c.	3	17
Spinach, boiled	½ c.	3	17
Tofu, firm	½ c.	3	17
Kidney beans	½ c.	2	11
Sardines	3 oz.	2	11

Copper

Copper, like iron, assists in electron transfer in the electron-transport chain. Furthermore, copper is a cofactor of enzymes essential for iron absorption and transport. The other important function of copper is as an antioxidant. Symptoms of mild to moderate copper deficiency are rare. More severe copper deficiency can cause anemia from the lack of iron mobilization in the body for red blood cell synthesis. Other signs and symptoms include growth retardation in children and neurological problems, because copper is a cofactor for an enzyme that synthesizes myelin, which surrounds many nerves.

Zinc

Zinc is a cofactor for over two hundred enzymes in the human body and plays a direct role in RNA, DNA, and protein synthesis. Zinc also is a cofactor for enzymes involved in energy metabolism. As the result of its prominent roles in anabolic and energy metabolism, a zinc deficiency in infants and children blunts growth. Cereal grains and some vegetables contain chemicals, one being phytate, which blocks the absorption of zinc and other minerals in the gut. It is estimated that half of the world's population has a zinc-deficient diet.

This is largely a consequence of the lack of red meat and seafood in the diet and reliance on cereal grains as the main dietary staple. In adults, severe zinc deficiency can cause hair loss, diarrhea, skin sores, loss of appetite, and weight loss. Zinc is a required cofactor for an enzyme that synthesizes the heme portion of hemoglobin and severely deficient zinc diets can result in anemia.

Selenium

Selenium is a cofactor of enzymes that release active thyroid hormone in cells and therefore low levels can cause similar signs and symptoms as iodine deficiency. The other important function of selenium is as an antioxidant.

Selenium Functions and Health Benefits

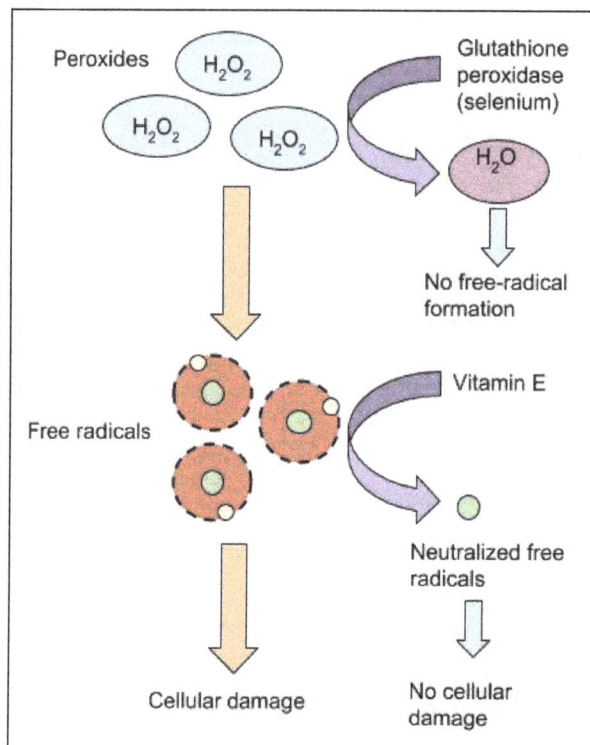

Selenium's Role in Detoxifying Free Radicals

Around twenty-five known proteins require selenium to function. Some are enzymes involved in detoxifying free radicals and include glutathione peroxidases and thioredoxin reductase. As an integral functioning part of these enzymes, selenium aids in the regeneration of glutathione and oxidized vitamin C. Selenium as part of glutathione peroxidase also protects lipids from free radicals, and, in doing so, spares vitamin E. This is just one example of how antioxidants work together to protect the body against free-radical induced damage. Other functions of selenium-containing proteins include protecting endothelial cells that line tissues, converting the inactive thyroid hormone to the active form in cells, and mediating inflammatory and immune system responses.

Dietary Reference Intakes for Selenium

The IOM has set the RDAs for selenium based on the amount required to maximize the activity of glutathione peroxidases found in blood plasma. The RDAs for different age groups are listed in Table "Dietary Reference Intakes for Selenium".

Table: Dietary Reference Intakes for Selenium.

Age Group	RDA Males and Females mcg/day	UL
Infants (0–6 months)	15	45
Infants (7–12 months)	20	65
Children (1–3 years)	20	90
Children (4–8 years)	30	150
Children (9–13 years)	40	280
Adolescents (14–18 years)	55	400
Adults (> 19 years)	55	400

Selenium at doses several thousand times the RDA can cause acute toxicity, and when ingested in gram quantities can be fatal. Chronic exposure to foods grown in soils containing high levels of selenium (significantly above the UL) can cause brittle hair and nails, gastrointestinal discomfort, skin rashes, halitosis, fatigue, and irritability. The IOM has set the UL for selenium for adults at 400 micrograms per day.

Dietary Sources of Selenium

Organ meats, muscle meats, and seafood have the highest selenium content. Plants do not require selenium, so the selenium content in fruits and vegetables is usually low. Animals fed grains from selenium-rich soils do contain some selenium. Grains and some nuts contain selenium when grown in selenium-containing soils.

Table: Selenium Contents of Various Foods.

Food	Serving	Selenium (mcg)	Percent Daily Value
Brazil nuts	1 oz.	544	777
Shrimp	3 oz.	34	49
Crab meat	3 oz.	41	59
Ricotta cheese	1 c.	41	59
Salmon	3 oz.	40	57

Pork	3 oz.	35	50
Ground beef	3 oz.	18	26
Round steak	3 oz.	28.5	41
Beef liver	3 oz.	28	40
Chicken	3 oz.	13	19
Whole-wheat bread	2 slices	23	33
Couscous	1 c.	43	61
Barley, cooked	1 c.	13.5	19
Milk, low-fat	1 c.	8	11
Walnuts, black	1 oz.	5	7

Iodine

Iodine is essential for the synthesis of thyroid hormone, which regulates basal metabolism, growth, and development. Low iodine levels and consequently hypothyroidism has many signs and symptoms including fatigue, sensitivity to cold, constipation, weight gain, depression, and dry, itchy skin and paleness. The development of goiter may often be the most visible sign of chronic iodine deficiency, but the consequences of low levels of thyroid hormone can be severe during infancy, childhood, and adolescence as it affects all stages of growth and development. Thyroid hormone plays a major role in brain development and growth and fetuses and infants with severe iodine deficiency develop a condition known as cretinism, in which physical and neurological impairment can be severe. The World Health Organization (WHO) estimates iodine deficiency affects over two billion people worldwide and it is the number-one cause of preventable brain damage worldwide.

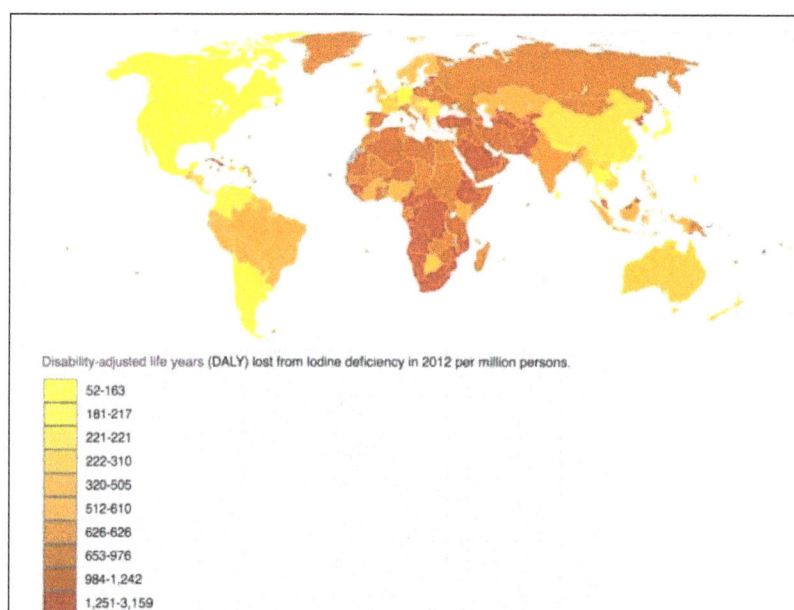

Disability-adjusted life years (DALY) lost from Iodine deficiency in 2012 per million persons.

- 52-163
- 181-217
- 221-221
- 222-310
- 320-505
- 512-610
- 626-626
- 653-976
- 984-1,242
- 1,251-3,159

Deaths Due to Iodine Deficiency Worldwide in 2012.

Dietary Sources of Iodine

The mineral content of foods is greatly affected by the soil from which it grew, and thus geographic location is the primary determinant of the mineral content of foods. For instance, iodine comes mostly from seawater so the greater the distance from the sea the lesser the iodine content in the soil.

Table: Iodine Content of Various Foods.

Food	Serving	Iodine (mcg)	Percent Daily Value
Seaweed	1 g.	16 to 2,984	11 to 1,989
Cod fish	3 oz.	99	66
Yogurt, low fat	8 oz.	75	50
Iodized salt	1.5 g.	71	47
Milk, reduced fat	8 oz.	56	37
Ice cream, chocolate	½ c.	30	20
Egg	1 large	24	16
Tuna, canned	3 oz.	17	11
Prunes, dried	5 prunes	13	9
Banana	1 medium	3	2

Chromium

The functioning of chromium in the body is less understood than that of most other minerals. It enhances the actions of insulin so plays a role in carbohydrate, fat, and protein metabolism. Currently, the results of scientific studies evaluating the usefulness of chromium supplementation in preventing and treating Type 2 diabetes are largely inconclusive. More research is needed to better determine if chromium is helpful in treating certain chronic diseases and, if so, at what doses. Dietary sources of chromium include nuts, whole grains, and yeast. The recommended intake for chromium is 35 mcg per day for adult males and 25 mcg per day for adult females. There is insufficient evidence to establish an UL for chromium.

Manganese

Manganese is a cofactor for enzymes that are required for carbohydrate and cholesterol metabolism, bone formation, and the synthesis of urea. The recommended intake for manganese is 2.3 mg per day for adult males and 1.8 mg per day for adult females. Manganese deficiency is uncommon. The best food sources for manganese are whole grains, nuts, legumes, and green vegetables.

Molybdenum

Molybdenum also acts as a cofactor that is required for the metabolism of sulfur-containing amino acids, nitrogen-containing compounds found in DNA and RNA, and various other functions. The recommended intake for molybdenum is 46 mcg per day for both adult males and females. The food sources of molybdenum is varies depending on the content in the soil in the specific region.

Fluoride

Fluoride's Functional Role

Fluoride is known mostly as the mineral that combats tooth decay. It assists in tooth and bone development and maintenance. Fluoride combats tooth decay via three mechanisms:

- Blocking acid formation by bacteria

- Preventing demineralization of teeth

- Enhancing remineralization of destroyed enamel.

The optimal fluoride concentration in water to prevent tooth decay ranges between 0.7–1.2 milligrams per liter. Exposure to fluoride at three to five times this concentration before the growth of permanent teeth can cause fluorosis, which is the mottling and discoloring of the teeth.

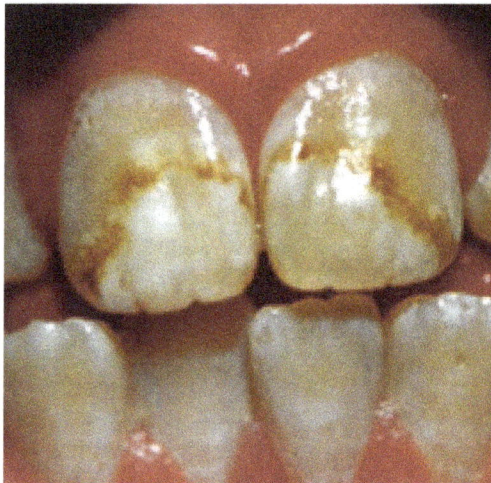

A Severe Case of Fluorosis.

Fluoride's benefits to mineralized tissues of the teeth are well substantiated, but the effects of fluoride on bone are not as well known. Fluoride is currently being researched as a potential treatment for osteoporosis. The data are inconsistent on whether consuming fluoridated water reduces the incidence of osteoporosis and fracture risk. Fluoride does stimulate osteoblast bone building activity, and fluoride therapy in patients with osteoporosis has been shown to increase BMD. In general, it appears that at low doses, fluoride treatment increases BMD in people with osteoporosis and is more effective in increasing bone quality when the intakes of calcium and vitamin D are adequate. The Food and Drug Administration has not approved fluoride for the treatment of osteoporosis mainly because its benefits are not sufficiently known and it has several side effects including frequent stomach upset and joint pain. The doses of fluoride used to treat osteoporosis are much greater than that in fluoridated water.

Dietary Sources of Fluoride

Greater than 70 percent of a person's fluoride comes from drinking fluoridated water when they live in a community that fluoridates the drinking water. Other beverages with a high amount of fluoride include teas and grape juice. Solid foods do not contain a large amount of fluoride. Fluoride content in foods depends on whether it was grown in soils and water that contained fluoride or cooked with fluoridated water. Canned meats and fish that contain bones do contain some fluoride.

Table: Fluoride Content of Various Foods.

Food	Serving	Fluoride (mg)	Percent Daily Value*
Fruit Juice	3.5 fl oz.	0.02-2.1	0.7-70
Crab, canned	3.5 oz.	0.21	7
Rice, cooked	3.5 oz.	0.04	1.3
Fish, cooked	3.5 oz.	0.02	0.7
Chicken	3.5 oz.	0.015	0.5

References

- Carbohydrate, science: britannica.com, Retrieved 8 May, 2019
- Protein, science: britannica.com, Retrieved 14 January, 2019
- Steroid-hormones, science: britannica.com, Retrieved 15 July, 2019
- Vitamin: newworldencyclopedia.org, Retrieved 5 February, 2019
- Vitamin, science: britannica.com, Retrieved 20 August, 2019

Chapter 4
Digestion and Absorption

The biological process through which food is converted into small water-soluble food molecules which can be absorbed into the blood is known as digestion. The chapter closely examines the processes related to the digestion and absorption of carbohydrates, proteins, lipids and vitamins to provide an extensive understanding of the subject.

Digestion is the mechanical and chemical break down of food into small organic fragments. Mechanical digestion refers to the physical breakdown of large pieces of food into smaller pieces which can subsequently be accessed by digestive enzymes. In chemical digestion, enzymes break down food into the small molecules the body can use.

It is important to break down macromolecules into smaller fragments that are of suitable size for absorption across cell membranes. Large, complex molecules of proteins, polysaccharides, and lipids must be reduced to simpler particles before they can be absorbed by the digestive epithelial cells. Different organs play specific roles in the digestive process. The animal diet needs carbohydrates, protein, and fat, as well as vitamins and inorganic components for nutritional balance.

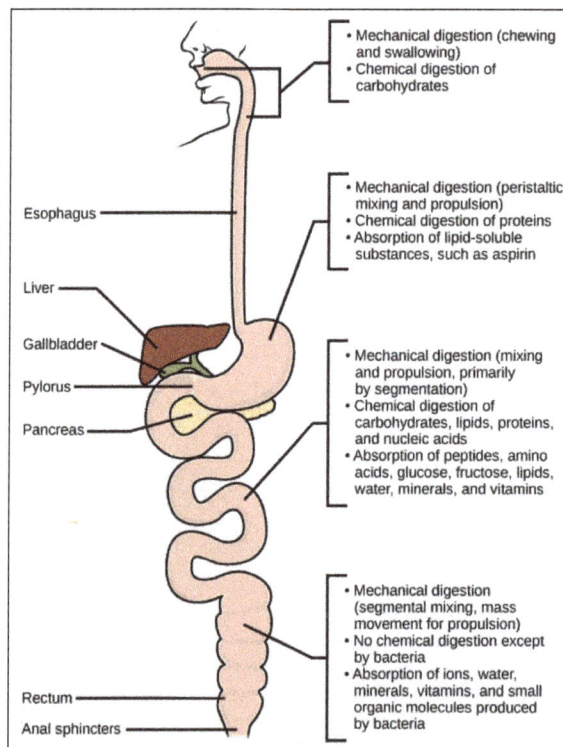

Mechanical and chemical digestion: Mechanical and chemical digestion of food takes place in many steps, beginning in the mouth and ending in the rectum.

Digestive enzymes are enzymes that break down polymeric macromolecules into their smaller building blocks, in order to facilitate their absorption by the body. Digestive enzymes are found in the digestive tracts of animals. Digestive enzymes are diverse and are found in the saliva secreted by the salivary glands, in the stomach secreted by cells lining the stomach, in the pancreatic juice secreted by pancreatic exocrine cells, and in the intestinal (small and large) secretions, or as part of the lining of the gastrointestinal tract.

Intestinal microflora benefit the host by gleaning the energy from the fermentation of undigested carbohydrates and the subsequent absorption of short-chain fatty acids. Intestinal bacteria also play a role in synthesizing vitamin B and vitamin K as well as metabolizing bile acids, sterols and xenobiotics.

Importance of Digestion

When we eat such things as bread, meat, and vegetables, they are not in a form that the body can use as nourishment. Our food and drink must be changed into smaller molecules of nutrients before they can be absorbed into the blood and carried to cells throughout the body. Digestion is the process by which food and drink are broken down into their smallest parts so that the body can use them to build and nourish cells and to provide energy.

The digestive system is a series of hollow organs joined in a long, twisting tube from the mouth to the anus. Inside this tube is a lining called the mucosa. In the mouth, stomach, and small intestine, the mucosa contains tiny glands that produce juices to help digest food.

Digestion involves the mixing of food, its movement through the digestive tract, and chemical breakdown of the large molecules of food into smaller molecules. Digestion begins in the mouth, when we chew and swallow, and is completed in the small intestine. The chemical process varies somewhat for different kinds of food.

Movement of Food through the System:

- Mouth: Seconds
- Esophagus: Seconds
- Stomach: Up to 3 ½ hours
- Small Intestine: Minutes
- Large Intestine: Hours

The large, hollow organs of the digestive system contain muscle that enables their walls to move. The movement of organ walls can propel food and liquid and also can mix the contents within each organ. Typical movement of the esophagus, stomach, and intestine is called peristalsis. The action of peristalsis looks like an ocean wave moving through the muscle. The muscle of the organ produces a narrowing and then propels the narrowed portion slowly down the length of the organ. These waves of narrowing push the food and fluid in front of them through each hollow organ.

The first major muscle movement occurs when food or liquid is swallowed. Although we are able to start swallowing by choice, once the swallow begins, it becomes involuntary and proceeds under the control of the nerves.

The esophagus is the organ into which the swallowed food is pushed. It connects the throat above with the stomach below. At the junction of the esophagus and stomach, there is a ringlike valve closing the passage between the two organs. However, as the food approaches the closed ring, the surrounding muscles relax and allow the food to pass.

The food then enters the stomach, which has three mechanical tasks to do. First, the stomach must store the swallowed food and liquid. This requires the muscle of the upper part of the stomach to relax and accept large volumes of swallowed material. The second job is to mix up the food, liquid, and digestive juice produced by the stomach. The lower part of the stomach mixes these materials by its muscle action. The third task of the stomach is to empty its contents slowly into the small intestine.

Several factors affect emptying of the stomach, including the nature of the food (mainly its fat and protein content) and the degree of muscle action of the emptying stomach and the next organ to receive the stomach contents (the small intestine). As the food is digested in the small intestine and dissolved into the juices from the pancreas, liver, and intestine, the contents of the intestine are mixed and pushed forward to allow further digestion.

Glands of the digestive system are crucial to the process of digestion. They produce both the juices that break down the food and the hormones that help to control the process. The glands that act first are in the mouth-the salivary glands. Saliva produced by these glands contains an enzyme that begins to digest the starch from food into smaller molecules.

The next set of digestive glands is in the stomach lining. They produce stomach acid and an enzyme that digests protein. One of the unsolved puzzles of the digestive system is why the acid juice of the stomach does not dissolve the tissue of the stomach itself. In most people, the stomach mucosa is able to resist the juice, although food and other tissues of the body cannot.

After the stomach empties the food and its juice into the small intestine, the juices of two other digestive organs mix with the food to continue the process of digestion. One of these organs is the pancreas. It produces a juice that contains a wide array of enzymes to break down the carbohydrates, fat, and protein in our food. Other enzymes that are active in the process come from glands in the wall of the intestine or even a part of that wall.

The liver produces yet another digestive juice-bile. The bile is stored between meals in the gallbladder. At mealtime, it is squeezed out of the gallbladder into the bile ducts to reach the intestine and mix with the fat in our food. The bile acids dissolve the fat into the watery contents of the intestine, much like detergents that dissolve grease from a frying pan. After the fat is dissolved, it is digested by enzymes from the pancreas and the lining of the intestine.

Control of Digestive Process

Hormone Regulators

A fascinating feature of the digestive system is that it contains its own regulators. The major hormones that control the functions of the digestive system are produced and released by cells in the mucosa of the stomach and small intestine. These hormones are released into the blood of the digestive tract, travel back to the heart and through the arteries, and return to the digestive system, where they stimulate digestive juices and cause organ movement. The hormones that control digestion are gastrin, secretin, and cholecystokinin (CCK):

- Gastrin causes the stomach to produce an acid for dissolving and digesting some foods. It is also necessary for the normal growth of the lining of the stomach, small intestine, and colon.

- Secretin causes the pancreas to send out a digestive juice that is rich in bicarbonate. It stimulates the stomach to produce pepsin, an enzyme that digests protein, and it also stimulates the liver to produce bile.

- CCK causes the pancreas to grow and to produce the enzymes of pancreatic juice, and it causes the gallbladder to empty.

Nerve Regulators

Two types of nerves help to control the action of the digestive system. Extrinsic (outside) nerves come to the digestive organs from the unconscious part of the brain or from the spinal cord. They release a chemical called acetylcholine and another called adrenaline. Acetylcholine causes the muscle of the digestive organs to squeeze with more force and increase the "push" of food and juice through the digestive tract. Acetylcholine also causes the stomach and pancreas to produce more digestive juice. Adrenaline relaxes the muscle of the stomach and intestine and decreases the flow of blood to these organs.

Even more important, though, are the intrinsic (inside) nerves, which make up a very dense network embedded in the walls of the esophagus, stomach, small intestine, and colon. The intrinsic nerves are triggered to act when the walls of the hollow organs are stretched by food. They release many different substances that speed up or delay the movement of food and the production of juices by the digestive organs.

Digestion and Absorption of Carbohydrates

From the Mouth to the Stomach

The mechanical and chemical digestion of carbohydrates begins in the mouth. Chewing, also known as mastication, crumbles the carbohydrate foods into smaller and smaller pieces. The salivary glands in the oral cavity secrete saliva that coats the food particles. Saliva contains the enzyme, salivary amylase. This enzyme breaks the bonds between the monomeric sugar units of disaccharides, oligosaccharides, and starches. The salivary amylase breaks down amylose and amylopectin into smaller chains of glucose, called dextrins and maltose. The increased concentration of maltose in the mouth that results from the mechanical and chemical breakdown of starches in whole grains is what enhances their sweetness. Only about five percent of starches are broken down in the mouth. (This is a good thing as more glucose in the mouth would lead to more tooth decay.) When carbohydrates reach the stomach no further chemical breakdown occurs because the amylase enzyme does not function in the acidic conditions of the stomach. But mechanical breakdown is ongoing—the strong peristaltic contractions of the stomach mix the carbohydrates into the more uniform mixture of chyme.

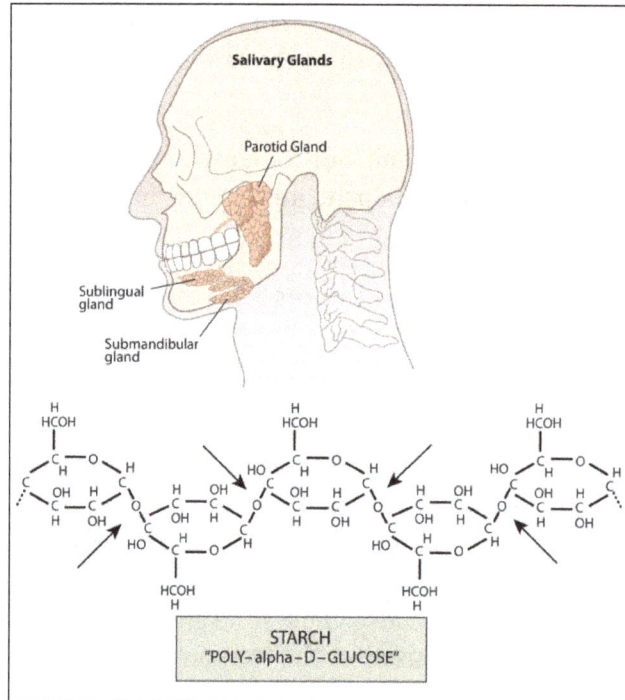

Slalivary Glands in the Mouth: Salivary glands secrete salivary amylase, which begins the chemical breakdown of carbohydrates by breaking the bonds between monomeric sugar units.

From the Stomach to the Small Intestine

The chyme is gradually expelled into the upper part of the small intestine. Upon entry of the chyme into the small intestine, the pancreas releases pancreatic juice through a duct. This pancreatic juice contains the enzyme, pancreatic amylase, which starts again the breakdown of dextrins into shorter and shorter carbohydrate chains. Additionally, enzymes are secreted by the intestinal cells that line the villi. These enzymes, known collectively as disaccharidase, are sucrase, maltase, and lactase. Sucrase breaks sucrose into glucose and fructose molecules. Maltase breaks the bond between the two glucose units of maltose, and lactase breaks the bond between galactose and glucose. Once carbohydrates are chemically broken down into single sugar units they are then transported into the inside of intestinal cells.

When people do not have enough of the enzyme lactase, lactose is not sufficiently broken down resulting in a condition called lactose intolerance. The undigested lactose moves to the large intestine where bacteria are able to digest it. The bacterial digestion of lactose produces gases leading to symptoms of diarrhea, bloating, and abdominal cramps. Lactose intolerance usually occurs in adults and is associated with race. The National Digestive Diseases Information Clearing House states that African Americans, Hispanic Americans, American Indians, and Asian Americans have much higher incidences of lactose intolerance while those of northern European descent have the least. Most people with lactose intolerance can tolerate some amount of dairy products in their diet. The severity of the symptoms depends on how much lactose is consumed and the degree of lactase deficiency.

Absorption: Going to the Blood Stream

The cells in the small intestine have membranes that contain many transport proteins in order to get the monosaccharides and other nutrients into the blood where they can be distributed to the rest of the body. The first organ to receive glucose, fructose, and galactose is the liver. The liver takes them up and converts galactose to glucose, breaks fructose into even smaller carbon-containing units, and either stores glucose as glycogen or exports it back to the blood. How much glucose the liver exports to the blood is under hormonal control and you will soon discover that even the glucose itself regulates its concentrations in the blood.

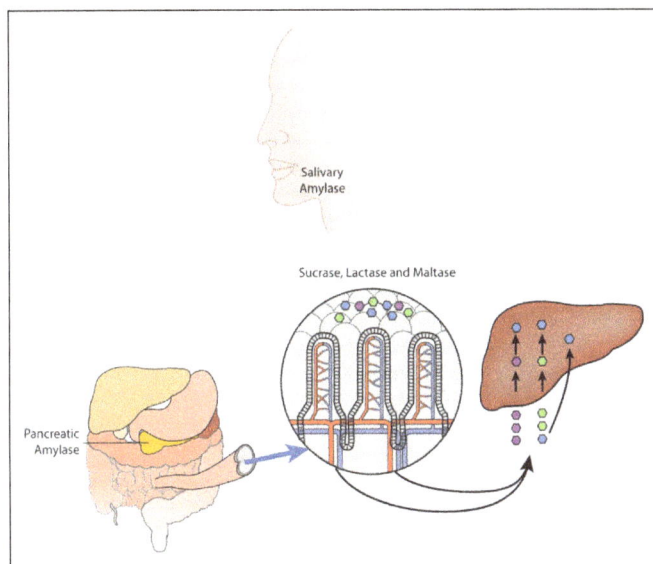

Carbohydrate Digestion: Carbohydrate digestion begins in the mouth and is most extensive in the small intestine. The resultant monosaccharides are absorbed into the bloodstream and transported to the liver.

Maintaining Blood Glucose Levels: The Pancreas and Liver

Glucose levels in the blood are tightly controlled, as having either too much or too little glucose in the blood can have health consequences. Glucose regulates its levels in the blood via a process called negative feedback. An everyday example of negative feedback is in your oven because it contains a thermostat. When you set the temperature to cook a delicious homemade noodle casserole at 375 °F the thermostat senses the temperature and sends an electrical signal to turn the elements on and heat up the oven. When the temperature reaches 375 °F the thermostat senses the temperature and sends a signal to turn the element off. Similarly, your body senses blood glucose levels and maintains the glucose "temperature" in the target range. The glucose thermostat is located within the cells of the pancreas. After eating a meal containing carbohydrates glucose levels rise in the blood.

Insulin-secreting cells in the pancreas sense the increase in blood glucose and release the hormone, insulin, into the blood. Insulin sends a signal to the body's cells to remove glucose from the blood by transporting it into different organ cells around the body and using it to make energy. In the case of muscle tissue and the liver, insulin sends the biological message to store glucose away as glycogen. The presence of insulin in the blood signifies to the body that glucose is available for fuel. As glucose is transported into the cells around the body, the blood glucose levels decrease. Insulin has an opposing hormone called glucagon. Glucagon-secreting cells in the pancreas sense the drop in glucose and, in response, release glucagon into the blood. Glucagon communicates to the cells in the body to stop using all the glucose. More specifically, it signals the liver to break down glycogen and release the stored glucose into the blood, so that glucose levels stay within the target range and all cells get the needed fuel to function properly.

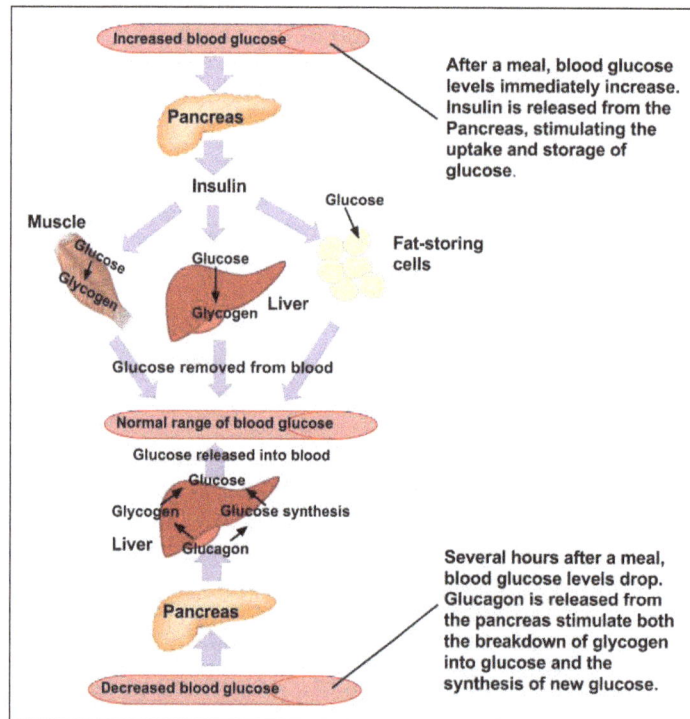

The Regulation of Glucose

Leftover Carbohydrates: The Large Intestine

Almost all of the carbohydrates, except for dietary fiber and resistant starches, are efficiently digested and absorbed into the body. Some of the remaining indigestible carbohydrates are broken down by enzymes released by bacteria in the large intestine. The products of bacterial digestion of these slow-releasing carbohydrates are short-chain fatty acids and some gases. The short-chain fatty acids are either used by the bacteria to make energy and grow, are eliminated in the feces, or are absorbed into cells of the colon, with a small amount being transported to the liver. Colonic cells use the short-chain fatty acids to support some of their functions. The liver can also metabolize the short-chain fatty acids into cellular energy. The yield of energy from dietary fiber is about 2 kilocalories per gram for humans, but is highly dependent upon the fiber type, with soluble fibers and resistant starches yielding more energy than insoluble fibers. Since dietary fiber is digested much less in the gastrointestinal tract than other carbohydrate types (simple sugars, many starches) the rise in blood glucose after eating them is less, and slower. These physiological attributes of high-fiber foods (i.e. whole grains) are linked to a decrease in weight gain and reduced risk of chronic diseases, such as Type 2 diabetes and cardiovascular disease.

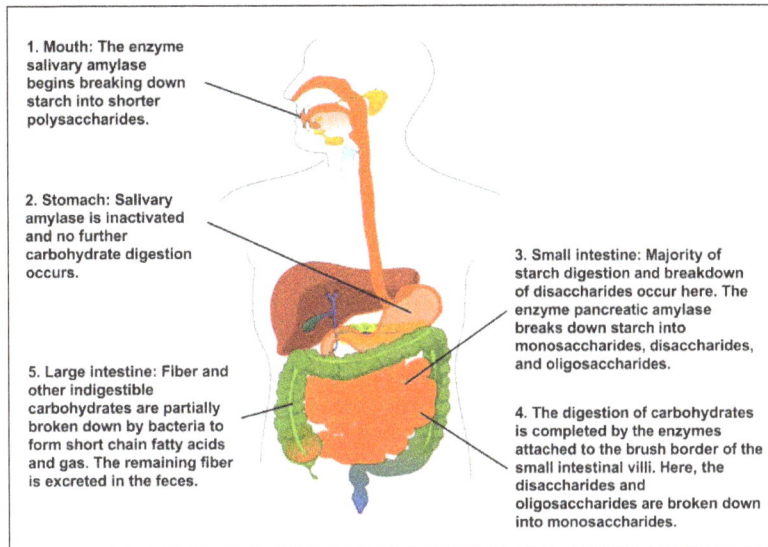

Overview of Carbohydrate Digestion

Digestion and Absorption of Proteins

Protein Digestion in Stomach

Protein → Metaprotein → Proteone → Peptone → Peptide

As the food passes from the stomach to small intestine the low pH of the food triggers the secretion of the hormone 'secretin' into the blood. It stimulates the pancreas to secrete HCO3 into the small intestine in order to neutralize HCl. The secretion of HCO_3 into the intestine abruptly raises the pH from 2.5 to 7.0. The entry of amino acids into the duodenum releases the hormone 'cholecystokinin' which in turn triggers the release of pancreatic juice (that contains many pancreatic enzymes like trypsinogen, chymotrypsinogen, procarboxypeptidases) by the exocrine cells of the pancreas (ecbolic and hydrolatic). Most of these enzymes are produced as zymogens (inactive enzymes) by the pancreas in order to protect the exocrine cells from being digested.

Subsequent to the entry of trypsinogen into the small intestine it is activated to trypsin by enterokinase secreted by the intestinal cells. Trypsin is formed from trypsinogen by the removal of hexapeptide from the N-terminal end.

The newly formed trypsin activates the remaining trypsinogen, Trypsin is an endopeptidase, specific for (acts on) the peptide bonds contributed by the basic amino acids like arginine, histidine and lysine. Chymotrypsin is secreted in an inactive from called chymotrypsinogen which is activated by trypsin. Chymotrypsin is an endopeptidase specific to aromatic amino acids i.e. phenylalanine, tyrosine, tryptophan.

Carboxypeptidase secreted as procarboxypeptidase is activated again by trypsin. It is an exopeptidase that cleaves the amino acids from the carboxy terminal end. Amino peptidase secreted as pro-aminopeptidase is once again activated by trypsin. It is an exopeptidase that cleaves the amino acids from the free amino terminal end. Dipeptides acts only on dipeptides and hydrolyses it into 2 amino acids.

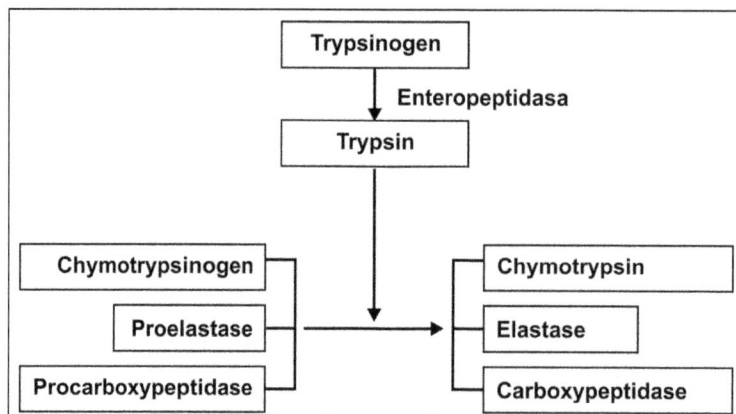

```
                    ┌─────────────────┐
                    │  Trypsinogen    │
                    └─────────────────┘
                             │  Enteropeptidasa
                             ▼
                    ┌─────────────────┐
                    │    Trypsin      │
                    └─────────────────┘
                             │
  ┌──────────────────┐       │        ┌──────────────────┐
  │ Chymotrypsinogen │───┐   │    ┌───│   Chymotrypsin   │
  └──────────────────┘   │   │    │   └──────────────────┘
     ┌──────────────┐    ├───┼───▶├──│     Elastase     │
     │  Proelastase │────┤        │  └──────────────────┘
     └──────────────┘    │        │  ┌──────────────────┐
  ┌──────────────────┐   │        └──│ Carboxypeptidase │
  │Procarboxypeptidase│──┘           └──────────────────┘
  └──────────────────┘
```

Proteolytic Enzymes and their Action

Secreted in	Enzymes secreted	Action
Stomach	Pepsin	Converts complex Proteins to small peptides
Pancreas	Trypsin	• Specifically acts on peptide bonds contributed by basic amino acids like arg, lys & his • Activates trypsinogen to trypsin • Procarboxypeptidase to carboxypeptidase, proelastase to elastase and proaminopeptidase to aminopeptidase
	Chymotrypsin	Specifically acts on peptide bondas contributed by aromatic amino acids like phe, tyr, trp
Small intestine	Carboxypeptidase	Carboxy Terminal amino Acids
	elastase	
	Amino peptidase	Amino terminal amino acids
	Dipeptidase	Acts on dipeptides and releases free amino acids

Even after the action of all these enzymes most of the proteins remain undigested. Protein like collagen, fibrin etc., escape digestion and are excreted out.

Celiac Disease

This is a rare disease caused due to genetic defect/absence of the enzyme required to hydrolyze the proteins containing N-glutamyl amino acids. Due to this the intestinal enzymes are unable to digest the water insoluble proteins present in wheat called gliadin which is injurious to the cells lining the small intestine.

In rare instances the inactive zymogen forms of the enzymes stored in the pancreas are pre-matured to active forms in the pancreas itself, which may be fatal to the pancreas. Antagonists called trypsin inhibitor, a protein secreted by the pancreas can be used to avoid such disaster.

Absorption of the Digested Proteins

There are four distinct carrier systems in the intestinal epithelium for the absorption of the digested proteins. These are:

- Carrier system for neutral amino acids
- Carrier system for basic amino acids
- Carrier system for acidic amino acids
- Carrier system for glycine and imino acid (proline).

The digested amino acids are carried across the mucosal cell membrane from the intestinal lumen to the cytoplasm of the cell by one of the above carrier systems specific to that particular amino acid. Absorption of amino acids is an up-hill process (i.e. against gradient as compared to the Na^+ absorption which is downhill i.e. along the gradient).

There are four systems that operate to absorb amino acids from the mucosal cells into the blood. They are:

- A — system (alanine system)
- L — system (leucine system)
- Ly – system (lysine system)
- Ala-ser-cyst – system.

Amino acids are taken up by the blood capillaries of the mucosa and are transported in the plasma to the liver. Some amounts of amino acids are also absorbed through the lymph. Glucagon stimulates the absorption of amino acids through 'A' system mediated by cAMP. Insulin stimulates the trans cellular transport of amino acids to minimize the loss in the urine. The proximal tubule cells reabsorb and return them to the blood stream. It is done by glutathione, a tripeptide. Three ATPs are utilized for the absorption of each amino acid.

Absorbed amino acids do not stimulate antibody production whereas an intact protein absorbed becomes antigenic. Intestinal membranes allow the transport of proteins across them ex.—In a neonate the intestinal mucosa is permeable to y-globulin (immunoglobulin) of colostrum.

The immune system in a neonate is not well developed thus absorption of intact y-globulin into the blood does not elicit any immune response instead it results in the defence of the neonate against infections. In adults, some proteins may be absorbed intact through the intestinal mucosa leading to the formation of antibodies and anaphylactic reactions or other such immunological phenomena after the absorption of those proteins. Thus in such cases allergies to food proteins occur.

Protein Turnover

Protein turnover is a continuous process of degradation and re-synthesis of all cellular proteins. Each day, human beings turn over 1 to 2% of their total body proteins i.e., about 2% of the body proteins are degraded and resynthesized every day. 75-80% of the amino acids released from the degraded proteins are reutilized for new protein synthesis and the nitrogen of the remaining 20-25% forms urea leaving the carbon backbone to be oxidized to intermediates of TCA or other metabolites.

The rate at which proteins degrade depends upon the physiological state of the individual. The time required to reduce the concentration of a given protein to 50% of its original concentration is termed as 'half-life (t½)'. The half-life of liver proteins ranges from 30 minutes to 150 hours. The half-life of HMG CoA reductase is 0.5-2 hours whereas aldolase, lactate dehydrogenase and cytochromes have a half-life of 100 hours. Hence it can be said that, almost all the proteins of the body are degraded within a span of 6-9 months and are replaced by new proteins.

Role of Lysosomes in Protein Turnover

Lysosomes play an important role in the degradation of intracellular and extracellular proteins. The proteins from the circulation and those within the cell lose the oligosaccharides and are then internalized by the lysosomes and are degraded by proteases called cathepsins. The non-glycosylated proteins are degraded in the cytosol by ubiquitin, a small protein of 8.5 kDa in all eukaryotic cells.

Ubiquitin forms a non-peptide bond with the N-terminal amino acid in the protein with conversion of ATP to AMP. Thus, the life of the protein depends upon the type of amino acid present at the N-terminal end. If serine and methionine are present as the N-terminal amino acid then the life of the proteins is long and if aspartate and arginine are present then the life is short because ubiquitin acts fast on these amino acids.

Digestion and Absorption of Lipids

Lipids are large molecules and generally are not water-soluble. Like carbohydrates and protein, lipids are broken into small components for absorption.

From the Mouth to the Stomach

The first step in the digestion of triglycerides and phospholipids begins in the mouth as lipids encounter saliva. Next, the physical action of chewing coupled with the action of emulsifiers enables the digestive enzymes to do their tasks. The enzyme lingual lipase, along with a small amount of phospholipid as an emulsifier, initiates the process of digestion. These actions cause the fats to become more accessible to the digestive enzymes. As a result, the fats become tiny droplets and separate from the watery components.

In the stomach, gastric lipase starts to break down triglycerides into diglycerides and fatty acids. Within two to four hours after eating a meal, roughly 30 percent of the triglycerides are converted to diglycerides and fatty acids. The stomach's churning and contractions help to disperse the fat molecules, while the diglycerides derived in this process act as further emulsifiers. However, even amid all of this activity, very little fat digestion occurs in the stomach.

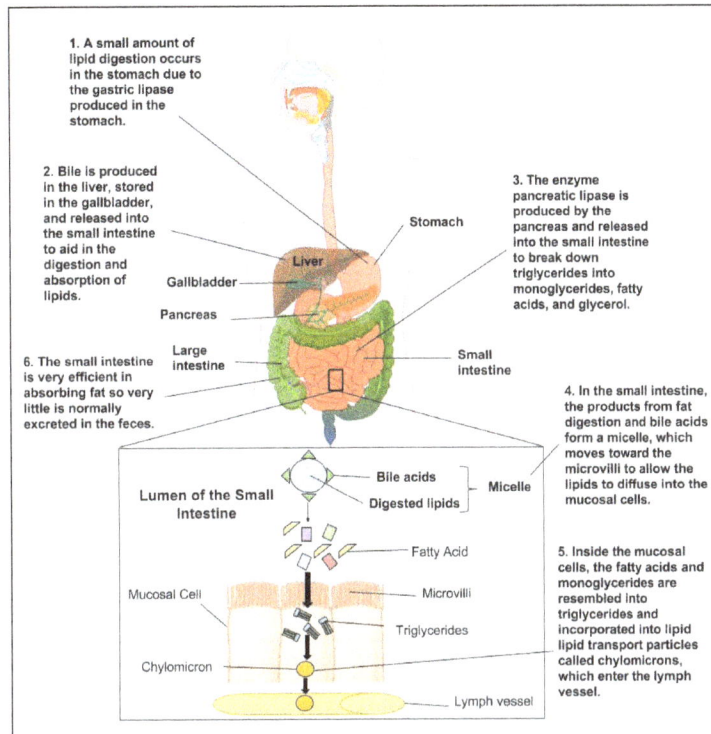

Lipid Digestion and Absorption.

Going to the Bloodstream

As stomach contents enter the small intestine, the digestive system sets out to manage a small hurdle, namely, to combine the separated fats with its own watery fluids. The solution to this hurdle is bile. Bile contains bile salts, lecithin, and substances derived from cholesterol so it acts as an emulsifier. It attracts and holds onto fat while it is simultaneously attracted to and held on to by water. Emulsification increases the surface area of lipids over a thousand-fold, making them more accessible to the digestive enzymes.

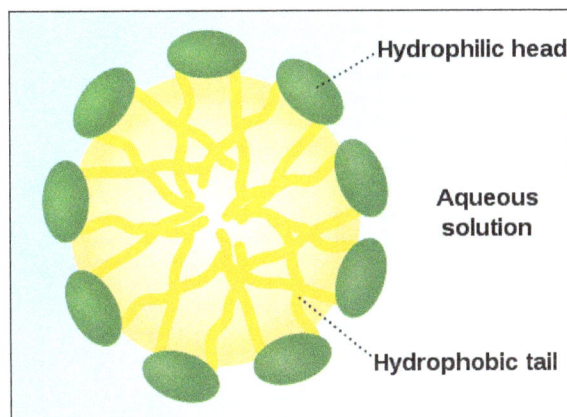

Micelle Formation

Once the stomach contents have been emulsified, fat-breaking enzymes work on the triglycerides and diglycerides to sever fatty acids from their glycerol foundations. As pancreatic lipase enters the small intestine, it breaks down the fats into free fatty acids and monoglycerides. Bile salts envelop the fatty acids and monoglycerides to form micelles. Micelles have a fatty acid core with a water-soluble exterior. This allows efficient transportation to the intestinal microvillus. Here, the fat components are released and disseminated into the cells of the digestive tract lining.

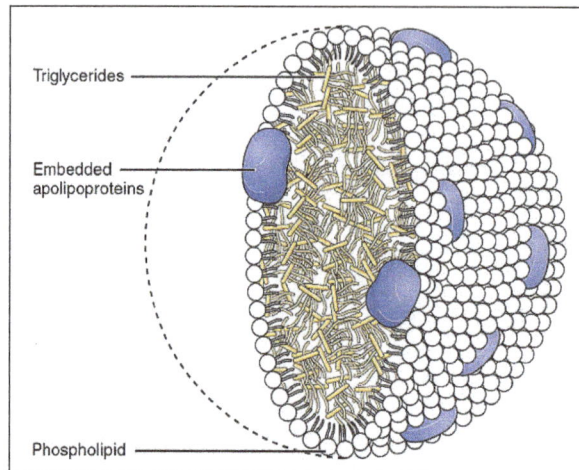

Schematic Diagram of a Chylomicron

Just as lipids require special handling in the digestive tract to move within a water-based environment, they require similar handling to travel in the bloodstream. Inside the intestinal cells, the monoglycerides and fatty acids reassemble themselves into triglycerides. Triglycerides, cholesterol, and phospholipids form lipoproteins when joined with a protein carrier. Lipoproteins have an inner core that is primarily made up of triglycerides and cholesterol esters (a cholesterol ester is a cholesterol linked to a fatty acid). The outer envelope is made of phospholipids interspersed with proteins and cholesterol. Together they form a chylomicron, which is a large lipoprotein that now enters the lymphatic system and will soon be released into the bloodstream via the jugular vein in the neck. Chylomicrons transport food fats perfectly through the body's water-based environment to specific destinations such as the liver and other body tissues.

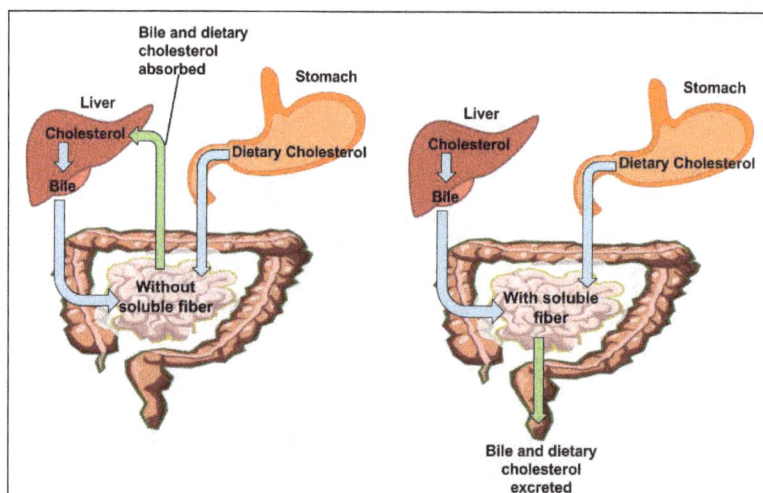

Cholesterol and Soluble Fiber

Cholesterols are poorly absorbed when compared to phospholipids and triglycerides. Cholesterol absorption is aided by an increase in dietary fat components and is hindered by high fiber content. This is the reason that a high intake of fiber is recommended to decrease blood cholesterol. Foods high in fiber such as fresh fruits, vegetables, and oats can bind bile salts and cholesterol, preventing their absorption and carrying them out of the colon.

If fats are not absorbed properly as is seen in some medical conditions, a person's stool will contain high amounts of fat. If fat malabsorption persists the condition is known as steatorrhea. Steatorrhea can result from diseases that affect absorption, such as Crohn's disease and cystic fibrosis.

Digestion of Vitamins and Minerals

Vitamins and minerals are digested, broken down and absorbed similarly in your body. There are a variety of vitamins and minerals you need in your diet to support each and every function. Vitamins are organic compounds made by plants, animals and humans. Minerals are inorganic elements, occurring naturally in soil and water. Plants absorb minerals through their roots and you absorb the minerals when you eat the plant food. Animals also eat plants, so you can also get some minerals indirectly by consuming foods originating from animal sources.

All minerals are stored in your body, but only some vitamins actually stay in your body. Vitamins are broken up into two categories: fat soluble, such as A, D, E or K, and water soluble, including all of the B vitamins and vitamin C. Fat-soluble vitamins stay in your body, whereas water-soluble vitamins are absorbed immediately, with any excess being excreted in urine. Organic compounds are considered vitamins when lacking that particular nutrient results in a deficiency, causing negative health effects, explains the Linus Pauling Institute. Minerals can also be broken up into two categories: trace and macro-minerals. Trace minerals include iron, copper and zinc; and some of the macro-minerals are calcium, phosphorous and magnesium. While these categories of minerals are equally important, trace minerals are needed in smaller amounts than macro-minerals.

Digestion of vitamins and minerals begins in your mouth, when you chew your food. When food enters the stomach, hydrochloric acid and other stomach enzymes help release its nutrients. Your pancreas helps by releasing bile that aids with digestion. From this point, the vitamins and minerals travel to the small intestine, where they are absorbed into the bloodstream. Your blood carries the nutrients to your liver, where they are used up immediately, stored for later use or sent to the kidneys for excretion through urine.

Factors Affecting Absorption

Damage to organs from heavy alcohol use can affect your body's ability to absorb and store vitamins and minerals. Years of excessive alcohol consumption can damage liver, stomach and intestinal cells that aid in vitamin and mineral digestion, the National Institute on Alcohol Abuse and Alcoholism explains. Additionally, having an intestinal disorder, such as Crohn's disease, irritable bowel syndrome or diverticulitis, can inhibit the absorption of vitamins and minerals. These types of intestinal problems cause food to rapidly pass through your digestive tract before it fully has a chance to absorb. Even if you consume adequate amounts of each nutrient, your body may not get a chance to absorb them.

Absorption of Vitamins

Vitamins are organic molecules necessary for normal metabolism in animals, but either are not synthesized in the body or are synthesized in inadequate quantities and must be obtained from the diet. Essentially all vitamin absorption occurs in the small intestine.

Absorption of vitamins in the intestine is critical in avoiding deficiency states, and impairment of intestinal vitamin absorption can results from a number of factors, including intestinal disease, genetic disorders in transport molecules, excessive alcohol consumption and interactions with drugs.

Absorption of Water-soluble Vitamins

Most water soluble vitamins are available for intestinal absorption from two sources: 1) the diet, and 2) synthesis by microbes in the large intestine or, in the case of ruminants, the rumen. These dual-origin vitamins include biotin, folic acid, pantothenic acid, riboflavin and thiamin. Ascorbic acid can be synthesized by many animals, but not by primates or guinea pigs, in which it is a true vitamin and must be obtained from dietary sources. Niacin is also a bit different - it can be synthesized within the body from tryptophan but is also absorbed in the intestine from dietary sources.

Water soluble vitamins of dietary origin are absorbed predominantly in the small intestine, whereas those synthesized by microbes in the large intestine are absorbed there. For most of these vitamins, specific carrier-mediated transport systems have been identified that allow uptake from the intestinal lumen into the enterocyte and for export from the basolateral surface of the enterocyte. Some of these transporters are sodium-dependent, while others are not.

Absorption of Fat-soluble Vitamins

The fat soluble vitamins A, D, E and K are absorbed from the intestinal lumen using the same mechanisms used for absorption of other lipids. In short, they are incorporated into mixed micelles with other lipids and bile acids in the lumen of the small intestine and enter the enterocyte largely by diffusion. Within the enterocytge, they are incorporated into chylomicrons and exported via exocytosis into lymph.

Absorption of Minerals and Metals

The vast bulk of mineral absorption occurs in the small intestine. The best-studied mechanisms of absorption are clearly for calcium and iron, deficiencies of which are significant health problems throughout the world.

Minerals are clearly required for health, but most also are quite toxic when present at higher than normal concentrations. Thus, there is a physiologic challenge of supporting efficient but limited absorption. In many cases intestinal absorption is a key regulatory step in mineral homeostasis.

Calcium

Calcium is absorbed from the intestinal luman by two distinct mechanims, and their relative magnitude of importance is determined by the amount of free calcium available for absorption:

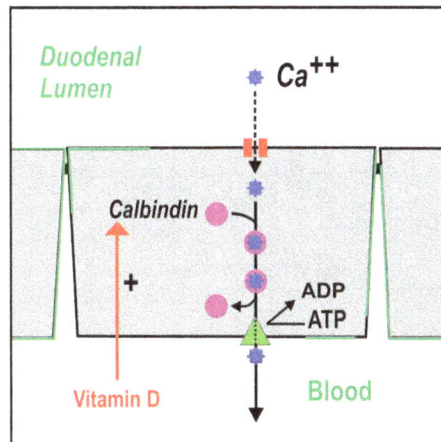

1. Active, transcellular absorption occurs only in the duodenum when calcium intake is low. This process involves import of calcium into the enterocyte, transport across the cell, and export into extracellular fluid and blood. Calcium enters the intestinal epithelial cells through voltage-insensitive (TRP) channels and is pumped out of the cell via a calcium-ATPase.

   The rate limiting step in transcellular calcium absorption is transport across the epithelial cell, which is greatly enhanced by the carrier protein calbindin, the synthesis of which is totally dependent on vitamin D.

2. Passive, paracellular absorption occurs in the jejunum and ileum, and, to a much lesser extent, in the colon when dietary calcium levels are moderate or high. In this case, ionized calcium diffuses through tight junctions into the basolateral spaces around enterocytes, and hence into blood. When calcium availability is high, this pathway responsible for the bulk of calcium absorption, due to the very short time available for active transport in the duodenum.

Phosphorus

Phosphorus is predominantly absorbed as inorganic phosphate in the upper small intestine. Phosphate is transported into the epithelial cells by contransport with sodium, and expression of this (or these) transporters is enhanced by vitamin D.

Iron

Iron homeostasis is regulated at the level of intestinal absorption, and it is important that adequate but not excessive quantities of iron be absorbed from the diet. Inadequate absorption can lead to iron-deficiency disorders such as anemia. On the other hand, excessive iron is toxic because mammals do not have a physiologic pathway for its elimination.

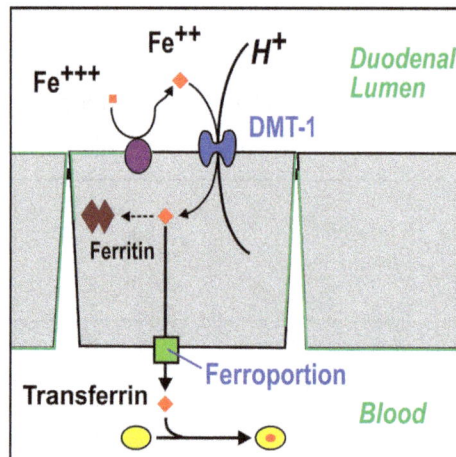

Iron is absorbed by villus enterocytes in the proximal duodenum. Efficient absorption requires an acidic environment, and antacids or other conditions that interfere with gastric acid secretion can interfere with iron absorption.

Ferric iron (Fe^{+++}) in the duodenal lumen is reduced to its ferrous form through the action of a brush border ferrireductase. Iron is the cotransported with a proton into the enterocyte via the divalent metal transporter DMT-1. This transporter is not specific for iron, and also transports many divalent metal ions.

Once inside the enterocyte, iron follows one of two major pathways. Which path is taken depends on a complex programming of the cell based on both dietary and systemic iron loads:

- Iron abundance states: Iron within the enterocyte is trapped by incorporation into ferritin and hence, not transported into blood. When the enterocyte dies and is shed, this iron is lost.

- Iron limiting states: Iron is exported out of the enterocyte via a transporter (ferroportin) located in the basolateral membrane. It then binds to the iron-carrier transferrin for transport throughout the body.

Iron in the form of heme, from ingestion of hemoglobin or myoglobin, is also readily absorbed. In this case, it appears that intact heme is taking up by the small intestinal enterocyte by endocytosis. Once inside the enterocyte, iron is liberated and essentially follows the same pathway for export as absorbed inorganic iron. Some heme may be transported intact into the circulation.

Copper

There appear to be two processes responsible for copper absorption - a rapid, low capacity system and a slower, high capacity system, which may be similar to the two processes seen with calcium absorption. Many of the molecular details of copper absorption remain to be elucidated. Inactivating mutations in the gene encoding an intracellular copper ATPase have been shown responsible for the failure of intestinal copper absorption in Menkes disease.

A number of dietary factors have been shown to influence copper absorption. For example, excessive dietary intake of either zinc or molybdenum can induce secondary copper deficiency states.

Zinc

Zinc homeostasis is largely regulated by its uptake and loss through the small intestine. Although a number of zinc transporters and binding proteins have been identified in villus epithelial cells, a detailed picture of the molecules involved in zinc absorption is not yet in hand.

Intestinal excretion of zinc occurs via shedding of epithelial cells and in pancreatic and biliary secretions.

A number of nutritional factors have been identified that modulate zinc absorption. Certain animal proteins in the diet enhance zinc absorption. Phytates from dietary plant material (including cereal grains, corn and rice) chelate zinc and inhibit its absorption. Subsistance on phytate-rich diets is thought responsible for a considerable fraction of human zinc deficiencies.

References

- Digestive-system-processes, biology: lumenlearning.com, Retrieved 11 March, 2019

- Digestion: nutristrategy.com, Retrieved 2 August, 2019

- Digestion-and-absorption-of-carbohydrates, humannutrition: hawaii.edu, Retrieved 17 April, 2019

- Protein-digestion-and-absorption-process-protein-metabolism, metabolism-proteins, proteins: biologydiscussion.com, Retrieved 23 July, 2019

- Digestion-and-absorption-of-lipids, humannutrition: hawaii.edu, Retrieved 21 January, 2019

- Digestion-of-vitamins-minerals: livestrong.com, Retrieved 17 May, 2019

- Absorb-vitamins, digestion: colostate.edu, Retrieved 28 February, 2019

- Absorb-minerals, digestion: colostate.edu, Retrieved 14 June, 2019

Chapter 5

Nutritional Deficiencies and Diseases

Nutritional deficiency occurs when the body does not receive the required amount of nutrients from food. It can cause a number of different diseases such as osteoporosis, rickets, goiter, anemia and beriberi. The topics elaborated in this chapter will help in gaining a better perspective about the deficiency of different nutrients and the diseases caused by their deficiency.

Malnutrition

Malnutrition involves a dietary deficiency. People may eat too much of the wrong type of food and have malnutrition.

Poor diet may lead to a lack of vitamins, minerals, and other essential substances. Too little protein can lead to kwashiorkor, symptoms of which include a distended abdomen. A lack of vitamin C can result in scurvy.

Scurvy is rare in industrialized nations, but it can affect older people, those who consume excessive quantities of alcohol, and people who do not eat fresh fruits and vegetables. Some infants and children who follow a limited diet for any reason may be prone to scurvy.

Malnutrition during childhood can lead not only to long-term health problems but also to educational challenges and limited work opportunities in the future. Malnourished children often have smaller babies when they grow up.

It can also slow recovery from wounds and illnesses, and it can complicate diseases such as measles, pneumonia, malaria, and diarrhea. It can leave the body more susceptible to disease.

Symptoms

Signs and symptoms of undernutrition include:

- Lack of appetite or interest in food or drink.
- Tiredness and irritability.
- Inability to concentrate.
- Always feeling cold.
- Loss of fat, muscle mass, and body tissue.
- Higher risk of getting sick and taking longer to heal.

- Longer healing time for wounds.

- Higher risk of complications after surgery.

- Depression.

- Reduced sex drive and problems with fertility.

In more severe cases:

- Breathing becomes difficult.

- Skin may become thin, dry, inelastic, pale, and cold.

- The cheeks appear hollow and the eyes sunken, as fat disappears from the face.

- Hair becomes dry and sparse, falling out easily.

Eventually, there may be respiratory failure and heart failure, and the person may become unresponsive. Total starvation can be fatal within 8 to 12 weeks.

Children may show a lack of growth, and they may be tired and irritable. Behavioral and intellectual development may be slow, possibly resulting in learning difficulties.

Protein-Energy Malnutrition Diseases

Protein-energy undernutrition (PEU), previously called protein-energy malnutrition, is an energy deficit due to deficiency of all macronutrients. It commonly includes deficiencies of many micronutrients. PEU can be sudden and total (starvation) or gradual. Severity ranges from subclinical deficiencies to obvious wasting (with edema, hair loss, and skin atrophy) to starvation.

Kwashiorkor

Kwashiorkor is a form of protein-energy malnutrition caused by the inadequate intake of protein with reasonable caloric (energy) intake. The other form of protein-energy malnutrition is the condition known as marasmus. Marasmus involves inadequate intake of both protein and calories. Hence, protein-calorie malnutrition encompasses a group of related disorders that include kwashiorkor, marasmus, and intermediate or mixed states of kwashiorkor and marasmus.

Kwashiorkor is also known as protein malnutrition, protein-energy (calorie) malnutrition and malignant malnutrition.

Signs and Symptoms of Kwashiorkor

Early signs of kwashiorkor present as general symptoms of malnutrition and include fatigue, irritability and lethargy. As protein deprivation continues the following abnormalities become apparent.

- Failure to thrive (failure to put on height and weight).

- Loss of muscle mass.

- Generalised swelling (oedema).

- Large protuberant belly (pot belly).

- Fatty liver.

- Failing immune system so prone to infections and increased severity of normally mild infections.

- Skin and hair changes.

Cutaneous Features of Kwashiorkor

Characteristic skin and hair changes occur in kwashiorkor and develop over a few days.

- Skin lesions are at first erythematous before turning purple and reddish-brown in colour with marked exfoliation (skin peeling and sloughing).

- Where the skin becomes dark and dry, it splits open when stretched to reveal pale areas between the cracks ("lacquered flaky paint", "crazy pavement dermatosis").

- Irregular or patchy discolouration of the skin caused by pigmentary changes.

- Hair becomes dry and lustreless and may turn reddish yellow to white in colour. It becomes sparse and brittle and can be pulled out easily.

- Nail plates are thin and soft and may be fissured or ridged.

Causes of Kwashiorkor

Kwashiorkor is the commonest and most widespread nutritional disorders in developing countries. It occurs in areas of famine or areas of limited food supply, and particularly in those countries where the diet consists mainly of corn, rice and beans. It has also been reported in children following very restricted diets for cultural reasons or in the context of presumed food allergy. It is more common in children than in adults. The onset in infancy is during the weaning or post-weaning period where protein intake has not been sufficiently replaced.

Marasmus

Marasmus is a form of malnutrition. It happens when the intake of nutrients and energy is too low for a person's needs. It leads to wasting, or the loss of body fat and muscle. A child with marasmus may not grow as children usually do.

Malnutrition happens when a lack of nutrients causes health problems, usually because a person's diet does not contain all the vitamins and nutrients that the body needs to function. When an individual does not get the right nutrients, it is harder for their body to carry out routine processes that enable them to grow new cells or fight disease. More serious health problems can then result.

In many parts of the world, marasmus happens because people do not have enough food. In developed countries, it can occur as a result of the eating disorder anorexia nervosa.

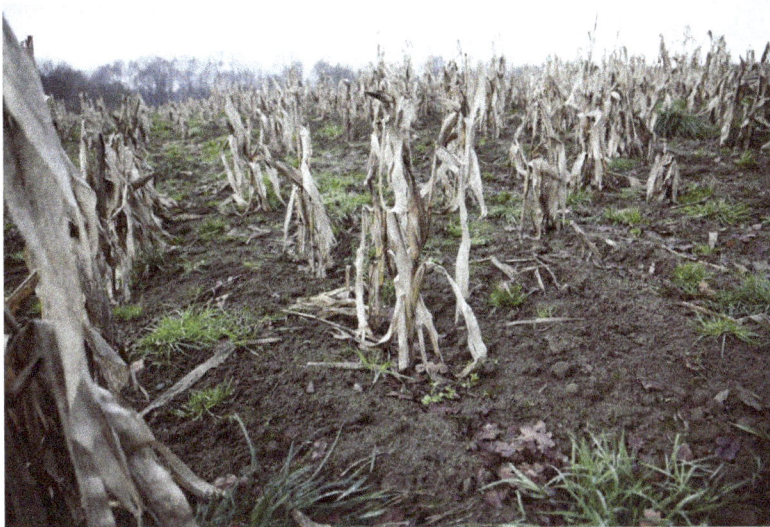

When crops fail, food supplies can drop, leading to malnutrition and marasmus in some places.

Marasmus is a severe form of protein-energy malnutrition that results when a person does not consume enough protein and calories. Without these vital nutrients, energy levels become dangerously low and vital functions begin to stop.

Both adults and children can have marasmus, but it most often affects young children in developing countries.

UNICEF estimate that nearly half of all deaths in children under the age of 5 years, or around 3 million each year, resulting from a lack of nutrition.

Causes and Risk Factors

Causes of marasmus include:

- Not having enough nutrition or having too little food.

- Consuming the wrong nutrients or too much of one and not enough of another.

- Having a health condition that makes it difficult to absorb or process nutrients correctly.

While consuming the wrong nutrients and having a health condition can contribute to marasmus, each of these alone would probably not be enough to cause it, as long as calories are available. In places where food can be scarce, breastfeeding infants for as long as possible may help reduce the risk of malnutrition.

However, if breastfeeding continues for longer than 6 months without an infant receiving solid food, the risk of marasmus can also increase, especially if the mother is malnourished herself. Those born preterm or with low birth weight may also have a predisposition to malnutrition afterward. Appropriate support and nutrition during pregnancy and in a child's early years are essential for preventing malnutrition.

Symptoms

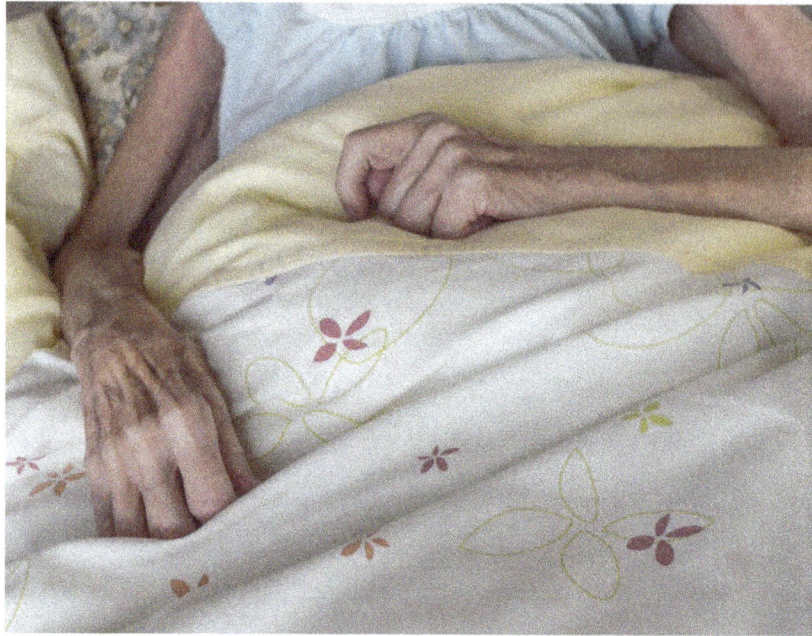

A loss of muscle and body weight are key symptoms of marasmus.

The primary symptom of marasmus is an acute loss of body fat and muscle tissues, leading to an unusually low body mass index (BMI). Marasmus is a type of wasting. In a child, the main symptom of marasmus is a failure to grow, known as stunted growth.

In adults and older children, the main symptom may be wasting, or a loss of body tissue and fat. An older child with wasting may have standard height for their age. A child with marasmus may also be very hungry and suck on their clothes or hands as if looking for something to eat. But some people with marasmus will have anorexia, and they will not want or be able to eat.

Over time, a person with marasmus will lose body tissue and fat in their face. Similarly, their bones become visible under their skin, and folds of skin develop from the loss of body mass. Their eyes may appear sunken.

Other symptoms include:

- Persistent dizziness
- Lack of energy
- Dry skin
- Brittle hair.

Apart from weight loss, long-term effects of marasmus in children include slow growth and repeated infections. Diarrhea, measles, or a respiratory infection are serious complications that can be fatal in a child with marasmus. Diarrhea can also be a contributing cause of marasmus. Other complications include bradycardia, hypotension and hypothermia.

Calcium Deficiency Diseases

Hypocalcemia, commonly known as calcium deficiency disease, occurs when calcium levels in the blood are low. A long-term deficiency can lead to dental changes, cataracts, alterations in the brain, and osteoporosis, which causes the bones to become brittle.

Osteoporosis

Osteoporosis is a condition characterized by a decrease in the density of bone, decreasing its strength and resulting in fragile bones. Osteoporosis literally leads to abnormally porous bone that is compressible, like a sponge. This disorder of the skeleton weakens the bone and results in frequent fractures (breaks) in the bones. Osteopenia, by definition, is a condition of bone that is slightly less dense than normal bone but not to the degree of bone in osteoporosis.

Normal bone is composed of protein, collagen, and calcium, all of which give bone its strength. Bones that are affected by osteoporosis can break (fracture) with relatively minor injury that normally would not cause a bone to fracture. The fracture can be either in the form of cracking (as in a hip fracture) or collapsing (as in a compression fracture of the vertebrae of the spine). The spine, hips, ribs, and wrists are common areas of bone fractures from osteoporosis although osteoporosis-related fractures can occur in almost any skeletal bone.

Causes and Risk Factors of Osteoporesis

The following are factors that will increase the risk of developing osteoporosis:

- Female gender.
- Caucasian or Asian race.
- Thin and small body frame.
- Family history of osteoporosis (for example, having a mother with an osteoporotic hip fracture doubles your risk of hip fracture).
- Personal history of fracture as an adult.
- Cigarette smoking.
- Excessive alcohol consumption.
- Lack of exercise.
- Diet low in calcium.
- Poor nutrition and poor general health, especially associated with chronic inflammation or bowel disease.
- Malabsorption (nutrients are not properly absorbed from the gastrointestinal system) from bowel diseases, such as celiac sprue that can be associated with skin diseases, such as dermatitis herpetiformis.

- Low estrogen levels in women (which may occur in menopause or with early surgical removal of both ovaries).

- Low testosterone levels in men (hypogonadism).

- Chemotherapy that can cause early menopause due to its toxic effects on the ovaries.

- Amenorrhea (loss of the menstrual period) in young women is associated with low estrogen and osteoporosis; amenorrhea can occur in women who undergo extremely vigorous exercise training and in women with very low body fat (for example, women with anorexia nervosa).

- Chronic inflammation, due to chronic inflammatory arthritis or diseases, such as rheumatoid arthritis or liver diseases.

- Immobility, such as after a stroke, or from any condition that interferes with walking.

- Hyperthyroidism, a condition wherein too much thyroid hormone is produced by the thyroid gland (as in Grave's disease) or is ingested as thyroid hormone medication.

- Hyperparathyroidism is a disease wherein there is excessive parathyroid hormone production by the parathyroid gland, a small gland located near or within the thyroid gland. Normally, parathyroid hormone maintains blood calcium levels by, in part, removing calcium from the bone. In untreated hyperparathyroidism, excessive parathyroid hormone causes too much calcium to be removed from the bone, which can lead to osteoporosis.

- When vitamin D is lacking, the body cannot absorb adequate amounts of calcium from the diet to prevent osteoporosis. Vitamin D deficiency can result from dietary deficiency, lack of sunlight, or lack of intestinal absorption of the vitamin such as occurs in celiac sprue and primary biliary cirrhosis.

- Certain medications can cause osteoporosis. These medicines include long-term use of heparin (a blood thinner), antiseizure medicine such as phenytoin (Dilantin) and phenobarbital, and long-term use of oral corticosteroids (such as prednisone).

- Inherited disorders of connective tissue, including osteogenesis imperfecta, homocystinuria, osteoporosis-pseudoglioma syndrome and skin diseases, such as Marfan syndrome and Ehlers-Danlos syndrome (These causes of hereditary secondary osteoporosis each are treated differently.)

Rickets

- Rickets is a bone disorder caused by a deficiency of vitamin D, calcium, or phosphate.

- There are several different types of rickets.

- There are different bony abnormalities associated with rickets, but all are due to poor mineralization with calcium and phosphate.

- The active form of vitamin D is synthesized by skin cells when exposed to sunlight.

- Vitamin D *IQ* is found in small amounts in some foods.

- Infants who are exclusively breastfed should receive vitamin D supplements.

- Children and adolescents who do not obtain enough vitamin D though milk and foods should receive vitamin D supplements *IQ*.

What is Rickets?

Rickets is a bone disorder caused by a deficiency of vitamin D, calcium, or phosphate. Rickets leads to softening and weakening of the bones and is seen most commonly in children 6-24 months of age. There are several subtypes of rickets, including hypophosphatemic rickets (vitamin-D-resistant rickets), renal or kidney rickets (renal osteodystrophy), and most commonly, nutritional rickets (caused by dietary deficiency of vitamin D, calcium, or phosphate). Classic nutritional rickets is also medically termed osteomalacia.

Risk Factors for the Development of Rickets

Rickets risk factors include:

- Premature birth (low levels of vitamin D, calcium, and phosphorus);

- Limited sun exposure (especially in high and low latitudes);

- Hereditary metabolic diseases (for example, X-linked hypophosphotemic rickets);

- Darkly pigmented individuals;

- Infants born to vitamin D-deficient mothers;

- Renal (kidney) diseases that affect calcium and phosphorus absorption; and

- Nutrition - suboptimal calcium and phosphorus intake or low vitamin D intake (seen in certain vegan diets due to avoidance of milk/dairy products). Soy milk and breakfast cereals fortified with vitamin D are helpful.

Types of Rickets

Nutritional Rickets

Nutritional rickets, also called osteomalacia, is a condition caused by vitamin D deficiency. Vitamin D is a fat-soluble vitamin that is essential for the normal formation of bones and teeth and necessary for the appropriate absorption of calcium and phosphorus from the bowels. It occurs naturally in very small quantities in some foods such as saltwater fish (salmon, sardines, herring, and fish-liver oils). Vitamin D is also naturally synthesized by skin cells in response to sunlight exposure. It is necessary for the appropriate absorption of calcium from the gut.

Infants and children most at risk for developing nutritional rickets include dark-skinned infants, exclusively breastfed infants, and infants who are born to mothers who are vitamin D deficient. In addition, older children who are kept out of direct sunlight or who have vegan diets may also be at risk.

Hypophosphatemic Rickets

Hypophosphatemic rickets is caused by chronically low levels of phosphate in the blood. The bones become painfully soft and pliable. This is caused by a genetic dominant X-linked defect in the ability for the kidneys to control the amount of phosphate excreted in the urine. The individual affected is able to absorb phosphate and calcium from the gut, but the phosphate is lost through the kidneys into the urine. This is not caused by a vitamin D deficiency. Patients with hypophosphatemic rickets typically have obvious symptoms by 1 year of age. Treatment is generally through nutritional supplements of phosphate and calcitriol (the activated form of vitamin D).

Renal (Kidney) Rickets

Similar to hypophosphatemic rickets, renal rickets is caused by a number of kidney disorders. Individuals suffering from kidney disease *IQ* often have decreased ability to regulate the amounts of electrolytes lost in the urine. This includes calcium and phosphate, and therefore the affected individuals develop symptoms almost identical to severe nutritional rickets. Treatment of the underlying kidney problem and nutritional supplementation are recommended for these patients.

Iron Deficiency Diseases

Iron deficiency occurs when the body doesn't have enough of the mineral iron. This leads to abnormally low levels of red blood cells. That's because iron is needed to make hemoglobin, a protein in red blood cells that enables them to carry oxygen around the body.

If your body doesn't have enough hemoglobin, your tissues and muscles won't get enough oxygen and be able to work effectively. This leads to a condition called anemia. Although there are different types of anemia, iron-deficiency anemia is the most common worldwide.

Common causes of iron deficiency include inadequate iron intake due to poor diet or restrictive diets, inflammatory bowel disease, increased requirements during pregnancy and blood loss through heavy periods or internal bleeding.

Goiter

A goiter is an enlarged thyroid gland. The thyroid gland is situated in front of the windpipe and is responsible for producing and secreting hormones that regulate growth and metabolism.

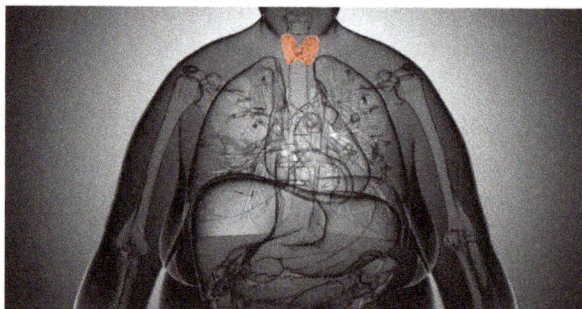

The thyroid gland: An underactive gland can cause weight gain.

Most cases are categorized as 'simple' goiters that do not involve inflammation or any detriment to thyroid function, produce no symptoms, and often have no obvious cause.

Some people experience a small amount of swelling. Others can have considerable swelling that constricts the trachea and causes breathing problems.

Symptoms

The degree of swelling and the severity of symptoms produced by the goiter depends on the individual.

Most goiters produce no symptoms. When symptoms do occur, the following are most common:

- Throat symptoms of tightness, cough, and hoarseness.
- Trouble swallowing.
- In severe cases, difficulty breathing, possibly with a high-pitch sound.

Other symptoms may be present because of the underlying cause of the goiter, but they are not because of the goiter itself. For example, an overactive thyroid can cause symptoms such as:

- Nervousness
- Palpitations
- Hyperactivity
- Increased sweating
- Heat hypersensitivity
- Fatigue
- Increased appetite
- Hair loss
- Weight loss

In cases where goiter is a result of hypothyroidism, the underactive thyroid can cause symptoms such as:

- Cold intolerance
- Constipation
- Forgetfulness
- Personality changes
- Hair loss
- Weight gain

Aside from the swelling itself, many people with goiter present no symptoms or signs at all.

Causes

Goiter can be caused by a number of different conditions:

Iodine Deficiency

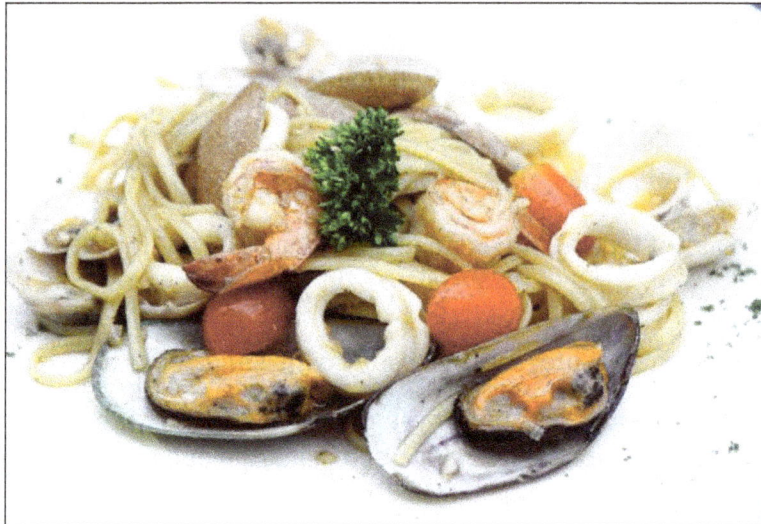

Deficiency of iodine - found in seafood - is a major cause of goiter.

Iodine deficiency is the major cause of goiter worldwide, but this is rarely a cause in more economically developed countries where iodine is routinely added to salt. As iodine is less commonly found in plants, vegan diets may lack sufficient iodine. This is less of a problem for vegans who live in countries such as the United States that add iodine to salt.

Dietary iodine is found in:

- Seafood
- Plant food grown in iodine-rich soil
- Cow's milk.

In some parts of the world, the prevalence of goiters can be as high as 80 percent, such as in the remote mountainous regions of southeast Asia, Latin America, and central Africa. In these places, daily intake of iodine can fall below 25 micrograms (mcg) per day, and children are often born with hypothyroidism. The thyroid gland needs iodine to manufacture thyroid hormones, which regulate the metabolism.

Autoimmune Disease

The main cause of goiter in developed countries is autoimmune disease. Women over the age of 40 are at greater risk of goiter, as are people with a family history of the condition. Hypothyroidism is the result of an underactive thyroid gland, and this causes goiter. Because the gland produces too little thyroid hormone, it is stimulated to produce more, leading to the swelling.

This usually results from Hashimoto's thyroiditis, a condition in which the body's immune system attacks its own tissue and causes inflammation of the thyroid gland.

Hyperthyroidism

Hyperthyroidism, or an overactive thyroid gland, is another cause of goiter. Too much thyroid hormone is produced. This usually happens as a result of Graves' disease, an autoimmune disorder where the body's immunity turns on itself and attacks the thyroid gland, causing it to swell.

Other Causes

Less common causes of goiter include the following:

- Smoking: Thiocyanate in tobacco smoke interferes with iodine absorption.

- Hormonal changes: Pregnancy, puberty, and menopause can affect thyroid function.

- Thyroiditis: Inflammation caused by infection, for example, can lead to goiter.

- Lithium: This psychiatric drug can interfere with thyroid function.

- Overconsumption of iodine: Too much iodine can cause a goiter.

- Radiation therapy: This can trigger a swollen thyroid, particularly when administered to the neck.

Types of Goiter

There are several main types of goiter:

- Diffuse smooth goiter: This occurs when the entire thyroid swells.

- Nodular goiter: A lump develops on the thyroid. These are extremely common. If many lumps develop, this is known as multinodular goiter.

- Retrosternal goiter: This type of goiter can grow behind the breastbone. This can constrict the windpipe, neck veins, or esophagus, and sometimes requires surgery.

Anemia

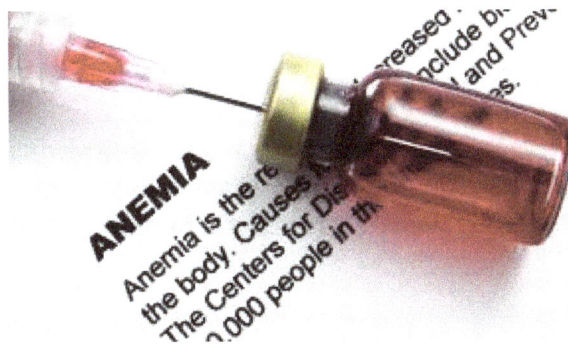

When there are not enough healthy red blood cells or hemoglobin present in the body, this is called anemia.

Anemia is a blood condition characterized by a lack of healthy red blood cells or hemoglobin. Hemoglobin is the part of the red blood cells that binds to oxygen. When the body does not have enough hemoglobin circulating, not enough oxygen gets to all parts of the body either.

As a result, organs and tissues may not function properly, and a person may feel fatigued. Iron deficiency anemia occurs when the body does not have enough iron to produce the hemoglobin it needs.

Causes of Anemia

Iron deficiency anemia relates directly to a lack of iron in the body. The cause of the iron deficiency varies, however.

Some common causes include:

- Poor diet or not enough iron in the diet

- Blood loss

- A decreased ability to absorb iron

- Pregnancy.

Poor Diet

Diets that lack iron are a leading cause of iron deficiency. Foods rich in iron, such as eggs and meat, supply the body with much of the iron it needs to produce hemoglobin. If a person does not eat enough to maintain their iron supply, an iron deficiency can develop.

Blood Loss

Iron is found primarily in the blood, as it is stored in red blood cells. An iron deficiency may result when a person loses a lot of blood from an injury, giving birth, or heavy menstruation. In some cases, slow loss of blood from chronic diseases or some cancers can lead to an iron deficiency.

Decreased Ability to Absorb Iron

Some people are not able to absorb enough iron from the food they eat. This may be due to a problem with the small intestine, such as celiac disease or Crohn's disease, or if a portion of the small intestine has been removed.

Pregnancy

Low iron levels are a common problem for pregnant women. The growing fetus needs a lot of iron, which can lead to an iron deficiency. Also, a pregnant woman has an increased amount of blood in her body. This larger volume of blood demands more iron to meet its needs.

Risk Factors of Anemia

Some groups of people have a higher risk of developing iron deficiency anemia. Groups that are at risk include:

- Vegetarians: People, such as vegetarians, who eat a plant-based diet, may be lacking in iron. To combat this, they should be sure to include foods rich in iron, such as beans or fortified cereals. Vegetarians who also eat seafood should consider oysters or salmon, as a part of their regular diet.

- Women: Monthly menstrual cycles can put women and teenage girls at an increased risk of iron deficiency.

- Blood donors: People who give blood regularly increase their chances of developing an iron deficiency. This is because of the frequent blood loss.

- Infants and children: Premature babies and those with a low birth weight can be at risk of iron deficiencies. Also, infants who do not get enough iron through breast milk are at a greater risk. A doctor may advise a breast-feeding woman to add iron-rich formula to their baby's diet if their iron levels are low.

Similarly, children going through growth spurts have an increased risk of iron deficiency. It is important for children to eat a varied and nutrient-rich diet to help avoid iron deficiencies.

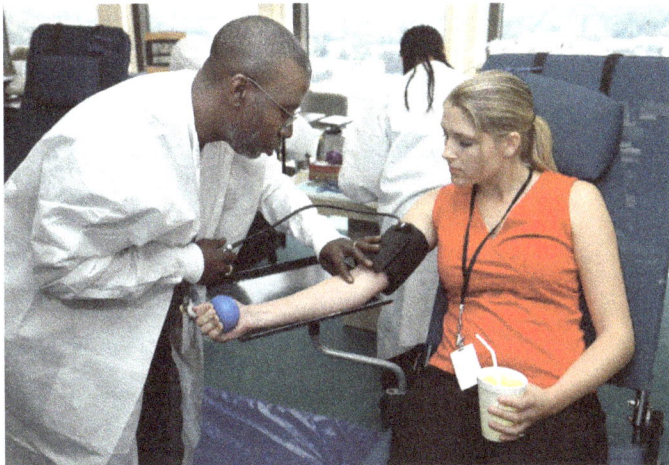

Frequent blood donation may increase the risk of developing an iron deficiency.

Symptoms of Anemia

Iron deficiency anemia often takes a long time to develop. People may not know they have it until the symptoms are severe. In some cases, an iron deficiency may improve with no intervention, as a person's situation changes, such as after a woman has given birth.

However, if a person has any symptoms of iron deficiency anemia, they should talk to their doctor. A person with an iron deficiency can have some of the following symptoms:

- General weakness

- Dizziness or lightheadedness

- Extreme fatigue

- Fast heartbeat

- Easily broken and brittle nails

- Paler than normal skin

- Chest pain

- Shortness of breath

- Headaches

- Cold hands and feet

- Soreness or inflammation of the tongue

- Cravings for non-nutritive things, such as dirt, starch, or ice

- Poor appetite, especially in children.

Thiamine Deficiency Disease

Thiamin deficiency is most common among people subsisting on white rice or highly refined carbohydrates in developing countries and among alcoholics. Symptoms include diffuse polyneuropathy, high-output heart failure, and Wernicke-Korsakoff syndrome. Thiamin is given to help diagnose and treat the deficiency.

Beriberi

Beriberi is a disease caused by a deficiency of thiamine (vitamin B_1) that affects many systems of the body, including the muscles, heart, nerves, and digestive system. In adults, there are different forms of beriberi, classified according to the body systems most affected. Dry beriberi involves the nervous system; wet beriberi affects the heart and circulation. Both types usually occur in the same patient, with one set of symptoms predominating.

A less common form of cardiovascular, or wet beriberi, is known as "shoshin." This condition involves a rapid appearance of symptoms and acute heart failure. It is highly fatal and is known to cause sudden death in young migrant laborers in Asia whose diet consists of white rice.

Cerebral beriberi, also known as Wernicke-Korsakoff syndrome, usually occurs in chronic alcoholics and affects the central nervous system (brain and spinal cord). It can be caused by a situation that aggravates a chronic thiamine deficiency, like an alcoholic binge or severe vomiting. Infantile beriberi is seen in breastfed infants of thiamine-deficient mothers, who live in developing nations.

Causes and Symptoms of Beriberi

Thiamine is one of the B vitamins and plays an important role in energy metabolism and tissue building. It combines with phosphate to form the coenzyme thiamine pyrophosphate (TPP), which is essential in reactions that produce energy from glucose or that convert glucose to fat for storage in the tissues. When there is not enough thiamine in the diet, these basic energy functions are disturbed, leading to problems throughout the body.

Special situations, such as an over-active metabolism, prolonged fever, pregnancy, and breastfeeding, can increase the body's thiamine requirements and lead to symptoms of deficiency. Extended periods of diarrhea or chronic liver disease can result in the body's inability to maintain normal levels of many nutrients, including thiamine. Other persons at risk are patients with kidney failure on dialysis and those with severe digestive problems who are unable to absorb nutrients. Alcoholics are susceptible because they may substitute alcohol for food and their frequent intake of alcohol decreases the body's ability to absorb thiamine.

The following systems are most affected by beriberi:

- Gastrointestinal system: When the cells of the smooth muscles in the digestive system and glands do not get enough energy from glucose, they are unable to produce more glucose from the normal digestion of food. There is a loss of appetite, indigestion, severe constipation, and a lack of hydrochloric acid in the stomach.

- Nervous System: Glucose is essential for the central nervous system to function normally. Early deficiency symptoms are fatigue, irritability, and poor memory. If the deficiency continues, there is damage to the peripheral nerves that causes loss of sensation and muscle weakness, which is called peripheral neuropathy. The legs are most affected. The toes feel numb and the feet have a burning sensation; the leg muscles become sore and the calf muscles cramp. The individual walks unsteadily and has difficulty getting up from a squatting position. Eventually, the muscles shrink (atrophy) and there is a loss of reflexes in the knees and feet; the feet may hang limp (footdrop).

- Cardiovascular system: There is a rapid heartbeat and sweating. Eventually the heart muscle weakens. Because the smooth muscle in the blood vessels is affected, the arteries and veins relax, causing swelling, known as edema, in the legs.

- Musculoskeletal system: There is widespread muscle pain caused by the lack of TPP in the muscle tissue.

Infants who are breastfed by a thiamine-deficient mother usually develop symptoms of deficiency between the second and fourth month of life. They are pale, restless, unable to sleep, prone to diarrhea, and have muscle wasting and edema in their arms and legs. They have a characteristic, sometimes silent, cry and develop heart failure and nerve damage.

Diagnosis

A physical examination will reveal many of the early symptoms of beriberi, such as fatigue, irritation, nausea, constipation, and poor memory, but the deficiency may be difficult to identify. Information about the individual's diet and general health is also needed.

Niacin Deficiency Disease

Niacin deficiency is a condition that occurs when a person doesn't get enough or can't absorb niacin or its amino acid precursor, tryptophan.

Also known as vitamin B3 or nicotinic acid, niacin is one of eight B vitamins. Like all B vitamins, niacin plays a role in converting carbohydrates into glucose, metabolizing fats and proteins, and keeping the nervous system working properly. Niacin also helps the body make sex- and stress-related hormones and improves circulation and cholesterol levels.

Tryptophan is one of the amino acids that makes up protein. Your liver can convert tryptophan from high-protein foods like meats and milk into niacin.

Pellagra

Pellagra is a condition that occurs when a person develops a deficiency in Vitamin B3, also called niacin. There are two types of deficiency a person can have. A primary deficiency occurs when a person is not getting enough niacin in his/her diet, and a secondary deficiency is when the body isn't able to use the nutrient properly.

Pellagra used to be a very common condition, especially in parts of the world that were dependent on corn-based diets. Today, most cases of pellagra occur in poverty-stricken areas, in people with health conditions that impair the body's ability to absorb nutrients, and also people with chronic alcoholism. While the condition can be cured if diagnosed, pellagra can be fatal if left untreated.

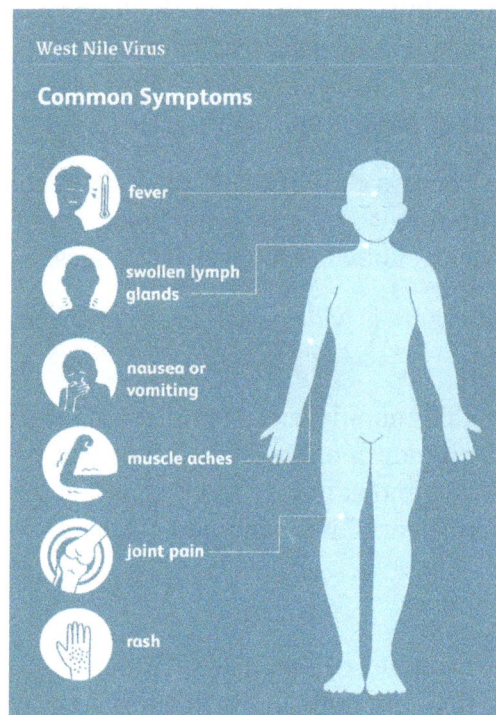

Symptoms

Vitamin B3 (also known as niacin) is essential to good health. Niacin helps our bodies convert the food we eat into energy. Two coenzymes produced by niacin, nicotinamide adenine dinucleotide (NAD) and nicotinamide adenine dinucleotide phosphate (NADP), also have important roles in the body. These coenzymes are integral to functions like gene expression and cellular processes such as cholesterol synthesis.

Niacin can be consumed directly through the foods we eat—these are either foods that are fortified or naturally-rich in vitamin B3, such as meat, dairy, and nuts. Our body can also convert an amino acid protein called tryptophan into niacin. Turkey is a very rich dietary source of tryptophan and therefore can help stave off niacin deficiency.

The adult Dietary Reference Intakes (DRIs) recommendations for niacin is 14 to 16 milligrams of niacin equivalents (mg/NE). If a person does not get enough niacin, or if they have a health condition that impairs the body's ability to use niacin or convert tryptophan into niacin, they are at risk for developing a deficiency. Severe niacin deficiency results in a disorder called pellagra.

There are three common symptoms of pellagra referred to as the "three Ds." Untreated pellagra will lead to death, sometimes called the "fourth D," within a few years.

Common Symptoms of Pellagra:

- Diarrhea

- Dermatitis

- Dementia

In the early stages, pellagra symptoms may be vague. Patients with the condition may only have one or two of the "Ds" along with other nonspecific symptoms. The rash and diarrhea, however, are seen in the majority of cases.

Watery diarrhea is usually the first symptom and is the result of inflammation of the gastrointestinal mucosa. Sometimes diarrhea may have blood or mucus, especially if a patient has a condition like Crohn's disease. In some cases, pellagra may lead to the diagnosis of inflammatory bowel disease.

As the condition goes on, people with pellagra also tend to have no appetite (sometimes leading to anorexia), feel sick to their stomach (nauseated), or have stomach pain. These symptoms can cause a cycle where a person who is already in a state of malnourishment leading to nutritional deficiency does not feel well enough to eat, or the person has a health condition that impacts their ability to adhere to a well-rounded diet.

In turn, the person will become more malnourished. A weakened state may predispose them to other health problems, such as viral illness, that their body can not effectively fight against due to lowered immunity.

Dermatitis, or skin inflammation, typically appears in the form of a rash in sun-exposed areas of the body. In fact, it often looks like a sunburn. The rash may become more intense, with skin peeling and changing in skin color (pigmentation) that can be permanent.

As the rash begins to blister, the skin may become rough and scaly, especially on the bottom part of the hands and feet, as well as on the race (a pattern known as a butterfly or malar rash). Areas of affected skin may be itchy, painful, and sensitive to the sun.

The neurological signs and symptoms occur later when the deficiency has become severe and has been going on for a prolonged period of time. At first, a person may experience memory loss, trouble sleeping, and mood changes.

As the deficiency gets worse, the neurological symptoms can be severe: a person may become disoriented or not know where they are, begin to have hallucinations, or even be in a stupor, failing to respond to their surroundings.

In extreme cases, the neurological symptoms of pellagra appear dementia-like or even stroke-like.

As the condition worsens and body systems begin to shut down, other symptoms may develop, including:

- Loss of coordination

- Glossitis (tongue swelling) that can obstruct a person's airway

- Dementia

- Paralysis

- Heart conditions such as dilated cardiomyopathy

- Stupor

- Coma.

Left untreated, multi-organ failure from pellagra can be fatal in three to five years.

Causes

People have been suffering the effects of niacin deficiency for centuries. The name pellagra (from the Italian pelle agra for "rough skin") was used to describe the condition by scholars in the early 18th century. At first, people were not sure what caused pellagra.

They noticed that one thing many people who became sick with the condition had in common was that their diet was primarily maize (corn). For many years, people believed that corn crops carried a pest or toxin that was making people sick.

As people began to travel to other cultures around the world, it became clear that many communities were able to subsist on corn crops without getting pellagra. The key was in how corn was prepared, which seemed to determine how nutritious the diet was. When the corn crops were treated with a certain alkalizing process, called nixtamalization, it allowed the niacin to be released.

As long as people were eating corn that had been prepared this way, such as corn tortillas, they wouldn't develop pellagra.

However, in some cases, even though a person is getting enough niacin from the food they eat, their body is not able to use it properly. This may be due to an underlying condition or caused by a medication. Reasons people develop secondary pellagra include:

- Genetic conditions like Hartnup disease, which inhibits the body's ability to absorb tryptophan from the intestines.

- Treatment with drugs that affect how the body uses B vitamins, such as the antituberculosis drug isoniazid or phenobarbital.

- Types of tumors that produce excessive serotonin (carcinomas) leading to a condition called carcinoid syndrome.

- Adhering to very restricted diets ("fad diets") or maize-based diets that have not been nixtamalized.

Additionally, conditions that put stress on the body (thereby increasing nutritional needs) can also lead to pellagra. Patients may be at increased risk of developing the deficiency if they have:

- A prolonged febrile illness.

- Diabetes mellitus.

- Human Immunodefiecney Virus (HIV).

- Chronic alcoholism and drug abuse.

- Anorexia nervosa.

- Liver cirrhosis.

- Patients receiving long-term dialysis.

A person's socioeconomic circumstances can also place them at risk for developing pellagra. People living in poverty who don't have adequate access to nutritious food, those living in famine conditions, and refugees are more likely to become severely malnourished.

While pellagra mostly develops in adults, children who are living in countries experiencing famine, whose families are homeless, or who are being neglected may also be at risk.

In many parts of the world where pellagra still occurs, it follows a predictable seasonal pattern. People tend to develop pellagra in the late spring or summer months after having limited access to food over the winter. More exposure to sunlight during the lighter months of the year can also make the characteristic rash of pellagra more apparent.

Often, people will recover from pellagra during the months of the year when they have access to nutritious food, only to have the condition recur when the season changes.

Pellagra occurs equally in men and women. It primarily occurs in adults but in some cases, infants and children may be at risk. People of all races can develop pellagra, though it is seen more often in developing countries and poverty-stricken regions of developed nations.

Vitamin C Deficiency Disease

vitamin C deficiency can occur as part of general undernutrition, but severe deficiency (causing scurvy) is uncommon. Symptoms include fatigue, depression, and connective tissue defects (eg, gingivitis, petechiae, rash, internal bleeding, impaired wound healing). In infants and children, bone growth may be impaired.

Scurvy

Scurvy is better known as severe vitamin C deficiency. Vitamin C, or ascorbic acid, is an essential dietary nutrient. It plays a role in the development and functioning of several bodily structures and processes, including:

- The proper formation of collagen, the protein that helps give the body's connective tissues structure and stability.

- Cholesterol and protein metabolism.

- Iron absorption.

- Antioxidant action.

- Wound healing.

- Creation of neurotransmitters like dopamine and epinephrine.

Symptoms of Scurvy

Vitamin C plays many different roles in the body. A deficiency in the vitamin causes widespread symptoms. Typically signs of scurvy begin after at least four weeks of severe, continual vitamin C deficiency. Generally, however, it takes three months or more for symptoms to develop.

Early Warning Signs

Early warning signs and symptoms of scurvy include:

- Weakness

- Unexplained exhaustion

- Reduced appetite

- Irritability

- Aching legs

- Low-grade fever.

Symptoms After one to Three Months

Common symptoms of untreated scurvy after one to three months include:

- Anemia, when the blood lacks enough red blood cells or haemoglobin.

- gingivitis, or red, soft, and tender gums that bleed easily.

- Skin hemorrhages, or bleeding under the skin.

- Bruise-like raised bumps at hair follicles, often on the shins, with central hairs that appear corkscrewed, or twisted, and break easily.

- Large areas of reddish-blue to black bruising, often on the legs and feet.

- Tooth decay.

- Tender, swollen joints.

- Shortness of breath.

- Chest pain.

- Eye dryness, irritation, and hemorrhaging in the whites of the eyes (conjunctiva) or optic nerve.

- Reduced wound healing and immune health.

- Light sensitivity.

- Blurred vision.

- Mood swings, often irritability and depression.

- Gastrointestinal bleeding.

- Headache.

Left untreated, scurvy can cause life-threatening conditions.

Severe Complications

Symptoms and complications associated with long-term, untreated scurvy include:

- Severe jaundice, which is yellowing of the skin and eyes.

- Generalized pain, tenderness, and swelling.

- Hemolysis, a type of anemia where red blood cells break down.

- Fever.

- Tooth loss.

- Internal hemorrhaging.

- Neuropathy, or numbness and pain usually in the lower limbs and hands.

- Convulsions.

- Organ failure.

- Delirium.

- Coma.

- Death.

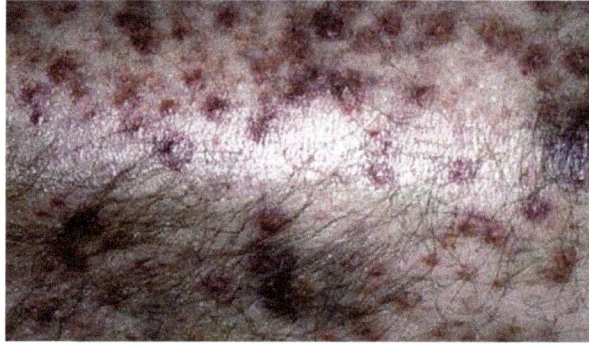

Scurvy in Infants

Infants with scurvy will be irritable, anxious, and difficult to soothe. They may also appear to be paralyzed, lying with their arms and legs extended halfway out. Infants with scurvy may also develop weak, brittle, bones prone to fractures and hemorrhaging, or bleeding.

Risk factors for scurvy in infants include:

- Malnourished mothers

- Being fed evaporated or boiled milk

- Difficulty nursing

- Restrictive or special dietary needs

- Digestive or absorption disorders.

Risk Factors and Causes

Your body can't make vitamin C. That means you have to consume all of the vitamin C your body needs through food or drinks, or by taking a supplement.

Most people with scurvy lack access to fresh fruits and vegetables, or don't have a healthy diet. Scurvy impacts many people in the developing world. Recent public health surveysTrusted Source have shown that scurvy may be far more prevalent in developed nations than once thought, especially in at-risk segments of the population. Medical conditions and lifestyle habits also increase the risk of the condition.

Risk factors for malnutrition and scurvy include:

- Being a child or 65 years of age and over.

- Daily alcohol consumption.

- Use of illegal drugs.

- Living alone.

- Restrictive or specified diets.

- Low income, reduced access to nutritious foods.

- Being homeless or a refugee.

- Living in areas with limited access to fresh fruits and vegetables.

- Eating disorders or psychiatric conditions that involve a fear of food.

- Neurological conditions.

- Disabilities.

- Forms of inflammatory bowel disease (ibd), including irritable bowel syndrome (ibs), crohn's disease, or ulcerative colitis.

- Digestive or metabolic conditions.

- Immune conditions.

- Living in a place where the cultural diet consists almost entirely of carbohydrates like breads, pastas, and corn.

- Chronic diarrhea.

- Dehydration.

- Smoking.

- Chemotherapy and radiation therapy.

- Dialysis and kidney failure.

References

- Protein-energy-undernutrition-peu, undernutrition, nutritional-disorders: msdmanuals.com, Retrieved 9 March, 2019

- Kwashiorkor: dermnetnz.org, Retrieved 19 June, 2019

- Osteoporosis: medicinenet.com, Retrieved 22 August, 2019

- What-is-the-history-of-rickets: medicinenet.com, Retrieved 27 March, 2019

- Iron-deficiency-signs-symptoms, nutrition: healthline.com, Retrieved 30 April, 2019

- Thiamin-deficiency, dependency-and-toxicity, vitamin-deficiency, nutritional-disorders: msdmanuals.com, Retrieved 21 January, 2019

- Beriberi, pathology, diseases-and-conditions, medicine: encyclopedia.com, Retrieved 25 May, 2019

- Niacin-deficiency-symptoms-and-treatments: webmd.com, Retrieved 20 April, 2019

- Pellagra: verywellhealth.com, Retrieved 11 July, 2019

- Scurvy, health: healthline.com, Retrieved 25 February, 2019

Permissions

We would like to thank the editorial team for lending their expertise to make the book truly unique. They have played a crucial role in the development of this book. Without their invaluable contributions this book wouldn't have been possible. They have made vital efforts to compile up to date information on the varied aspects of this subject to make this book a valuable addition to the collection of many professionals and students.

This book was conceptualized with the vision of imparting up-to-date and integrated information in this field. To ensure the same, a matchless editorial board was set up. Every individual on the board went through rigorous rounds of assessment to prove their worth. After which they invested a large part of their time researching and compiling the most relevant data for our readers.

The editorial board has been involved in producing this book since its inception. They have spent rigorous hours researching and exploring the diverse topics which have resulted in the successful publishing of this book. They have passed on their knowledge of decades through this book. To expedite this challenging task, the publisher supported the team at every step. A small team of assistant editors was also appointed to further simplify the editing procedure and attain best results for the readers.

Apart from the editorial board, the designing team has also invested a significant amount of their time in understanding the subject and creating the most relevant covers. They scrutinized every image to scout for the most suitable representation of the subject and create an appropriate cover for the book.

The publishing team has been an ardent support to the editorial, designing and production team. Their endless efforts to recruit the best for this project, has resulted in the accomplishment of this book. They are a veteran in the field of academics and their pool of knowledge is as vast as their experience in printing. Their expertise and guidance has proved useful at every step. Their uncompromising quality standards have made this book an exceptional effort. Their encouragement from time to time has been an inspiration for everyone.

The publisher and the editorial board hope that this book will prove to be a valuable piece of knowledge for students, practitioners and scholars across the globe.

Index

www.ingramcontent.com/pod-product-compliance
Lightning Source LLC
Chambersburg PA
CBHW082036190326
41458CB00010B/3378